RA
644
.A25
P7534
1994

Preventing AIDS.

$49.50

DATE			

Preventing AIDS
Theories and Methods of Behavioral Interventions

AIDS Prevention and Mental Health

Series Editors:

David G. Ostrow, M.D., Ph.D. and Jeffrey A. Kelly, Ph.D.
Medical College of Wisconsin
Milwaukee, Wisconsin

Methodological Issues in AIDS Behavioral Research
Edited by David G. Ostrow, M.D., Ph.D., and Ronald C. Kessler, Ph.D.

Preventing AIDS: Theories and Methods of Behavioral Interventions
Edited by Ralph J. DiClemente, Ph.D., and John L. Peterson, Ph.D.

A Continuation Order Plan is available for this series. A continuation order will bring delivery of each new volume immediately upon publication. Volumes are billed only upon actual shipment. For further information please contact the publisher.

Preventing AIDS
Theories and Methods of Behavioral Interventions

Edited by

Ralph J. DiClemente, Ph.D.

University of Alabama
Birmingham, Alabama

and

John L. Peterson, Ph.D.

Georgia State University
Atlanta, Georgia

Foreword by
Jonathan Mann, M.D., M.P.H.

Plenum Press • New York and London

Library of Congress Cataloging-in-Publication Data

Preventing AIDS : theories and methods of behavioral interventions /
    edited by Ralph J. DiClemente and John L. Peterson ; foreword by
    Jonathan Mann.
        p.   cm.
    Includes bibliographical references and index.
    ISBN 0-306-44606-5
    1. HIV infections--Prevention. 2. Health behavior.
    I. DiClemente, Ralph J. II. Peterson, John L.
    RA644.A25P7534   1994
    614.5'993--dc20

                                                            94-2857
                                                            CIP

ISBN 0-306-44606-5

© 1994 Plenum Press, New York
A Division of Plenum Publishing Corporation
233 Spring Street, New York, N.Y. 10013

Printed in the United States of America

Contributors

Albert Bandura • Department of Psychology, Stanford University, Stanford, California 94305

Marshall H. Becker • Department of Health Behavior and Health Education, School of Public Health, University of Michigan, Ann Arbor, Michigan 48109-2029

James W. Dearing • Department of Communication, Michigan State University, East Lansing, Michigan 48824-1212

Don C. Des Jarlais • Chemical Dependency Institute, Beth Israel Medical Center, New York, New York 10003

Ralph J. DiClemente • School of Public Health, Department of Health Behavior and School of Medicine, Departments of Medicine and Pediatrics, and Center for AIDS Research, University of Alabama, Birmingham, Alabama 35294

Lynda S. Doll • Division of HIV/AIDS, National Center for Infectious Diseases, Centers for Disease Control and Prevention, Atlanta, Georgia 30333

Edward Dunne • Department of Psychiatry, College of Physicians and Surgeons, Columbia University, New York, New York, 10032

Julie Feldman • Division of Child Psychiatry, College of Physicians and Surgeons, Columbia University, New York, New York 10032

Martin Fishbein • Department of Psychology, University of Illinois, Champaign, Illinois 61820

Samuel R. Friedman • National Development and Research Institutes, 11 Beach Street, New York, New York, 10013

Joseph Guydish • Institute for Health Policy Studies, School of Medicine, University of California, San Francisco, San Francisco, California 94143-0936

Janet S. Harrison • Division of HIV/AIDS, National Center for Infectious Diseases, Centers for Disease Control and Prevention, Atlanta, Georgia 30333

Robert B. Hays • School of Medicine, University of California, San Francisco, San Francisco, California 94143, and Center for AIDS Prevention Studies, San Francisco, California 94105

Penelope J. Hitchcock • Sexually Transmitted Diseases Branch, National Institute of Allergy and Infectious Diseases, National Institutes of Health, Bethesda, Maryland 20892

John B. Jemmott III • Department of Psychology, Princeton University, Princeton, New Jersey 08544

Loretta Sweet Jemmott • College of Nursing, Rutgers, The State University of New Jersey, Newark, New Jersey 07112

Jeffrey A. Kelly • Department of Psychiatry and Mental Health Sciences, Medical College of Wisconsin, Milwaukee, Wisconsin 53226

Douglas Kirby • ETR Associates, P.O. Box 1830, Santa Cruz, California 95061-1830

Gary Meyer • Department of Communication, Michigan State University, East Lansing, Michigan 48824-1212

Susan E. Middlestadt • Social Development Program, Academy for Educational Development, Washington, DC 20037

Janet S. Moore • Division of HIV/AIDS, National Center for Infectious Diseases, Centers for Disease Control and Prevention, Atlanta, Georgia 30333

Thomas R. O'Brien • Viral Epidemiology Section, National Cancer Institute, Rockville, Maryland 20892

Nancy S. Padian • School of Medicine, University of California, San Francisco, and San Francisco General Hospital, San Francisco, California 94110

John L. Peterson • Department of Psychology, Georgia State University, Atlanta, Georgia 30303

Laurie Roehrich • Department of Psychiatry, University of California, San Francisco, and Substance Abuse Services, San Francisco General Hospital, San Francisco, California 94110

Everett M. Rogers • Department of Communication and Journalism, University of New Mexico, Albuquerque, New Mexico 87131-1171

Margaret Rosario • Department of Psychiatry, College of Physicians and Surgeons, and School of Public Health, Columbia University, New York, New York 10032

Irwin M. Rosenstock • Department of Health Behavior and Health Education, School of Public Health, University of Michigan, Ann Arbor, Michigan 48109-2029, and College of Health and Human Services, California State University, Long Beach, Long Beach, California 90840

Mary Jane Rotheram-Borus • Division of Social Psychiatry, Department of Psychiatry, UCLA Neuropsychiatric Institute, Los Angeles, California 90024-1759

James L. Sorensen • Department of Psychiatry, University of California, San Francisco, and Substance Abuse Services, San Francisco General Hospital, San Francisco, California, 94110

Victor J. Strecher • Department of Health Behavior and Health Education, School of Public Health, University of North Carolina at Chapel Hill, Chapel Hill, North Carolina, 17599

Tamara L. Wall • Department of Psychiatry, University of California, San Francisco, and Substance Abuse Services, San Francisco General Hospital, San Francisco, California 94110

Thomas P. Ward • National Development and Research Institutes, 11 Beach Street, New York, New York 10013

John K. Watters • Department of Family and Community Medicine and Institute for Health Policy Studies, School of Medicine, University of California, San Francisco, San Francisco, California 94143-1304

Janneke H. H. M. van de Wijgert • School of Medicine, University of California, San Francisco, and San Francisco General Hospital, San Francisco, California 94110

Foreword

Public health has a legacy of neglect regarding social and behavioral research. Too often, prompted by technical and scientific progress, we have ignored—even marginalized—the vital "human element" in health thinking and practice. Thus, for example, while family planning programs focused on providing a choice among safe and effective contraceptive methods (a supremely worthy goal), the central issue of sexuality and sexual behavior was generally neglected. Similarly, the enormous and important efforts to develop rapid and reliable diagnostic and treatment methods for sexually transmitted diseases helped divert attention away from the crucial issues of sexual practice. In short, we seem to have difficulty addressing the fundamental behaviors—including sex, drug taking and other intoxications, and violence—that are central to the major causes of preventable morbidity, disability, and premature mortality in the world today.

Our collective reluctance to examine and understand ourselves is also expressed in the oft-repeated pipedream that scientific progress will "take care of" the HIV/AIDS pandemic by delivering a preventive vaccine, an effective cure, or both. Yet even a cursory glance at the relationship between scientific/technical progress and health shows that meeting the scientific challenges is only one step toward effective application of the vaccine or drug. It is typical, not atypical, that hepatitis B vaccine is only now becoming relatively freely available to large populations in the developing world, more than a decade after the vaccine's licensure. It would be similarly naive to think that once the vials of an effective AIDS vaccine are in hand, our only concern will be how to make the vaccine truly available to all who need it. Simply stated, how we use the fruits of scientific research is as "behavioral"—albeit at a collective level—and as important in the future of the HIV/AIDS pandemic as the specific life activities, individually practiced, that are usually called "behavior."

HIV/AIDS has helped focus attention on our relatively primitive current capacity to describe usefully, understand, or modify effectively several basic behaviors, at either the individual or collective level. Therefore, this fine book, edited by Ralph DiClemente and John Peterson, offers a useful contribution by presenting both a range of conceptual frameworks and practical experiences in the efforts to prevent HIV infection.

But where do we go from here? Perhaps several breakthroughs are needed. First, we need a broad acknowledgment of the central, crucial, inextricable interdependence between health and behavior. Second, we need to support innovative and creative efforts to develop new conceptual frameworks where (as is most often the case) existing concepts seem inadequate. Third, we must be rigorously self-critical, to distinguish the workmanship-like efforts at routine KABP (Knowledge, Attitudes, Beliefs, Practices) surveys from research that can truly and concretely inform design and modification of prevention efforts. Fourth, we need to build bridges between the worlds of behavioral research and the world of public health.

Yet in the end, we will need to recognize that changing public and political attitudes toward behavioral research is part of a larger agenda that seeks to transform society in ways that promote health. Health, thanks to the World Health Organization's definition, is now understood to involve physical, mental, and social well-being. Accordingly, a society that denies its humanness, its basic nature as a human community, a community of people, and prefers to think in terms of social or environmental engineering or modification cannot be truly healthy. It may not be evident on a daily basis, but those working to understand and respond to human behavior—individual and collective— are the great pioneers upon whom the future of health—and our world— may well depend.

Jonathan Mann, MD, MPH

François-Xavier Bagnoud Professor
of Health and Human Rights
Harvard School of Public Health
Director, International AIDS Center,
Harvard AIDS Institute

Preface

Early in the acquired immunodeficiency syndrome (AIDS) epidemic, a number of authors predicted that the behavioral sciences would have an influential role in the prevention of human immunodeficiency virus (HIV) infection. These predictions have held true. Behavior change represents the only available strategy for HIV prevention. Despite this awareness, until recently only very little behavioral research has consisted of intervention studies. Within recent years, however, behavioral scientists have conducted substantially more studies designed to assess the efficacy of behavior change interventions. The current volume represents an effort to compile and examine this rapidly expanding body of research.

Preventing AIDS: Theories and Methods of Behavioral Interventions brings together a multidisciplinary group of behavioral researchers who have conducted major research interventions in HIV primary prevention. This volume identifies the principal theories and methods utilized in behavioral change interventions and examines their impact in a variety of populations.

In the first chapter, DiClemente and Peterson provide an overview of the role of behavioral interventions for HIV prevention. The five following chapters describe the major theoretical models used in behavior change interventions. First, Rosenstock, Strecher, and Becker discuss the health belief model and its application to HIV risk behavior change. Next, Bandura describes social cognitive theory and its influence on controlling HIV infection. Then, Fishbein, Middlestadt, and Hitchcock examine how the theory of reasoned action may be useful in changing high-risk sexual behaviors. Dearing, Meyer, and Rogers delineate diffusion theory and its appropriateness for developing community-level HIV prevention interventions. In the last chapter of this group, Friedman, Des Jarlais, and Ward consider the importance of social models for changing behaviors associated with HIV infection.

Several chapters specifically address risk-reduction interventions for adolescents. Kirby and DiClemente address behavior change interventions in school settings. Similarly, Jemmott and Jemmott consider the effect of community-based interventions as a behavior change strategy. Rotheram-

Borus, Feldman, Rosario, and Dunne discuss the approaches used for risk reduction among runaway adolescents.

The next group describes the behavior change interventions tailored to injection drug users. Roehrich, Wall, and Sorensen present intervention approaches for injection drug users who are in treatment. Conversely, Watters and Guydish discuss the utility of prevention approaches for drug users in natural settings.

Two chapters focus on behavioral interventions for heterosexual women—an understudied population—at increased risk for HIV infection. Padian, van de Wijgert, and O'Brien discuss the influence of behavior change interventions for female partners of HIV-infected or high-risk men. Moore, Harrison, and Doll describe the types of interventions employed to reduce high-risk behavior among sexually active, heterosexual women.

The next section delineates the techniques used to modify high-risk behavior among homosexual and bisexual men. Hays and Peterson consider the influence of behavior change interventions among gay and bisexual men in large metropolitan areas. Kelly addresses the influence of intervention strategies for HIV prevention among gay and bisexual men in small cities. Finally, Peterson and DiClemente provide a synopsis of major limitations and gaps in behavioral intervention research and the implications for future research.

Although behavioral science has contributed to preventing the spread of HIV, enormous challenges remain. Meeting these challenges will require continued use and evaluation of rigorous individual and community-level interventions. The clock is ticking, and time is running out to curtail the HIV/ AIDS epidemic.

Ralph J. DiClemente
John L. Peterson

Contents

Chapter 3. Social Cognitive Theory and Exercise of Control over HIV Infection

Albert Bandura

Chapter 4. Using Information to Change Sexually Transmitted Disease-Related Behaviors: An Analysis Based on the Theory of Reasoned Action

Martin Fishbein, Susan E. Middlestadt, and Penelope J. Hitchcock

Chapter 5. Diffusion Theory and HIV Risk Behavior Change
James W. Dearing, Gary Meyer, and Everett M. Rogers

Chapter 6. Social Models for Changing Health-Relevant Behavior
Samuel R. Friedman, Don C. Des Jarlais, and Thomas P. Ward

Chapter 7. School-Based Interventions to Prevent Unprotected Sex and HIV among Adolescents
Douglas Kirby and Ralph J. DiClemente

Chapter 8. Interventions for Adolescents in Community Settings

John B. Jemmott III and Loretta Sweet Jemmott

Chapter 9. Preventing HIV among Runaways: Victims and Victimization

Mary Jane Rotheram-Borus, Julie Feldman, Margaret Rosario, and Edward Dunne

Chapter 13. Interventions for Sexually Active, Heterosexual Women in the United States

Janet S. Moore, Janet S. Harrison, and Lynda S. Doll

Chapter 14. HIV Prevention for Gay and Bisexual Men in Metropolitan Cities

Robert B. Hays and John L. Peterson

Chapter 15. HIV Prevention among Gay and Bisexual Men in Small Cities
Jeffrey A. Kelly

Chapter 16. Lessons Learned from Behavioral Interventions: Caveats, Gaps, and Implications
John L. Peterson and Ralph J. DiClemente

Changing HIV/AIDS Risk Behaviors
The Role of Behavioral Interventions

RALPH J. DiCLEMENTE and
JOHN L. PETERSON

INTRODUCTION

In just over a decade, the acquired immunodeficiency syndrome (AIDS) has become the most serious infectious disease in contemporary history. Since 1981, more than a quarter of a million individuals have been diagnosed with AIDS and over one million Americans are estimated to have been infected with the human immunodeficiency virus (HIV), the pathogen found to cause AIDS (Centers for Disease Control, 1993). The HIV epidemic has disproportionately affected gay and bisexual men, injection drug users and their female sex partners, and the infants of these women, while rapidly becoming one of the top ten causes of death among men and women between 24 and 45 years of age (*Morbidity and Mortality Weekly Review*, 1991).

Despite advances in biomedical research, there is still no preventive vaccine or medical cure for this deadly disease. Consequently, efforts to change high-risk behaviors remain the only available means to prevent HIV infection. Because HIV is largely transmitted through sexual behavior and the sharing of drug injection equipment, it can be prevented through appropriate behavioral changes. The risk behaviors responsible for HIV infection, however, occur in the context of people's interpersonal relationships and pose many social, psychological, and cultural obstacles to curtailing the epidemic. In this

RALPH J. DiCLEMENTE • School of Public Health, Department of Health Behavior and School of Medicine, Departments of Medicine and Pediatrics, and Center for AIDS Research, University of Alabama, Birmingham, Alabama 35294.   *JOHN L. PETERSON* • Department of Psychology, Georgia State University, Atlanta, Georgia 30303.

Preventing AIDS: Theories and Methods of Behavioral Interventions, edited by Ralph J. DiClemente and John L. Peterson. Plenum Press, New York, 1994.

chapter we discuss the important role of behavioral interventions in promoting HIV risk behavior change.

REDUCING RISKY SEXUAL BEHAVIORS

While sexual abstinence is the most obvious method of preventing sexual transmission of HIV, a substantial proportion of adults and adolescents fail to adopt this strategy (Anderson et al., 1990; Catania et al., 1992; DiClemente, 1990; Hein, 1992; Kann et al., 1991; Peterson et al., 1992). In fact, the expectation that most sexually active adults and adolescents will routinely adopt sexual abstinence as an HIV prevention strategy is unrealistic. Consequently, for most people who are not celibate, appropriate and consistent use of condoms represents the most effective strategy to reduce their risk of exposure to HIV (Cates, 1990; Cates & Stone, 1992; Van de Perre, Jacobs, & Sprecher-Goldberg, 1987).

Changing high-risk sexual behavior is a particularly difficult problem, however, because the decision to use condoms occurs in the context of people's social relationships and life-styles. A number of factors may influence the decision to use condoms during sexual intercourse including age, gender, and cultural differences regarding sexuality and sex-role relationships. Consequently, this complex decision-making process is more likely to be understood if these multiple influences, and the interactions between them, are considered in developing and implementing interventions to reduce high-risk sexual behaviors.

REDUCING RISKY INJECTION DRUG USE BEHAVIORS

In addition to sexual transmission, HIV is largely transmitted through sharing contaminated drug injection equipment. Consequently, HIV risk reduction for injection drug users (IDUs) promotes the adoption of safer injection practices. Specifically, these practices include avoiding or reducing needle reuse or sharing, cleaning injection equipment with bleach, and seeking drug abuse treatment (Des Jarlais, Friedman, & Woods, 1990).

Despite the promise of these strategies for HIV prevention, efforts to promote needle cleaning or to avoid needle sharing among IDUs have encountered formidable obstacles. These include political concerns that needle exchange might increase or appear to condone drug use, the criminality of purchasing injection equipment, limited availability of drug treatment services, and overcoming the cultural–social factors related to needle sharing.

HIV/AIDS INTERVENTION STUDIES AND WHY THEY ARE NEEDED

Early HIV prevention efforts, primarily information based, were intended to meet the urgent need for risk education services. The assumption was that a greater understanding of the behaviors associated with HIV transmission would more likely result in the adoption of HIV-preventive behaviors. Despite a marked increase in public awareness of HIV transmission, however, there has not been a corresponding change in HIV high-risk behaviors (Hingson & Strunin, 1992; Memon, 1990). While HIV risk information may be necessary, it is not sufficient to motivate behavior change (Becker & Joseph, 1988). Therefore, future prevention efforts should depend less on demonstrating that people have improved their level of HIV risk information than on demonstrating that they have actually changed their HIV risk behaviors.

If HIV prevention efforts cannot rely on providing risk information alone, then the difficult task is to develop interventions that influence other factors which are more responsible for behavior change. These behavior change interventions are likely to be more successful if they are based on carefully controlled studies derived from behavioral science theory (Kelly, Murphy, Sikkemas, & Kalichman, 1993). Theoretically based intervention studies are necessary to identify precisely which factors or components of interventions produce behavioral change. Over a decade into the AIDS epidemic, however, there are few such studies available, and even fewer which demonstrate the impact of behavioral interventions to change behavior (Fisher & Fisher, 1992; Kelly & Murphy, 1992). Consequently, more rigorous behavioral intervention studies are needed to further our understanding of how best to modify people's HIV risk behaviors (Coates, 1990; Leviton & Valdiserri, 1990).

REFERENCES

Anderson, J. E., Kann, L., Holtzman, D., Arday, S., Truman, B., & Kolbe, L. (1990). HIV/AIDS knowledge and sexual behavior among high school students. *Family Planning Perspectives, 22,* 252–255.

Becker, M. H., & Joseph, J. G. (1988). AIDS and behavioral change to reduce risk: A review. *American Journal of Public Health, 78,* 394–410.

Catania, J. A., Coates, T. J., Stall, R., Turner, H., Peterson, J., Hearst, N., Dolcini, M. M., Hudes, E., Gagnon, J., Wiley, J., & Groves, R. (1992). Prevalence of AIDS-related risk factors and condom use in the United States. *Science, 258,* 1101–1106.

Centers for Disease Control and Prevention (1993, February). *HIV/AIDS Surveillance.* Atlanta: Department of Health and Human Services.

Cates, W. (1990). The epidemiology and control of sexually transmitted diseases in adolescents. In M. Schydlower & M. A. Shafer (Eds), *AIDS and other sexually transmitted diseases* (pp. 409–427). Philadelphia, PA: Hanley & Belfus.

Cates, W., & Stone, K. M. (1992). Family planning, sexually transmitted diseases and contraceptive choice: A literature update: Pt. 1. *Family Planning Perspectives, 24,* 75–84.

Coates, T. J. (1990). Strategies for modifying sexual behavior for primary and secondary prevention of HIV disease. *Journal of Consulting & Clinical Psychology, 58,* 57–69.

Des Jarlais, D. C., Friedman, S. R., & Woods, J. S. (1990). Intravenous Drug Use and AIDS. In D. G. Ostrow (Ed.), *Behavioral aspects of AIDS* (pp. 139–155). New York: Plenum.

DiClemente, R. J. (1990). The emergence of adolescents as a risk group for human immunodeficiency virus infection. *Journal of Adolescent Research, 5,* 7–17.

Fisher, J. D., & Fisher, W. A. (1992). Changing AIDS-risk behavior. *Psychological Bulletin, 111,* 455–474.

Hein, K. (1992). Adolescents at risk for HIV infection. In R. J. DiClemente (Ed.), *Adolescents and AIDS: A generation in jeopardy* (pp. 3–16). Newbury Park, CA: Sage.

Hingson, R., & Strunin, L. (1992). Monitoring adolescents' response to the AIDS epidemic: Changes in knowledge, attitudes, beliefs and behaviors. In R. J. DiClemente (Ed.), *Adolescents and AIDS: A generation in jeopardy* (pp. 17–33). Newbury Park, CA: Sage.

Kann, L., Anderson, J. E., Holtzman, D., Ross, J., Truman, B. I., Collins, J., & Kolbe, L. J. (1991). HIV-related knowledge, beliefs, and behaviors among high school students in the United States: Results from a national survey. *Journal of School Health, 61,* 397–401.

Kelly, J. A., Murphy, D. A., Sikkemas, K. J., & Kalichman, S. C. (1993). Psychological interventions are urgently needed to prevent HIV infection: New priorities for behavioral research in the second decade of AIDS. *American Psychologist, 48,* 1023–1034.

Kelly, J. A., & Murphy, D. A. (1992). Psychological interventions with AIDS and HIV: Prevention and treatment. *Journal of Consulting & Clinical Psychology, 60,* 476–485.

Leviton, L. C., & Valdiserri, R. O. (1990). Evaluating AIDS prevention: Outcome, implementation, and mediating variables. *Evaluation & Program Planning, 13,* 55–66.

Memon, A. (1990). Young people's knowledge, beliefs, and attitudes about HIV/AIDS: A review of the research. *Health Education Research, 5,* 327–335.

Morbidity & Mortality Weekly Review (1991, January 25). Mortality attributable to HIV infection in the United States, 1981–1990. Washington DC: U.S. Department of Health & Human Services, Public Health Service.

Peterson, J. L., Grinstead, O. A., Golden, E., Catania, J. A., Kegeles, S., & Coates, T. J. (1992). Correlates of HIV risk behaviors in black and white San Francisco heterosexuals: The population-based AIDS in multiethnic neighborhoods (AMEN) study. *Ethnicity & Disease, 2,* 361–370.

Van de Perre, P., Jacobs, D., & Sprecher-Goldberger, S. (1987). The latex condom, an efficient barrier against sexual transmission of AIDS-related viruses. *AIDS, 1,* 49–52.

2

The Health Belief Model and HIV Risk Behavior Change

IRWIN M. ROSENSTOCK,
VICTOR J. STRECHER, and
MARSHALL H. BECKER

INTRODUCTION

The Health Belief Model (HBM) was initially developed in the 1950s by a group of social psychologists in the U.S. Public Health Service in an effort to explain the widespread failure of people to participate in programs to prevent or to detect disease (Hochbaum, 1958; Rosenstock, 1960, 1966, 1974). Later, the model was extended to apply to people's responses to symptoms (Kirscht, 1974) and to their behavior in response to diagnosed illness, particularly compliance with medical regimens (Becker, 1974). Over three decades, the model has been one of the most widely used psychosocial approaches to explaining health-related behavior.

Although the model evolved gradually in response to very practical programmatic concerns that will be described later, its basis in psychological theory is provided as an aid to understanding its rationale as well as its strengths and weaknesses.

IRWIN M. ROSENSTOCK • Department of Health Behavior and Health Education, School of Public Health, University of Michigan, Ann Arbor, Michigan 48109-2029, and College of Health and Human Services, California State University, Long Beach, Long Beach, California 90840. *VICTOR J. STRECHER* • Department of Health Behavior and Health Education, School of Public Health, University of North Carolina at Chapel Hill, Chapel Hill, North Carolina 17599. *MARSHALL H. BECKER* • Department of Health Behavior and Health Education, School of Public Health, University of Michigan, Ann Arbor, Michigan 48109-2029.

Preventing AIDS: Theories and Methods of Behavioral Interventions, edited by Ralph J. DiClemente and John L. Peterson. Plenum Press, New York, 1994.

During the early 1950s, academic social psychology was engaged in developing an approach to understanding behavior that grew out of a confluence of learning theories derived from two major sources: Stimulus-response (S-R) theory (Hull, 1943; Thorndike, 1898; Watson, 1925) and "Cognitive Theory" (Kohler, 1925; Lewin, 1935, 1936, 1951; Lewin, Dembo, Festinger, & Sears, 1944; Tolman, 1932). Stimulus-response theory itself represents a marriage of classical conditioning theory (Pavlov, 1927) and instrumental conditioning theory (Thorndike, 1898).

In simple terms, S-R theorists believe that learning results from events ("reinforcements") which reduce physiological drives that activate behavior. In the case of punishment, behavior that avoids punishment is learned because it reduces the tension set up by the punishment. The concept of drive reduction, however, is not necessary to S-R theory. Skinner (1938) formulated the widely accepted hypothesis that the frequency of a behavior is determined by its consequences (or reinforcements). For Skinner, the mere temporal association between a behavior and an immediately following reward is sufficient to increase the probability that the behavior will be repeated. Such behaviors are termed operants; they operate on the environment to bring about changes resulting in reward or reinforcement. In this view, no mental concepts such as "reasoning" or "thinking" are required to explain behavior.

Cognitive theorists emphasize the role of subjective hypotheses or expectations held by the subject (e.g., Lewin et al., 1944). In this perspective, behavior is a function of the subjective *value* of an outcome and of the subjective probability or *expectation* that a particular action will achieve that outcome. Such formulations are generally termed "value-expectancy" theories. Mental processes such as thinking, reasoning, hypothesizing, or expecting are critical components of all cognitive theories. Cognitive theorists, along with behaviorists, believe that reinforcements, or consequences of behavior, are important, but for cognitive theorists, reinforcements operate by influencing expectations (or hypotheses) regarding the situation rather than by influencing behavior directly (Bandura, 1977a).

The HBM is a value-expectancy theory. When value-expectancy concepts were gradually reformulated in the context of health-related behavior, the translations were as follows: (1) the desire to avoid illness or to get well (value); and (2) the belief that a specific health action available to a person would prevent (or ameliorate) illness (expectation). The expectancy was further delineated in terms of the individual's estimate of personal susceptibility to and severity of an illness, and of the likelihood of being able to reduce that threat through personal action.

The development of the HBM grew out of real concerns with the limited success of various programs of the Public Health Service in the 1950s. One such early example was the failure of large numbers of eligible adults to participate in tuberculosis screening programs provided at no charge, in mobile X-ray units conveniently located in various neighborhoods. The concern of the program operators was with explaining people's behavior by illuminating those factors that were facilitating or inhibiting positive responses.

Beginning in 1952, Hochbaum (1958) studied probability samples of more than 1200 adults in three cities that had conducted recent TB screening programs in mobile X-ray units. He assessed their "readiness" to obtain X-rays, which included their beliefs that they were susceptible to tuberculosis and their beliefs in the personal benefits of early detection. Perceived susceptibility to tuberculosis itself comprised two elements: first, the respondents' beliefs about whether contracting tuberculosis was a realistic (not merely a mathematical) possibility for them personally; and second, the extent to which they accepted the fact that one may have tuberculosis in the absence of all symptoms.

The measure of perceived personal benefits of early detection also included two elements: whether respondents believed that X rays could detect tuberculosis prior to the appearance of symptoms and whether they believed that early detection and treatment would improve the prognosis. For the group of persons that exhibited both beliefs, that is, belief in their own susceptibility to tuberculosis and the belief that overall benefits would accrue from early detection, 82 percent had at least one voluntary chest X ray during a specified period preceding the interview. Of the group exhibiting neither of these beliefs, only 21 percent had obtained a voluntary X ray during the criterion period. In short, four out of five people who exhibited both beliefs (susceptibility and benefits) took the predicted action, while four of five people who accepted neither of the beliefs had not taken the action. Hochbaum thus demonstrated with considerable precision that a particular action to screen for a disease was strongly associated with the two interacting variables—perceived susceptibility and perceived benefits.

Hochbaum also thought that the readiness to take action (perceived susceptibility and perceived benefits) could only be potentiated by other factors, particularly by "cues" to instigate action, such as bodily events, or by environmental events, such as media publicity. He did not, however, study the role of cues empirically. Indeed, while the concept of cues as a trigger mechanism is appealing, it has been the most difficult concept to study in explanatory surveys, as a cue can be as fleeting as a sneeze, or the barely conscious perception of a poster.

COMPONENTS OF THE HEALTH BELIEF MODEL

Over the years since Hochbaum's survey, many investigations have helped to expand and clarify the model and to extend it beyond screening behaviors to include all preventive actions to illness behaviors and to sick-role behavior (see summaries in Becker, 1974; Becker & Maiman, 1980; Janz & Becker, 1984; Kirscht, 1974; Rosenstock, 1974). In general, it is now believed that individuals will take action to ward off, to screen for, or to control ill-health conditions if they regard themselves as susceptible to the condition. They will also take action if they believe the health condition to have potentially serious consequences; if they believe that a course of action available to them would be beneficial in reducing either their susceptibility to or the severity of the condition; and if they believe that the anticipated barriers to (or costs of) taking the action are outweighed by its benefits. Each component of the model is described in greater detail below.

Perceived Susceptibility

This dimension refers to one's subjective perception of the risk of contracting a health condition. In the case of medically established illness, the dimension has been reformulated to include acceptance of the diagnosis, personal estimates of resusceptibility, and susceptibility to illness in general.

Perceived Severity

Feelings concerning the seriousness of contracting an illness or of leaving it untreated include evaluations of both medical and clinical consequences (e.g., death, disability, and pain) and possible social consequences (such as effects of the conditions on work, family life, and social relations). We have come to label the combination of susceptibility and severity as "perceived threat."

Perceived Benefits

While acceptance of personal susceptibility to a condition also believed to be serious (perceived threat) produces a force leading to behavior, the particular course of action that will be taken depends upon beliefs regarding the effectiveness of the various available actions in reducing the disease threat, termed the perceived *benefits* of taking health action. Thus, an individual exhibiting an optimal level of beliefs in susceptibility and severity would not be expected to accept any recommended health action unless that action was perceived as potentially efficacious.

Perceived Barriers

The potential negative aspects of a particular health action, or perceived barriers, may act as impediments to undertaking the recommended behavior.

The individual engages in a cost-benefit analysis wherein the they weigh the action's effectiveness against perceptions that it may be expensive, dangerous (having negative side effects or iatrogenic outcomes), unpleasant (painful, difficult, upsetting), inconvenient, time-consuming, and so forth. Thus, the combined levels of susceptibility and severity provide the energy or force to act and the perception of benefits (less barriers) provides a preferred path of action (Rosenstock, 1974).

Cues to Action

In various early formulations of the HBM, the concept of cues which trigger action were discussed and may ultimately prove to be important, but they have not been systematically studied.

Other Variables

Diverse demographic, sociopsychological, and structural variables may affect the individual's perceptions and thus indirectly influence health-related behavior. Specifically, sociodemographic factors, particularly educational attainment, are believed to have an indirect effect on behavior by influencing the perception of susceptibility, severity, benefits, and barriers.

Self-Efficacy

In 1977, Bandura introduced the concept of self-efficacy, or efficacy expectation, as distinct from outcome expectation (Bandura, 1977a, 1977b, 1986), which we believe must be added to the HBM in order to increase its explanatory power (Rosenstock, Strecher, & Becker, 1988). Outcome expectation, defined as a person's estimate that a given behavior will lead to certain outcomes, is quite similar to the HBM concept of "perceived benefits." Self-efficacy is defined as "the conviction that one can successfully execute the behavior required to produce the outcomes" (Bandura, 1977a, p. 79). The role of self-efficacy is discussed in detail in Bandura's chapter in this book (see Chapter 3). The issue of how HBM constructs operate in relation to each other has never been adequately addressed. We propose a view of how HBM constructs may be interrelated and tested in our analysis of the model and its utility for understanding autoimmune deficiency syndrome (AIDS) protective behavior in a later section of this chapter.

It is not difficult to see why self-efficacy was never explicitly incorporated into early formulations of the HBM. The original focus of the early model was on circumscribed preventive actions, usually of a one-shot nature, such as accepting a screening test or an immunization, actions which generally were simple behaviors for most people to perform. Since it is likely that most prospective members of target groups for those programs had adequate self-efficacy for performing those simple behaviors (which often involved receiving a service), that dimension was not even recognized.

The situation is vastly different, however, when attempting to modify life-style behaviors which require long-term changes. The problems involved in modifying lifelong habits concerning eating, drinking, exercising, smoking, and sexual practices are obviously far more difficult to surmount than are those for accepting a one-time immunization or a screening test. It requires a good deal of confidence that one can, in fact, alter such life-styles before successful change is possible. Thus, for behavior change to succeed, people must (as the original HBM theorizes) feel threatened by their current behavioral patterns (perceived susceptibility and severity), and believe that change of a specific kind will be beneficial by resulting in a valued outcome at acceptable cost, but they must also feel themselves competent (self-efficacious) to implement that change. A growing body of literature supports the importance of self-efficacy in helping to account for initiation and maintenance of behavioral change (Bandura, 1977b, 1986; Marlatt & Gordon, 1985; Strecher, DeVellis, Becker, & Rosenstock, 1986).

The HBM, originally developed to explain health-related behavior, focused on cognitive variables. Efforts to change cognition about health matters, however, have often involved attempts to arouse affect (fear) through threatening messages (Leventhal, 1970). According to protection motivation theory (Rogers, 1975) the most persuasive communications are those that arouse fear while enhancing perceptions central to the HBM, of the severity of an event, the likelihood of exposure to that event, and the efficacy of responses to that threat. More recently, Rogers (1983) has incorporated self-efficacy into his theory. This view of the joint role of fear and reassurance in persuasive communications is generally accepted.

As a convenient way of summarizing the Health Belief Model components we may subsume the key variables under three categories, which are summarized in Figure 1.

EVIDENCE FOR AND AGAINST THE MODEL

In 1974, Health Education Monographs devoted an entire issue to "The Health Belief Model and Personal Health Behavior" (Becker, 1974). That monograph summarized findings from research on the HBM to understand why individuals did or did not engage in a wide variety of health-related actions. Considerable empirical support was found for the model in explaining

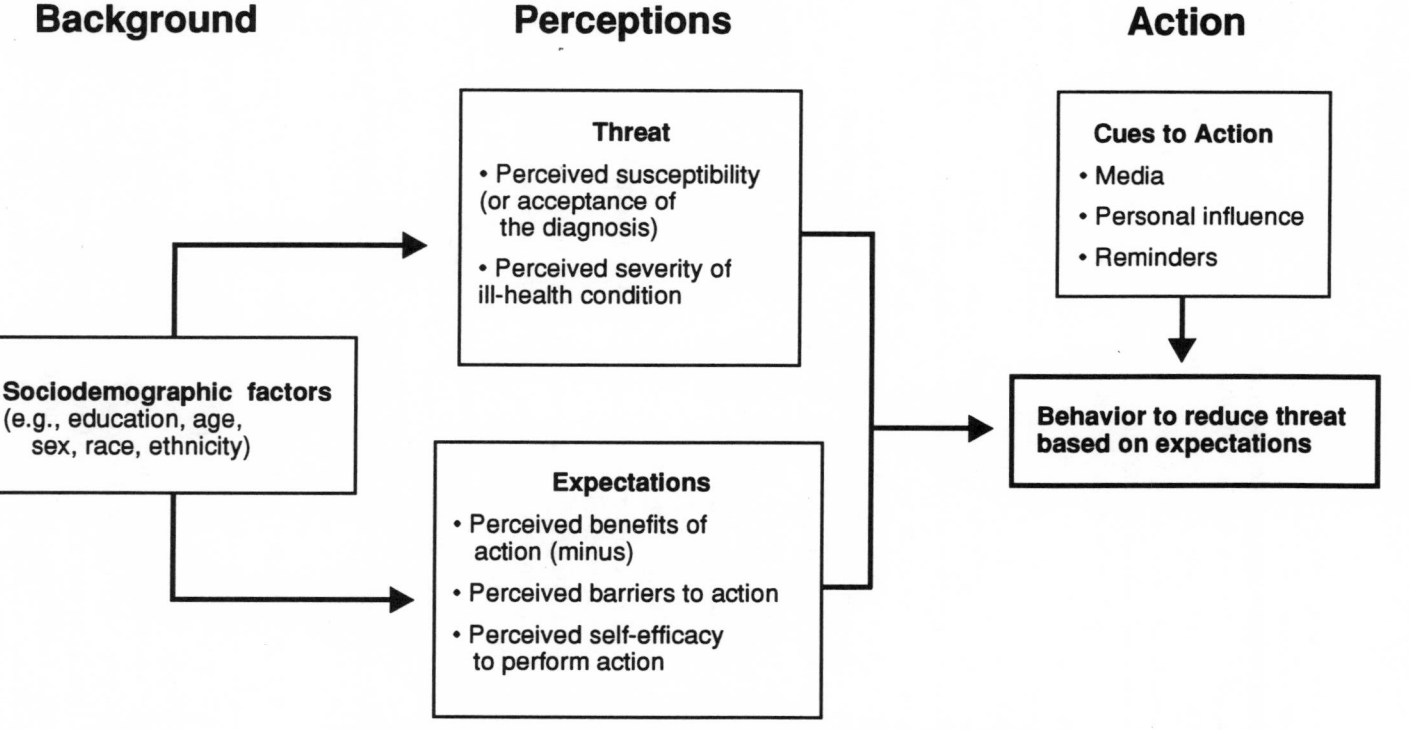

Figure 1. Schematic diagram of the components of the Health Belief Model

behavior pertinent to prevention and behavior in response to symptoms or to diagnosed disease.

During the following decade, the HBM continued to be a major organizing framework for explaining and predicting acceptance of health and medical care recommendations. Accordingly, an updated critical review was made of HBM studies conducted between 1974 and 1984, which also combined the new results with earlier findings to permit an overall assessment of the model's performance (Janz & Becker, 1984).

A brief summary of the findings of the detailed reviews of 1974 and 1984 is presented below. The interested reader should consult these sources directly for more detailed information.

Included in the 1984 review were such preventive health and screening behaviors as influenza inoculations, Tay-Sachs carrier status screening program, practice of breast self-examination, and attendance at screening programs for high blood pressure, seat-belt use, exercise, nutrition, smoking, visits to physicians for checkups, and fear of being apprehended while under the influence of alcohol. Sick-role behaviors included compliance with antihypertensive regimens, diabetic regimens, end-stage renal disease regimens, medication regimens for parents to give their children with otitis media, weight loss regimens, and medication regimens for parents to give to asthmatic children.

Summary results provide substantial empirical support for the HBM, with findings from prospective studies at least as favorable as those obtained from retrospective research.

"Perceived barriers" was the single most powerful predictor of behavior, relative to other HBM constructs, across different behaviors and type of studies. While both "perceived susceptibility" and "perceived benefits" were important overall, "perceived susceptibility" was a stronger predictor of preventive health behavior than sick-role behavior, while the reverse was true for "perceived benefits." Overall, "perceived severity" was the least powerful predictor; however, this construct was strongly related to sick-role behavior.

THE HEALTH BELIEF MODEL AND AIDS-PROTECTIVE BEHAVIORS

We preface this section with a number of caveats. First, this section is a selective, not comprehensive, review of the literature. Second, our focus was on research largely examining HBM constructs and safe-sex behavior. This decision was forced on us due to the paucity of research literature related to other HIV-transmission vectors (the most notable example being intravenous drug use). A number of studies include intravenous (IV) drug use in a composite dependent variable (a general AIDS-preventive behavior index), but the emphasis remained on safe-sex behavior. Third, while a few studies on adolescents were examined in our review, the vast majority of studies focused on gay and heterosexual adult populations. Finally, we examined both cross-sectional and longitudinal studies, but recognize the clear superiority of longitudinal designs in studies of belief–behavior relationships.

Ideally, we should have looked at the predictive utility of the HBM as a whole model. That is, we should have examined how individuals with various combinations of health beliefs were more or less likely to engage in higher- or lower-risk AIDS preventive behaviors. One would predict, for example, perceptions of susceptibility and severity to be associated largely with an intention to take action, similar to the predicted functions of attitudes in the theory of reasoned action (Ajzen & Fishbein, 1980). We agree with Catania and colleagues' (Catania, Kegeles, & Coates, 1990b) theoretical analysis that, for individuals who objectively exhibit high-risk behaviors, perceived susceptibility is a factor required before commitment to changing these risky behaviors can occur. The HBM goes on to hypothesize that those committed to taking action would then assess the benefits of taking a recommended health action and the barriers to taking the action. If the benefits outweigh the barriers, the individual would be more likely to take the recommended health action.

Unfortunately, none of the research we could find which examines the utility of the HBM in predicting AIDS-preventive behavior, analyzed the constructs in this manner. In fact, every study we found treated the constructs separately. Analyses that essentially incorporate all health belief constructs into a multiple regression model do not test the HBM in the manner we are advising here. One would hypothesize, for example, that among those with high perceived threat, perceptions of benefits and barriers would be more predictive of behavior change. Appropriate tests of this hypothesis would require analyses of subgroups (e.g., testing the effects of benefits and barriers only for those with high perceived threat) or multivariate analyses involving a carefully constructed series of interaction terms.

Perceived Susceptibility, Severity, and Perceived Threat

As previously mentioned, perceiving a threat of a particular illness or disease is seen, in the HBM, as a critical initial cognitive step in the process of taking a recommended action to reduce the threat. It will be recalled that the HBM views the perception of threat as a combination of two factors: individuals' perception that they are susceptible to the disease or illness and a perception that the illness is severe, where severity may include medical, clinical, financial, and social consequences.

How do perceptions of susceptibility and severity function to produce a state of heightened threat? Whether individuals actually separate the two concepts in their consideration of threat is unclear (Weinstein, 1988). Indeed, the relationship is not made clear in the HBM itself. Perceptions of threat could be made sequentially or multiplicatively.

An example may be illustrative. Suppose a person reporting, on a scale of 1 to 10 (where 1 represents a low value and 10 represents a high value), that their susceptibility to acquiring AIDS is a 4, but that the severity of AIDS, again on a scale of 1 to 10, is a 10. If the threat perception was based on a sequential assessment process, the person might first consider the severity of the disease. If the severity was low, there might be no subsequent consideration of susceptibility. If severity reaches a certain threshold, which in this case it has, the person then considers whether or not to take action. This is when the perception of susceptibility is considered. Perceived susceptibility is moderate, and the person takes precautions, in part, as a function of this perception. In the case of getting the flu, this same person might report that their susceptibility level is an 8, and that the severity is a 5. In this case, a sequential assessment process beginning with severity might pass the "severity threshold" to consider the susceptibility to getting the flu, and the overall perceived threat would be quite high. The sequential process could also move in the opposite way, beginning with an assessment of susceptibility, though this seems less likely. We would anticipate people first becoming alarmed at the severity of a disease or illness before considering their personal susceptibility.

If susceptibility and severity are multiplicative, the resultant threat perception could be very different. In the example outlined above, the multiplicative process, if linear, would result in a 40/100 measure of perceived threat for both the AIDS and flu examples. Note that in the sequential process, the person would be far more likely to take precautions against acquiring the flue than against acquiring AIDS. Also, the multiplicative process produced the same level of threat perception for both the AIDS and flu examples as would have been produced in the sequential process using the AIDS example.

How is this theoretical analysis relevant to the global problem of AIDS? The way in which an individual processes risk-based messages should have a large influence on the messages created in AIDS campaigns. For example, should a campaign attempt to see that everyone first understands and accepts the severity of AIDS and HIV? Will promoting the severity of AIDS and HIV enhance perceptions of threat in individuals who believe they are relatively low-risk individuals, or is susceptibility alone important to perceived threat once the high severity of AIDS is taken into account? Unfortunately, there is no empirical research available specifically addressing this issue. A relatively simple, though post hoc way to examine this problem would be to reexamine data that has both severity and susceptibility measures, comparing the amount of variance explained in high-risk AIDS-related behaviors using both multiplicative and sequential combinations.

One might argue that the entire issue of how one processes severity and susceptibility constructs is moot in the problem of AIDS because everyone perceives AIDS as an extremely severe disease. Indeed, if perceived severity was consistently high, the processing function would be irrelevant, because we would be essentially dealing with only one variable, that of susceptibility. However, as we will discuss later, individuals do appear to vary in their assessments of the severity of AIDS.

Perceived Susceptibility

When reviewing research examining a susceptibility–behavior association, we found very mixed results. In a longitudinal study of gay men's AIDS-protective behavior, Aspinwall, Kemeny, Taylor, Schneider, and Dudley (1991) found decreases in numbers of sexual partners (anonymous and known) chiefly among seronegative men, who had earlier perceived themselves to be at increased risk of contracting HIV. Cross-sectional studies (e.g., Hays, Kegeles, & Coates, 1990; Allard, 1989; Basen-Engquist, 1992; Hingson, Strunin, Berlin, & Heeren, 1990) also have found significant susceptibility–behavior associations. Countering these findings are a number of longitudinal studies (e.g., McKusick, Coates, Morin, Pollack, & Hoff, 1990; Montgomery et al., 1989) and cross-sectional studies (e.g., Brown, DiClemente, & Park, 1992; Catania et al., 1992; DiClemente, 1991; DiClemente et al., 1992; Durbin et al., in press; Walter et al., 1992).

We were particularly interested in whether trends in a susceptibility–behavior association differed among higher risk versus lower risk groups, in cross-sectional versus longitudinal study designs, and in various methods of measuring susceptibility. In this analysis, we found little to suggest a higher or lower susceptibility–behavior association among gay men, among the general adult population, or among adolescents. We also found no trend among longitudinal versus cross-sectional studies. We did, however, find variation in results by the methods used to measure susceptibility. A number of articles we reviewed used a behavioral anchor in their susceptibility measures; for example, asking the question: "*If you do not practice safer sex,* how likely are you to become infected with the AIDS virus?" as opposed to simply: "How likely are you to become infected with the AIDS virus?" Recent research by Ronis (1992) strongly suggests that susceptibility questions should be clearly conditional on action or inaction. Unconditional susceptibility measures can lead to a pattern of personalized interpretation—respondents who indicate that their risk of infection is great largely *because* they are not practicing safer sex.

Perceived Severity

Perceptions of AIDS severity must address the perceived costs of being HIV positive and of having AIDS. As mentioned previously, perceived seriousness refers to personal evaluations of the probable biomedical, financial, and social consequences of contracting HIV and having AIDS. Ostensibly, one would think that items reflecting this construct would focus on the life changes involved in an increasingly debilitative disease such as AIDS, interpersonal effects, the agony of the dying process, and the perceived impact of one's death. Then, as previously stated, this measure should interact with the perception of susceptibility to form a perception of AIDS threat.

Some might argue that AIDS severity would be perceived of as uniformly high—everyone would report that AIDS is an extremely severe disease. Unfortunately, most measures in the research literature did not focus directly on these elements of AIDS severity. Items that most closely related to perceived severity included a general measure of AIDS seriousness: "How serious a health problem is AIDS?" (Aspinwall et al., 1991), and a measure of the likelihood of dying from AIDS (Hingson et al., 1990). These measures, however, still did not directly address personal evaluations of the probable biomedical, financial, and social consequences of contracting HIV and having AIDS.

Would most individuals perceive that contracting HIV and dying from AIDS as "severe"? This would seem likely. However, fear of death or the perception of death as being severe may not always be the case for high-risk individuals. In a study of HIV risk taking among young men, Hays and colleagues (Hays, Kegeles, & Coates, 1990) cite a poignant statement of an HIV-positive respondent: "It seems like nobody cares if I die anyway" (p. 905). Consideration must also be given to the possibility that the perceived severity of rejection and of not being loved, may exceed the perceived severity of the infection and thus lead to unsafe sexual practices. These comments, in our opinion, speak to the need for sophisticated measurement of perceived severity of all aspects of AIDS, including dying from the disease.

Most measures of AIDS severity we found focused on the anxiety that AIDS produced. For example, the personal severity measure used by Montgomery and colleagues (1989) in a study of gay men in Chicago concerned the "stress of AIDS since beginning and past month." Anxiety and worry could certainly be found in those that perceive AIDS as a serious disease. Anxiety from AIDS is likely to be low, however, unless an individual also feels *susceptible* to the risk of acquiring AIDS. In other words, anxiety is not just a function of perceived severity.

Studies using AIDS anxiety measures have found mixed associations with AIDS-related behaviors. For example, Montgomery and colleagues (1989) found perceived severity to be the most consistent longitudinal predictor of AIDS-protective behavior changes out of all Health Belief Model constructs. Allard (1989) found cross-sectional associations between severity measures (many of which were related to AIDS anxiety) and AIDS-protective behaviors. Walter and colleagues (1992) and Catania and colleagues (1992), however, also in cross-sectional studies, did not find such associations. Catania and colleagues (Catania, Kegeles, & Coates, 1990a) found that among individuals seeking an HIV antibody test, those who reported greater AIDS anxiety were *less* likely to return for their test results.

Perceived Benefits minus Barriers to Behavior Change

For any level of perceived threat of AIDS beyond a threshold, the HBM would hypothesize that AIDS-protective behavior decisions become largely a function of perceptions of benefits minus perceived barriers to behavior change. If the perception of AIDS threat is not high, strong perceived benefits of AIDS-protective behavior may still influence behavior change. For example, a person who uses condoms because his partner prefers them may adopt and maintain condom-use behavior regardless of his perception of AIDS threat. Although there are perceived benefits in this example, they are not directly related to AIDS-protective behavior, but rather to the benefits of pleasing one's partner. If the perceptions of AIDS threat and benefits are not high, it is not likely that low perceived barriers would necessarily influence AIDS-preventive behavior.

Perceived Benefits

Of the possible benefits, "response efficacy," or the perception that adopting and maintaining AIDS-preventive behaviors will reduce AIDS risk, is one of the most commonly researched. Measures of response efficacy (e.g., Allard, 1989; Aspinwall et al., 1991; DiClemente et al., 1992; Hingson et al., 1990), although this relationship was found only among HIV-positive men without a primary sexual partner, have been associated with AIDS-preventive behaviors in cross-sectional and longitudinal studies. The HBM would hypothesize that these associations would be even stronger among those reporting strong perceptions of AIDS threat. This is consistent with Catania and colleagues' (1990b) theoretical analysis suggesting that response efficacy will be most relevant once a decision to commit to changing sexual behaviors has been made.

Other benefits of AIDS-preventive behaviors have been examined by Catania et al. (1991). Positive personal feelings resulting from condom use and positive regard from the respondent's sex partner for condom use, distinguished men who always used condoms from those who did not. A nearly significant trend ($p < .06$) was found for the effects of condom use on sexual pleasure. The perception that condoms enhanced sexual pleasure distinguished men who always did versus did not use condoms.

Perceived Barriers

In Catania et al. (1991), as well as others, condom use is generally perceived as a *barrier* to sexual pleasure. In one cross-sectional study, DiClemente and his colleagues (1992) found that among inner-city, predominantly minority adolescents, those whose perceived cost of condom use was lowest (low perceived barrier to using condoms), were markedly more likely to report being consistent condom users. However, the relationship between perceived barriers and AIDS-preventive behaviors have been mixed across both longitudinal and cross-sectional studies.

A number of the studies we reviewed included questionable measures of barriers. Montgomery et al. (1989), for example, used a "barriers" measure that included knowledge of the virus and modes of transmission, whether the respondent was ever paid for sex, and belief in a vaccine or a potential cure; the study did not include lack of sexual enjoyment as a barrier. These measures were unrelated to subsequent AIDS-protective behavior changes. Another negative study (Allard, 1989) used only two "barriers to [AIDS] treatment" items—not at all relevant to preventive practices.

Studies using more relevant barriers measures tended to find results in the expected direction. Basen-Engquist (1992) found strong associations in the expected direction between perceived barriers and both intention to use condoms and actual condom use. Seven barriers were aggregated to form a single scale; examples of barriers included "embarrassment caused by practicing safer sex, moral implications of condom use, and satisfaction involved in practicing safer sex" (p. 125). Aspinwall and colleagues (1991) used barrier measures that included importance, temptation, and difficulty of refraining from sex with numerous partners. This study found that gay men without primary partners who reported strong barriers reported higher numbers of anonymous sexual partners at follow-up. Baseline reports of strong barriers to changing unprotected anal receptive intercourse also predicted subsequent unprotected anal receptive intercourse with partners whose HIV status was unknown.

As these studies suggest, the concepts of benefits and barriers are rather open-ended, and can include wide domains of factors, including emotional, physical, and social. It should be noted here that one of the most important barriers to engaging in AIDS-preventive behaviors may be lack of self-efficacy. As noted earlier, this construct has been suggested for inclusion in the HBM.

Researchers must continue determining just which benefits and barriers exist and which have the greatest influence on AIDS-preventive behaviors. As with the construct of perceived susceptibility, we found that the adequacy of the benefits and barriers measures used, as judged by their face validity, often were the most important predictors of whether a positive or negative association with AIDS-protective behavior was found. Unfortunately, most studies we reviewed failed to specify the actual measures used.

Cues to Action

In the HBM, if perceived AIDS threat is high and perceived benefits outweigh perceived barriers, a cue-to-action can prompt or trigger an individual to adopt and maintain AIDS-preventive behavior, in effect stimulating the belief–action link. Again, we are suggesting that the cue-to-action construct be analyzed in concert with perceived threat. We hypothesize that cues-to-action will be more strongly associated with AIDS-preventive behavior among individuals who have a high perceived AIDS threat. None of the studies we could find analyzed the cue-to-action construct in this manner.

As indicated earlier, the cue-to-action construct is, in general and in the area of AIDS prevention, the least studied construct in the HBM. This is unfortunate, since a good deal of anecdotal evidence supports the importance of brief, though salient cues that stimulate a decision to act. Similar to perceived barriers and benefits, it is important to determine what cues-to-action exist as well as their relative efficacy in influencing AIDS-preventive behaviors.

Cues-to-action were examined in the Hingson et al. (1990) and the Aspinwall et al. (1991) studies. Among a general population of adolescents, Hingson and colleagues asked the respondent whether he or she had read or heard about AIDS from media sources; ever discussed AIDS with a family member, teacher, or physician; and whether they knew someone with AIDS. Having discussed AIDS with friends or with a physician was positively associated with condom use. However, knowledge of someone with AIDS was *negatively* associated with condom use. Aspinwall et al. (1991) asked how many close friends had AIDS-related complex (ARC), how many had AIDS, and how many had died from AIDS or ARC in the past year. A summed index of these potential cues-to-action did not predict AIDS-protective behavior changes.

RECOMMENDATION FOR FUTURE RESEARCH

We offer the following recommendations for researchers and reviewers of manuscripts submitted for publication that examine HBM variables:

1. Test the HBM as a model—not as a collection of equally weighted variables operating simultaneously. It makes little sense to include all the health belief constructs in a multivariate analysis, select the "strongest swimmers," and claim that these are the factors on which to intervene (Brown, DiClemente, & Reynolds, 1991). In the AIDS prevention area, we found *no* study that tested the HBM; we found many that tested individual HBM constructs. We offer the following hypotheses as a starting point for testing the Health Belief Model as a model:

   a. Perceived threat is a sequential function of perceived severity and perceived susceptibility. A heightened state of severity is required before perceived susceptibility becomes a powerful predictor. Perceived susceptibility, under the state of high perceived severity, will be a stronger predictor of intention to engage in AIDS-preventive behaviors than it will be a predictor of actual engagement in AIDS-preventive behaviors.

   b. Perceived benefits and barriers will be stronger predictors of behavior change when perceived threat is high rather than when it is low. Under conditions of low perceived threat, benefits of and barriers to engaging in AIDS-preventive behavior will not be salient. The only exception to this may be when certain benefits of the recommended behavior are perceived to be high (e.g., a partner's support and encouragement for safe sex), perceived threat may not need to be high.

   c. Self-efficacy, a factor now included in the HBM, will be a strong predictor of many AIDS-preventive behaviors. Self-efficacy will be a particularly strong predictor of behaviors that require significant skills to perform. As previously mentioned, self-efficacy is not addressed in this chapter, since an entire chapter in this book (Chapter 3) is devoted to the subject.

   d. Cues-to-action will have a greater influence on behavior in situations where perceived threat is great. The cue-to-action construct is a little-studied phenomenon: in the AIDS-prevention area, we know little about what cues-to-action exist or their relative impact.

2. Specify the measures used to study belief constructs in publications. We suspect that an important reason for variance in results between studies is due to large variations in the specific measures used. When the actual questions were included in the article or could be uncovered in some manner, a disconcertingly large proportion did not appear to be good measures of HBM constructs.

3. Researchers should delay aggregating items measuring benefits, barriers, and cue-to-action into general constructs; such items are often unrelated

to one another, and have low inter-item correlations. To the practitioner charged with creating programs that will contain AIDS prevention messages, analysis of single items can often offer more relevant information than a general grouped construct.

4. Include a behavioral anchor when measuring perceived susceptibility. A behaviorally anchored question would ask, "*If you do not practice safer sex,* how likely are you to become infected with the AIDS virus?" as opposed to, "How likely are you to become infected with the AIDS virus?" The reader is referred to recent research by Ronis (1992), which finds strong evidence for the importance of asking susceptibility questions that are conditional on action or inaction.

IMPLICATIONS FOR AIDS PREVENTION

This chapter has described both strengths and limitations in the HBM as formulated to date. It is hoped that future theory building or theory testing research will direct efforts more toward strengthening the HBM where it is weak than toward repeating what has already been established. More work is needed on experimental interventions to modify health beliefs and health behavior than on surveys to reconfirm already established correlations. More work is also needed to specify and measure factors that need to be added to the model to increase its predictive power. The addition of self-efficacy to the traditional HBM should improve explanation and prediction, particularly in the area of life-style practices.

This review has provided limited, but important, evidence that HBM variables are associated with health-related behavior and that manipulation of the health belief variables can lead to increased compliance with health recommendations. It is timely for professionals who are attempting to influence health-related behaviors to make use of the health belief variables, including self-efficacy in their program planning, both in needs assessment and in program strategies. Programs to deal with a health problem should be based, in part, on knowledge of how many and which members of a target population feel susceptible to AIDS, believe it to constitute a serious health problem, and believe that the threat could be reduced by changing their sexual practice at an acceptable psychological cost. Moreover, health professionals should also assess the extent to which clients possess adequate self-efficacy to carry out the prescribed actions, sometimes over long periods of time.

The collection of data on health beliefs, including self-efficacy, along with other data pertinent to the group or community setting permits the planning of more effective programs than would otherwise be possible. Interventions can then be targeted to the specific needs identified by such an assessment. This is true whether dealing with the problems of individual patients, with groups of clients or with entire communities. For example, if we find that people fear the consequence of AIDS and accept their susceptibility to the disease, but also believe that there are no preventives for AIDS or that the preventives may seem unacceptable, we can tailor interventions to increase perceived benefits, and to reduce perceived barriers. Other belief combinations would call for emphasizing different risk-reduction strategies.

Changes in knowledge and beliefs will surely continue to be required in efforts to achieve behavior change; however, an analysis of the literature linking self-efficacy to health behavior indicates that in the realm of chronic disease control, much more emphasis is likely to be needed on skill training to enhance self-efficacy. We leave discussion of this topic to the next chapter by Bandura.

In planning programs to influence the behavior of large groups of people for long periods of time, the role of the HBM (including self-efficacy) must be considered in context. Permanent changes in behavior can rarely be wrought solely by direct attacks on belief systems. Even more, where the behavior of large groups is the target, interventions at societal levels (e.g., social networks, work organizations, the physical environment, the legislature) along with interventions at the individual level will likely prove more effective than single-level interventions. Yet, we should never lose sight of the fact that a crucial way station on the road to improved health is in the beliefs and behavior of each of a series of individuals.

REFERENCES

Ajzen, I., & Fishbein, M. (1980). *Understanding attitudes and predicting social behavior.* NJ: Prentice-Hall.

Allard, R. (1989). Beliefs about AIDS as determinants of preventive practices and of support for coercive measures. *American Journal of Public Health,* 448–452.

Aspinwall, L., Kemeny, M., Taylor, S., Schneider, S., Dudley, J. (1991). Psychosocial predictors of gay men's AIDS risk-reduction behavior. *Health Psychology, 10,* 432–444.

Bandura, A. (1977a). *Social learning theory.* Englewood Cliffs, NJ: Prentice-Hall.

Bandura, A. (1977b). Self-efficacy: Toward a unifying theory of behavior change. *Psychological Review, 84,* 191–215.

Bandura, A. (1986). *Social foundations of thought and action.* Englewood Cliffs, NJ: Prentice-Hall.

Basen-Engquist, K. (1992). Psychosocial predictors of "safer sex" behaviors in young adults. *AIDS Education & Prevention, 4,* 120–134.

Becker, M. H. (Ed.) (1974). The health belief model and personal health behavior. *Health Education Monographs, 2,* 324–473.

Becker, M. H., & Maiman, L. A. (1980). Strategies for enhancing patient compliance. *Journal of Community Health, 6,* 113–135.

Brown, L. K., DiClemente, R. J., & Park, T. (1992). Predictors of condom use among sexually active adolescents. *Journal of Adolescent Health, 13,* 651–657.

Brown, L. K., DiClemente, R. J., & Reynolds, L. A. (1991). HIV prevention for adolescents: Utility of the Health Belief Model. *Journal of AIDS Education & Prevention, 3,* 50–59.

Catania, J., Coates, T., Kegeles, S., Fullilove, M., Peterson, J., Marin, B., Siegel, D., & Hulley, S. (1992). Condom use in multi-ethnic neighborhoods of San Francisco: The population-based AMEN (AIDS in multi-ethnic neighborhoods) study. *American Journal of Public Health, 182,* 284–287.

Catania, J., Coates, T., Stall, R., Bye, L., Kegeles, S., Capell, F., Henne, J., McKusick, L., Morin, S., Turner, H., Pollack, (1991). Changes in condom use among homosexual men in San Francisco. *Health Psychology, 10,* 190–199.

Catania, J., Kegeles, J., & Coates, T. (1990a). Psychosocial predictors of people who fail to return for their HIV test results. *AIDS, 4*(3), 261–262.

Catania, J., Kegeles, J., & Coates, T. (1990b). Towards an understanding of risk behavior: An AIDS risk reduction model (AARM). *Health Education Quarterly, 17,* 53–72.

DiClemente, R. J. (1991). Predictors of HIV-preventive sexual behavior in a high-risk adolescent population: The influence of perceived peer norms and sexual communication on incarcerated adolescents' consistent use of condoms. *Journal of Adolescent Health, 12,* 385–390.

DiClemente, R. J., Durbin, M., Siegel, D., Krasnovsky, F., Lazarus, N., & Comacho, T. (1992). Determinants of condom use among junior high school students in a minority, inner-city school district. *Pediatrics, 89,* 197–202.

Durbin, M., DiClemente, R. J., Siegel, D., Krasnovsky, F., Lazarus, N., & Comacho, T. (in press). Predictors of multiple-partnered sex among predominantly minority inner-city adolescents in an AIDS epicenter. *Journal of Adolescent Health.*

Hays, R., Kegeles, S., Coates, T. (1990). High HIV risk-taking among young gay men. *AIDS, 4,* 901–907.

Hingson, R., Strunin, L., Berlin, B., & Heeren, T. (1990). Beliefs about AIDS, use of alcohol and drugs, and unprotected sex among Massachusetts adolescents. *American Journal of Public Health, 80,* 295–299.

Hochbaum, G. M. (1958). *Public participation in medical screening programs: A sociopsychological study.* (Public Health Service, PHS Publication 572). Washington, DC: U. S. Government Printing Office.

Hull, C. L. (1943). *Principles of behavior.* New York: Appleton-Century-Crofts.

Janz, N. K., & Becker, M. H. (1984). The health belief model: A decade later. *Health Education Quarterly, 11,* 1–47.

Kirscht, J. P. (1974). The health belief model and illness behavior. *Health Education Monographs, 2,* 387–408.

Kohler, W. (1925). *The mentality of apes.* New York: Harcourt Brace.

Leventhal, H. (1970). Findings and theory in the study of fear communications. In L. Berkowitz (Ed.), *Advances in Experimental Social Psychology* (Vol 5). New York: Academic Press.

Lewin, K. (1935). *A dynamic theory of personality.* New York: McGraw-Hill.

Lewin, K. (1936). *Principles of topological psychology.* New York: McGraw-Hill.

Lewin, K. (1951). The nature of field theory. In M. H. Marx (Ed.), *Psychological Theory.* New York: Macmillan.

Lewin, K., Dembo, T., Festinger, L., & Sears, P. S. (1944). Level of aspiration. In J. Hunt (Ed.), *Personality and the Behavior Disorders.* New York: The Ronald Press.

Marlatt, G. A. & Gordon, J. R. (Eds.). (1985). *Relapse prevention.* New York: Guilford Press.

McKusick, L., Coates, T., Morin, S., Pollack, L., & Hoff, C. (1990). Longitudinal predictors of reductions in unprotected anal intercourse among gay men in San Francisco: The AIDS behavioral research project. *American Journal of Public Health, 80*(8), 978–983.

Montgomery, S., Joseph, J., Becker, M., Ostrow, D., Kessler, R., & Kirscht, J. (1989). The health belief model in understanding compliance with preventive recommendations for AIDS: How useful? *AIDS Education and Prevention, 1,* 303–323.

Pavlov, I. (1927). *Conditioned reflexes.* Oxford: Oxford University Press.

Rogers, R. W. (1975). A protection motivation theory of fear appeals and attitude change. *The Journal of Psychology, 91,* 93–114.

Rogers, R. W. (1983). Cognitive and psychological in fear appeals and attitude change: A revised theory of protection motivation. In J. Cacioppo & R. Petty (Eds.), *Social psychophysiology.* New York: Guilford Press.

Ronis, D. (1992). Conditional health threats: Health beliefs, decisions, and behaviors among adults. *Health Psychology, 11,* 127–134.

Rosenstock, I. M. (1960). What research in motivation suggests for public health. *American Journal of Public Health, 50,* 295–301.

Rosenstock, I. M. (1966). Why people use health services. *Milbank Memorial Fund Quarterly, 44,* 94–124.

Rosenstock, I. M. (1974). Historical origins of the health belief model. *Health Education Monographs, 2,* 328–335.

Rosenstock, I. M., Strecher, V. J., & Becker, M. H. (1988). Social learning theory and the health belief model. *Health Education Quarterly, 15,* 175–183.

Skinner, B. F. (1938). *The behavior of organisms.* New York: Appleton-Century-Crofts.

Strecher, V. J., DeVellis, B. M., Becker, M. H., & Rosenstock, I. M. The role of self-efficacy in achieving health behavior change. *Health Education Quarterly, 13,* 73–92.

Thorndike, E. L. (1898). Animal intelligence: an experimental study of the associative processes in animals. *Psychological Monographs, 2,* (Whole No. 8).

Tolman, E. C. (1932). *Purposive behavior in animals and men.* New York: Appleton-Century-Crofts.

Walter, H., Vaughan, R., Gladis, M., Ragin, D., Kasen, S., Cohall, A. (1992). Factors associated with AIDS risk behaviors among high school students in an AIDS epicenter. *American Journal of Public Health, 82,* 528–532.

Watson, J. B. (1925). *Behaviorism.* New York: Norton.

Weinstein, N. D. (1988). The precaution adoption process. *Health Psychology, 7,* 355–386.

3

Social Cognitive Theory and Exercise of Control over HIV Infection

ALBERT BANDURA

INTRODUCTION

Prevention of infection with the acquired immunodeficiency syndrome (AIDS) virus requires people to exercise influence over their own behavior and their social environment. Societal efforts designed to control the spread of AIDS have centered mainly on informing the public about how the human immunodeficiency virus (HIV) is transmitted and how to safeguard against such infection. It is widely assumed that if people are adequately informed about the AIDS threat they will take appropriate self-protective action. Heightened awareness and knowledge of health risks are important preconditions for self-directed change. Unfortunately, information alone does not necessarily exert much influence on refractory health-impairing habits. To achieve self-directed change, people need to be given not only reasons to alter risky habits but also the behavioral means, resources, and social supports to do so. Effective self-regulation of behavior is not achieved by an act of will. It requires certain skills in self-motivation and self-guidance (Bandura, 1986). Moreover, there is a major difference between possessing self-regulative skills and being able to use them effectively and consistently under difficult circumstances. Success,

This is a revised and updated chapter which appeared in R. DiClemente (Ed.), *Adolescents and AIDS: A generation in jeopardy* (pp. 89–116). Newbury Park, CA: Sage Publications, Inc., 1992.

ALBERT BANDURA • Department of Psychology, Stanford University, Stanford, California 94305.

Preventing AIDS: Theories and Methods of Behavioral Interventions, edited by Ralph J. DiClemente and John L. Peterson. Plenum Press, New York, 1994.

therefore, requires strong self-belief in one's efficacy to exercise personal control.

Perceived self-efficacy is concerned with people's beliefs that they can exert control over their own motivation, thought processes, emotional states, and patterns of behavior. People's beliefs about their capabilities affect what they choose to do, how much effort they mobilize, how long they will persevere in the face of difficulties, whether they engage in self-debilitating or self-encouraging thought patterns, and the amount of stress and depression they experience in taxing situations. When people lack a sense of self-efficacy, they do not manage situations effectively even though they know what to do and possess the requisite skills. Self-doubts override knowledge and self-protective action.

Numerous studies have been conducted linking perceived self-efficacy to health-promoting and health-impairing behavior (Bandura, 1991a; O'Leary, 1985). The results show that perceived self-efficacy can affect every phase of personal change; for example, whether people even consider changing their health habits, how hard they try should they choose to do so, how much they change, and how well they maintain the changes they have achieved. In addition to influencing health habits, a low sense of efficacy in coping with stressors activates autonomic, catecholamine, and endogenous opioid systems that can impair immune function (Bandura, 1991a; Maier, Laudenslager, & Ryan, 1985).

Translating health knowledge into effective self-protection action against AIDS infection requires social and self-regulative skills and a sense of personal power to exercise control over sexual and drug activities, the two major transmitter modes of the AIDS virus. As Gagnon and Simon (1973) have correctly observed, managing sexuality involves managing interpersonal relationships. Thus, risk reduction calls for enhancement of interpersonal efficacy rather than simply targeting a specific infective behavior for change. The major problem is not teaching people safer sex guidelines, which is easily achievable, but equipping them with skills and self-beliefs that enable them to put the guidelines consistently into practice in the face of counteracting influences. Difficulties arise in following safer sex practices because self-protection often conflicts with interpersonal pressures and sentiments. In these interpersonal situations the sway of coercive threat, allurements, desire for social acceptance, social pressures, situational constraints, fear of rejection, and personal embarrassment can override the influence of the best of informed judgment. Women have the lowest assurance in their power to exercise control over pressures by a desirable partner to engage in unprotected intercourse that potentially places them at risk of infection (Kasen, Vaughan, & Walter, 1992). Experiences of forced unwanted intercourse, which are not uncommon, lower women's sense of efficacy to negotiate safer sex (Heinrich, 1993). The weaker the perceived self-efficacy, the more such social and affective factors can increase the likelihood of risky sexual behavior.

Exercise of personal control over sexual behaviors that carry risk of infection calls on skills and self-efficacy in communicating frankly about sexual matters and protective sexual methods and ensuring their use. Some of the people who perceive a personal risk of sexually transmitted disease are reducing the number of sexual partners and are more wary of engaging in sex with casual partners. Ignorance of a partner's sexual and drug activities has become a new risk factor. To rest self-protection on partners' reports of their sexual and drug history, however, is a hazardous safeguard. Sexual ardor and impression management can readily expurgate risky histories in personal disclosures. Most people in steady relationships see little need for protective measures through belief in their partner being monogamous and having negative serostatus. Youth often go through a series of relationships resulting in exposure to multiple partners, however, usually of unknown serostatus. Moreover, survey studies reveal that a majority of "monogamous" relationships are so in name rather than in actual practice. Because the AIDS virus is transmittable heterosexually, occasional sex with partners outside a monogamous relationship, especially those who have had bisexual or drug involvements, expands the range of potential risk for heterosexuals as well.

Subjective risk appraisal for AIDS infection is highly unreliable because infected individuals remain asymptomatic for a long time and their sexual and drug history often remain a private matter. Lacking knowledge of the behavioral history and serostatus of sexual partners, people tend to make their risk appraisals on the basis of social and physical appearances, which can be highly misleading. Given evidence that most males would lie about their sexual history to gain sex (Keeling, 1989), seeking protection through probing inquiry provides illusory safety. Indeed, the more strongly people believe in their personal ability to assess by inquiry the risk status of a new partner, the more likely they are to engage in unprotected intercourse (O'Leary, Goodhart, Jemmott, & Boccher-Lattimore, 1992). Hence, the development of communicative efficacy should center on skills for negotiating safer sex practices rather than for history taking of highly suspect reliability.

Even people who are well informed on safer sex guidelines often err in their subjective appraisal of the extent to which they are putting themselves at risk of HIV infection. Bauman and Siegel (1987) found that gay men practicing hazardous sex underestimate the riskiness of their behavior as judged against epidemiologically established linkage to seropositivity. Misappraisals of riskiness of one's sexual practices tend to be associated with underestimation of personal susceptibility to infection, with misbeliefs that risky sex with a few regular partners is safe, and erroneous beliefs that behavioral precautions that actually have no protective value (showering before and after sexual contact, healthful regimens, inspecting partners for lesions) will render risky sex safe. Such findings underscore the need for risk-reduction messages not only to describe risky sexual practices but to correct common misbeliefs about irrelevant factors that invest risky practices with false safety.

In managing sexuality and intravenous drug use, people have to exercise influence over themselves as well as over others. This requires self-regulative skills in motivating and guiding one's actions. Self-regulation operates through internal standards, affective reactions to one's own conduct, use of motivating self-incentives, and other forms of cognitive self-guidance (Bandura, 1986, 1991b). Self-regulative skills thus form an integral part of risk-reduction capabilities. They partly determine the social situations into which people get themselves, how well they navigate through them, and how effectively they can resist social inducements to potentially risky behavior. It is not often that people deliberately set out to entangle themselves in highly risky activities. Rather, they make a series of seemingly innocuous choices that eventually culminates in risky involvements. Effective self-regulation, therefore, requires self-monitoring skills for recognizing and aborting potential entanglement scenarios early in the chain of portentous decisions. It is easier to wield control over preliminary choice behavior likely to lead to troublesome social situations than to try to extricate oneself from such situations while enmeshed in them. This is because the antecedent phase involves mainly anticipatory motivators which are amenable to cognitive control; the entanglement phase includes stronger social inducements to engage in high-risk behavior which are less easily manageable.

In some countries, such as those of Africa, Latin America, and the Caribbean, AIDS is almost exclusively a heterosexually transmitted disease, with untreated venereal diseases increasing susceptibility to HIV infection. In Europe and the United States, the route of heterosexual transmission is mainly via bisexuals and intravenous drug users infected by sharing contaminated needles. Southern Asian countries are witnessing a rapid spread of infection among intravenous drug users which then spreads to heterosexual partners and their newborns (Des Jarlais & Friedman, 1988b). Control of the spread of the AIDS virus by intravenous drug users requires risk-reduction strategies aimed at both drug and sexual practices. Relatively little effort has been devoted to developing interventions to prevent infection among intravenous drug users. This is a serious neglect because infected drug users are transmitting the virus heterosexually to their female sexual partners who, in turn, run a high chance of infecting their infants through perinatal transmission. As a result, AIDS is taking an increasingly heavy toll on women and children, especially among ethnic minorities in impoverished environs where drug use is prevalent. Those who continue to inject drugs intravenously, despite cognizance of the threat of AIDS infection, need access to sterile needles and knowledge on how to disinfect needles to safeguard against transmission of the virus. They need to be taught protective sexual practices to avoid infecting their sexual partners and be persuaded to use them consistently.

PERCEIVED SELF-EFFICACY AND ADOPTION OF HEALTH PRACTICES

People's beliefs that they can motivate themselves and regulate their own behavior plays a crucial role in whether they even consider altering habits detrimental to health. They see little point to even trying if they believe they cannot exercise control over their own behavior and that of others. Even people who believe their detrimental habits may be harming their health achieve little success in curtailing their behavior unless they believe they have sufficient power to resist those who instigate it. This observation is corroborated in a longitudinal study of gay men's sexual behavior conducted by McKusick, Wiley, Coates, and Morin (1986). Several psychological factors that could influence sexual risk-taking behavior were assessed. These included perceived threat that one is potentially at risk of exposure to the AIDS virus; degree of peer support for adopting safer sexual behavior; social skills necessary to negotiate protective sexual behavior; level of self-esteem; and perceived self-efficacy that one can take protective actions that lessen the risk of AIDS infection. Belief in one's personal efficacy to exercise control over one's sexual behavior emerged as the best predictor of sexual risk-taking behavior. The lower the perceived self-efficacy, the higher the likelihood of engagement in sexual practices that carry a high risk of AIDS infection. Men who frequented bars and bath houses had a lower sense of efficacy than those who were committed to a monogamous relationship. Social skill in negotiating self-protective sexual activity was also associated with low-risk sexual practices.

The role of perceived self-efficacy in the adoption and maintenance of self-protective behavior is corroborated in other lines of research. Even though individuals acknowledge that safer sex practices reduce risk of infection, they do not adopt them if they believe they cannot exercise control in sexual relations (Siegel, Mesagno, Chen, & Christ, 1989). Perceived self-efficacy to negotiate condom use predicts safer sex practices in adolescents (Basen-Engquist & Parcel, 1992; Jemmott, Jemmott, & Fong, 1992; Jemmott, Jemmott, Spears, Hewitt, & Cruz-Collins, 1991; Kasen et al., 1992) and adults (Brafford & Beck, 1991; Heinrich, 1993; O'Leary et al., 1992). Alcohol and drug use in the context of sexual activity foster sexual behaviors at high risk of infection. Drugs and alcohol lower a person's perceived ability to adhere to safer sex practices (Kasen et al., 1992; Rosenthal, Moore, & Flynn, 1991). Among drug users, perceived self-efficacy predicts success in regular use of clean needles and condoms with sexual partners (Kok, deVries, Mudd, & Strecher, 1991). Perceived self-efficacy is related to self-protective behavior both concurrently and longitudinally.

The spreading threat of AIDS has produced substantial changes in sexual practices in the gay community, as shown in reduction of high-risk sexual acts and number of sexual partners. In the study of longitudinal predictors, McKusick and his colleagues found that a strong sense of efficacy in exercising self-protective control, association with groups that made safer sex the norm, and knowledge of serostatus were the significant predictors of enduring reductions in high-risk sexual practices (McKusick, Coates, Morin, Pollack, & Hoff, 1990). The reductions in high-risk practices accompanying each of these three sources of influence are summarized in Figure 1. These longitudinal predictors underscore the importance of self-efficacy enhancement through skill development and alterations of subcommunity norms in programs designed to produce long-term behavior change.

COMPONENTS OF EFFECTIVE SELF-DIRECTED CHANGE

Social cognitive theory explains human functioning in terms of triadic reciprocal causation (Bandura, 1986). In this causal model, which is summarized schematically in Figure 2, (1) personal determinants in the form of cognitive, affective, and biological factors, (2) behavior, and (3) environmental influences, all operate as interacting determinants of each other. An effective program of widespread change in detrimental health practices includes four major components aimed at altering each of the three classes of interacting determinants. The first is informational, designed to increase people's awareness and knowledge of health risks. The second component is concerned with development of the social and self-regulative skills needed to translate informed concerns into effective preventive action. The third component is aimed at skill enhancement and building resilient self-efficacy by providing opportunities for guided practice and corrective feedback in applying the skills in high-risk situations. The final component involves enlisting and creating social supports for desired personal changes. Let us consider how each of these four components would apply to self-directed change of behaviors that pose a high risk of AIDS infection.

Informational Component

Efforts to encourage people to adopt health practices rely heavily on persuasive communications in health education campaigns. In such health messages, appeals to fear by depicting the ravages of disease are often used as

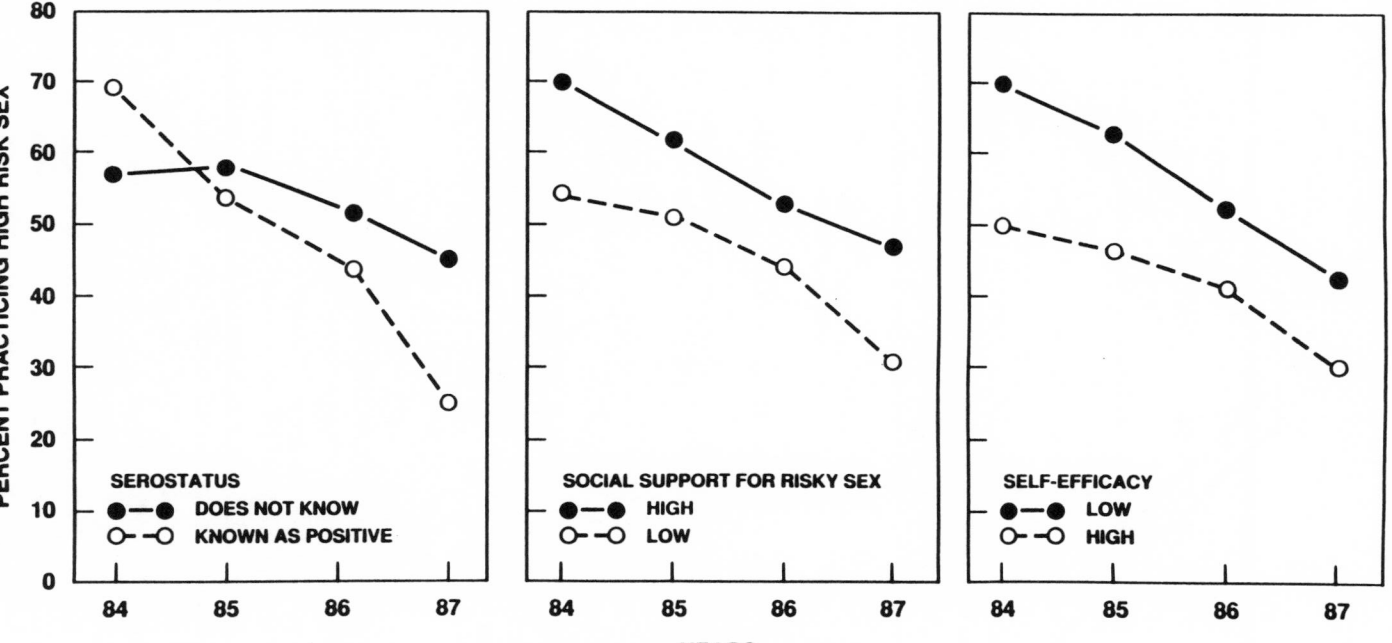

Figure 1. Changes in percent of homosexual respondents practicing high-risk sexual behavior over time as a function of knowledge of seropositive status, perceived self-efficacy to adhere to self-protective behavior, and perceived number of friends and acquaintances following a norm of risky sexual activities (McKusick, Coates, Morin, Pollack, & Hoff, 1990).

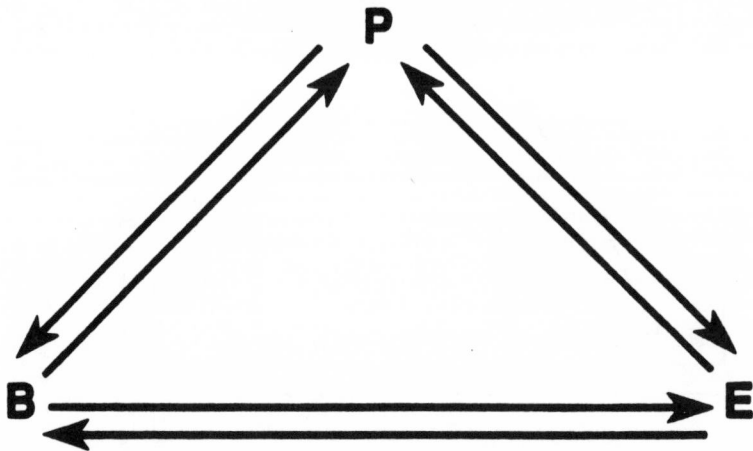

Figure 2. Schematization of triadic reciprocal causation. *B* signifies behavior; *P* the cognitive, biological, and other internal events that affect perceptions and action; and *E* the external environment.

motivators, and recommended preventive practices are provided as guides for action. People need enough knowledge of potential dangers to warrant action, but they do not have to be scared out of their wits to act, any more than homeowners have to be terrified to insure their households. Rather, what people need is sound information on how AIDS is transmitted, guidance on how to regulate their behavior, and firm belief in their personal ability to turn concerns into effective preventive actions. Responding to these needs requires a shift in emphasis from trying to scare people into healthy behavior to empowering them with the tools for exercising personal control over their health habits.

The influential role of people's beliefs in their personal efficacy in adopting preventive health practices is shown by Beck and Lund (1981). They studied the persuasiveness of health communications in which the seriousness of a disease and susceptibility to it were varied. Patients' perceived self-efficacy that they could stick to the required preventive behavior was a good predictor of whether they adopted the preventive practices. Fear arousal had little effect on whether or not they did so. Analyses of the mechanisms through which mass media health campaigns exert their effects similarly reveal that perceived self-efficacy plays an influential role in the adoption of health practices (Maibach, Flora, & Nass, 1991; Slater, 1989). The stronger the preexisting perceived self-efficacy, and the more the media campaigns enhance people's self-regulative power, the more likely they are to adopt the recommended practices.

The relationship remains even when multiple controls are applied for a host of other possible influences.

To be most effective, health communications should instill in people the belief that they have the capability to alter their health habits and should instruct them on how to do it. Communications that explicitly do so increase people's determination to modify habits detrimental to their health (Maddux & Rogers, 1983). Entrenched habits rarely yield to a single attempt at self-regulation. Success is usually achieved through renewed effort following failed attempts. To strengthen the staying power of self-beliefs, health communications should emphasize that success requires perseverant effort, so that people's sense of efficacy is not undermined by a few setbacks to the point where they get discouraged and give up. Faultless self-regulation is not easy to come by even for pliant habits, let alone for addictive and sexual behavior. A strong sense of controlling efficacy is built by overcoming setbacks through perseverant effort. Unfortunately, the possibility that the AIDS virus is transmittable to the immunologically vulnerable through a few sexual contacts with infected partners or sharing a few contaminated needles does not leave much room for carelessness or occasional reversions to risky habits.

An increased research effort is needed to determine how preventive health communications should be framed to maximize their impact on perceived self-regulative efficacy. Self-efficacy theory provides one set of guidelines (Bandura, 1986). I shall consider later how symbolic modeling influences should be structured to maximize their psychosocial impact. Decision theory regarding risk perception and risky decisions provides other suggestions (Tversky & Kahneman, 1981). For example, people interpret information regarding risky activities in terms of potential gains and potential losses. There is some evidence to suggest that health communications are more persuasive if framed in terms of health losses to get people to check for maladies, but in terms of health benefits to get them to adopt preventive behavior (Rothman, Salovey, Antone, Keough, & Drake, in press). Meyerowitz and Chaiken (1987) found that health communications framed in terms of health benefits had less impact on perceived self-efficacy and behavior designed to detect maladies than communications framed in terms of health losses. They examined four alternative mechanisms through which health communications could alter health habits: by transmission of factual information, fear arousal, change in risk perception, and enhancement of perceived self-efficacy. The health communications fostered adoption of preventive health practices mainly by their effect on perceived self-efficacy. National education campaigns need to exploit more fully our knowledge of social influence processes, and the cognitive and affective mechanisms governing human motivation and behavior.

The preconditions for change are created by increasing people's awareness and knowledge of the profound threat of AIDS. They need to be provided with a great deal of factual information about the nature of AIDS, its modes of transmission, what constitutes high-risk sexual and drug practices, and how to achieve protection from infection. This is easier said than done. Our society does not provide much in the way of treatment of drug addiction, nor is it about to provide refractory drug users with easy access to sterile needles and other drug paraphernalia. It has little experience in how to reach and educate drug users on how to disinfect needles to reduce the risk of AIDS infection.

In the sexual domain, our society has always had difficulty talking frankly about sex and imparting sexual information to the public at large. Because parents generally do a poor job of it as well, most youngsters pick up their sex education from other, often less trustworthy and reputable, sources outside the home or from the consequences of uninformed sexual experimentation. To complicate matters further, some sectors of the society lobby actively for maintaining a veil of silence regarding protective sexual practices on the belief that such information will promote indiscriminate sexuality. In their view, the remedy for the spreading AIDS epidemic is a national celibacy campaign for unweds and gays and faithful monogamy among the wedded. They oppose educational programs in the schools that talk about sex methods that provide protection against AIDS infection.

The net result is that many of our public education campaigns regarding AIDS are couched in desexualized generalities that leave some ignorance in their wake. To those most at risk, such sanitized expressions as "exchange of bodily fluids" is not only uninformative but can be misinformative by investing safe bodily substances with perceived infective properties. Even those more skilled in deciphering medical locutions do not always know what the preventive messages are talking about. For example, an intensive campaign spanning a full week, conducted at a university campus, included public lectures, numerous panel discussions, presentations in dormitories, and condom distribution, all of which were widely reported in the campus newspaper. A systematic assessment of students' beliefs and sexual practices conducted several weeks later revealed that more than a quarter of the students did not know what constitutes "safer sex," and some of them had misconceptions of safer sex practices that, in fact, would present high risk of infection (Chervin & Martinez, 1987). Other findings of this study, which will be reviewed later, document the severe limitations of efforts to change sexual practices by information alone.

The informational component of the model of self-directed change includes two main factors, the informational content of the health communications and the mechanisms of social diffusion. Detailed factual information about AIDS must be socially imparted in an understandable, credible, and persuasive manner. Social cognitive theories provide a number of guidelines on how this might be best accomplished (Bandura, 1986; McGuire, 1984;

Zimbardo, Ebbesen, & Maslach, 1977). However, developing effective AIDS prevention programs is only the first step; they must also be disseminated. Unlike other health risk-reduction campaigns which involve relatively prosaic habits, the risky habits for AIDS infection are laden with matters of illegalities and what are judged to be immoralities.

Informative health messages, however well designed, cannot have much social impact without effective means of dissemination. Because of their wide reach and influence, the mass media, especially television, can serve as major vehicles of social diffusion of information regarding health guidelines. For several reasons, however, a variety of diffusion vehicles must be enlisted in a public health campaign. High costs and restricted access to television limit its availability. Moreover, television networks typically adopt a conservative stance on controversial matters. They have resisted getting into the act for fear that talk of protective sex practices will jeopardize advertising revenue by arousing the wrath of some sectors of their viewing audience. This resistance would have weakened if the AIDS virus had spread rapidly through the heterosexual population across all sectors of society, thus making it a general societal problem rather than one confined to gays and drug users. It is unlikely that the television industry will offer much help as long as AIDS remains mainly a disease of poor minorities. Existing social, religious, recreational, occupational, and educational organizations can serve as highly effective disseminators of preventive health guidelines. Wide cultural diversity requires that the messages of risk-reduction campaigns for AIDS be tailored to socioeconomic, racial, and ethnic differences in value orientations and disseminated through multiple sources to ensure adequate exposure (Mantell, Schinke, & Akabas, 1988).

Nontraditional social networks must be enlisted for high-risk groups who are beyond the reach of the usual community organizations. For example, in outreach programs, "streetwise" counselors have been highly successful in reaching drug populations (Watters et al., 1990). After they become known in the social circles of drug users, the counselors help them with referrals to drug treatment programs. They offer them explicit instruction in safer sex practices. They teach intravenous drug users how to reduce the risk of AIDS by disinfecting needles with ordinary household bleach which kills the HIV virus. The disinfection procedure, which had been rarely used before, was widely adopted and consistently applied. Although this outreach program also increased the use of condoms, the drug users were much more conscientious in disinfecting needles than in protecting their sexual partners against sexually transmitted infection. Such findings underscore the need for sexual partners to exercise personal control in protecting their own health.

A comprehensive national program regarding the growing AIDS threat must address broader social issues as well as risky health practices. This is because the AIDS epidemic has far-reaching social repercussions. One of these issues concerns the widespread public fear of AIDS infection. Many people continue to believe that the AIDS virus can be transmitted by casual contact or by insect transmission and food handling, despite evidence to the contrary. Efforts by health professionals to dispel misapprehensions are discounted by many of those who are alarmed on the grounds that what is proclaimed safe currently may be discovered to be risky later. Recurrent disputes among researchers in the public media regarding risk factors for other diseases have eroded some of the credibility of medical expertise. Widespread public fear gets translated into advocacy of laws requiring sweeping mandatory blood testing and identification and social restriction of those with antibodies to the HIV virus.

In public perceptions of the AIDS threat, risky behavior gets transformed to risky groups. As AIDS imposes mounting financial burdens on society and strains medical and social service systems, members of high-risk groups tend to become targets of growing public hostility. Once entire groups get stigmatized because some of their members behave in risky ways, those who do not also become the objects of fear and hostility. The way in which they are treated socially may be dictated more by group identity than by their personal characteristics. Public alarm fueled by many misbeliefs enhances such stigmatization. Policy debates on how to control the spread of AIDS have become highly politicized. Prohibitionists argue that public health campaigns promote indiscriminate sex. Their critics argue that knowledge does not foster sexuality and that prohibitionists are intent at curtailing sex practices they find morally objectionable rather than at increasing the safety of sex. Uninformed public reactions to the AIDS threat require serious attention as do the risky health practices themselves, because they help to shape public policies and impose constraints on health education programs. Even societies that possess the necessary scientific knowledge, resources, and expertise can be immobilized by conflicts of values and morals from establishing psychosocial programs that can help to stem the tide of infection.

Development of Self-Protective Skills and Controlling Self-Efficacy

It is not enough to convince people that they should alter risky habits. Despite a high level of knowledge, many continue risky sexual and drug practices. People also need guidance on how to translate their concerns into efficacious actions. In the campus survey mentioned earlier (Chervin & Martinez, 1987), after exposure to the intensive educational campaign less than half of the students who were sexually active used safer sex methods designed to prevent infection with sexually transmitted diseases. Most of them even avoided talking about the matter with their sexual partners. Studies conducted on other campuses similarly reveal that most sexually active students who are knowledgeable about AIDS do not adopt safer sex practices (Edgar, Freimuth, & Hammond, 1988). Among inner-city youth, neither a high level of factual knowledge about HIV transmission nor even knowing someone who was infected or had died of AIDS reduce behaviors that carry high risk of infection (Stiffman, Earls, Dore, & Cunningham, 1992). McKusick, Horstman, and Coates (1985) similarly found that gay men were uniformly well informed about safer sex methods for protecting against AIDS infection, but those who had a low sense of efficacy that they could manage their behavior and sexual relationships were unable to act on their knowledge.

The ability to learn by social modeling provides a highly effective method for increasing human knowledge and skills. A special power of modeling is that it can simultaneously transmit knowledge and valuable skills to large numbers of people through the medium of videotape modeling. Knowledge of modeling processes identifies a number of factors that can be used to enhance the instructive power of modeling (Bandura, 1986). Applications of modeling principles to AIDS prevention would focus on how to manage interpersonal situations and one's own behavior in ways that afford protection against infection with the AIDS virus. Both self-regulative and risk-reduction strategies for dealing with a variety of situations that promote risky behavior should be modeled to convey general guides that can be applied and adjusted to fit changing circumstances.

We saw earlier that human competency requires not only skills but also self-belief in one's capability to use those skills well. Indeed, results of numerous studies of diverse health habits and physical dysfunctions reveal that the impact of different methods of influence on health behavior is partly mediated through their effects on perceived self-efficacy (Bandura, 1992). The stronger the self-efficacy beliefs they instil, the more likely are people to enlist and sustain the effort needed to change habits detrimental to health. Modeling influences should, therefore, be designed to build self-assurance as well as to convey strategies for how to deal effectively with coerciveness for risky practices. The influence of modeling on beliefs about one's capabilities relies on comparison with others. People judge their own capabilities, in part, from how well those whom they regard as similar to themselves exercise control over situations. People develop stronger belief in their capabilities and more readily adopt modeled ways if they see models similar to themselves solve problems successfully with the modeled strategies, than if they see the models as very different from themselves (Bandura, 1986). To increase the impact of modeling, the characteristics of models such as their age, sex, and status, the type of problems with which they cope, and the situation in which they apply their skills, should be made to appear similar to the people's own circumstances.

Enhancement of Social Proficiency and Resiliency of Self-Efficacy

Proficiency requires extensive practice and this is no less true of managing the interpersonal aspects of sexuality. After people gain knowledge of new skills and social strategies, they need guidance and opportunities to perfect those skills. Initially, people practice in simulated situations where they need not fear making mistakes or appearing inadequate. This is best achieved by role-playing in which they practice handling the types of situations they have to manage in their social environment. They receive informative feedback on how they are doing and the corrective changes that need to be made. The simulated practice is continued until the skills are performed proficiently and spontaneously.

Not all the benefits of guided practice are due to skill improvement. Some of the gains result from raising people's beliefs in their capabilities (Bandura, 1988b). Experiences in exercising control over social situations serve as self-efficacy builders. This is an important aspect of self-directed change because if people are not fully convinced of their personal efficacy they undermine their efforts in situations that tax capabilities and readily abandon the skills they have been taught when they fail to get quick results or suffer reverses. The important matter is not that difficulties rouse self-doubts, which is a natural immediate reaction, but rather the degree and speed of recovery from setbacks. It is resiliency in perceived self-efficacy that counts in maintenance of changes in health habits. The higher the perceived self-efficacy, the greater is the success in maintenance of health-promoting behavior (Bandura, 1992).

The influential role played by perceived self-efficacy in the management of sexual activities is documented in studies of contraceptive use by teenage women at high risk because they often engage in unprotected intercourse (Kasen et al., 1992; Levinson, 1986). Such research shows that perceived self-efficacy in managing sexual relationships is associated with more effective use of contraceptives. The predictive relation remains when controls are applied for demographic factors, knowledge, and sexual experience.

Gilchrist and Schinke (1983) applied the main features of the multicomponent model of personal change to teach teenagers how to exercise self-protective control over sexual situations. They received essential factual information about high-risk sexual behavior and self-protective measures. Through modeling they were taught how to communicate frankly about sexual matters and contraceptives, how to deal with conflicts regarding sexual activities, and how to resist unwanted sexual advances. They practiced applying these social skills by role-playing in simulated situations and received instructive feedback. The self-regulative program significantly enhanced perceived self-efficacy and skill in managing sexuality. Botvin and his associates provide a comprehensive school-based program that teaches generative self-regulative skills for managing sexual activities and social pressures for alcohol and drug use (Botvin & Dusenbury, 1992).

The Jemmotts have developed and tested an AIDS prevention program incorporating the major elements of the self-regulative model, with additional features designed to dispel beliefs that condom use reduces sexual pleasure. Participants are provided with information about the cause, transmission, and prevention of AIDS. They receive guided mastery training to enhance their sense of efficacy to negotiate and manage condom use. They are taught how to eroticize condom use to remove the attitudinal barrier to using them (Jemmott & Jemmott, 1992). The program produced significant AIDS risk reduction in African-American male adolescents (Jemmott et al., 1992). Those who had the benefit of the program were more knowledgeable about infective risks, less accepting of risky practices, and reported engaging in lower levels of risky sexual behavior with fewer sexual partners in follow-up assessments than did those in a control condition. Jemmott and his colleagues compared their social cognitive program with informational interventions that increased knowledge either about AIDS prevention or general health promotion (Jemmott et al., 1991). The participants were sexually active African-American female adolescents recruited from a family planning clinic serving a low-income community. Compared to the information-only interventions, the sociocognitive program produced a greater sense of efficacy to negotiate condom use, more positive outcome expectations regarding sexual enjoyment with condoms, and stronger intentions to use condoms. These diverse effects were replicated with sexually active African-American female adolescents drawn from the inner city (Jemmott & Jemmott, 1992). The stronger the instilled sense of efficacy and eroticization of condoms the stronger the intention to use them. AIDS knowledge, in itself, did not affect intentions to use condoms. These reproducible benefits of the sociocognitive model are of particular interest because they are achieved with both male and female adolescents at high risk of HIV infection through frequent unprotected sexual activity.

Research by Kelly and his colleagues further attests to the substantial value of self-regulative programs for AIDS risk reduction (Kelly, St. Lawrence, Hood, & Brasfield, 1989). Gay men were taught through modeling, role-playing, and corrective feedback how to exercise self-protective control in sexual relationships and to resist coercions to engage in high-risk sex. Multifaceted assessments showed that they became more skillful in handling sexual relationships and coercions, they markedly reduced risky sexual practices, and used condoms on a regular basis. As shown in Figure 3, these self-protective practices were maintained in follow-up assessments. In contrast, a matched control group of gay men continued to engage in unprotected high-risk sexual practices. In an extended follow-up, the majority of participants continued to adhere to safer sex practices, whereas the remainder, who had an earlier history of high-level risky behaviors, reported some behavioral lapses (Kelly, St. Lawrence, & Brasfield, 1991). The highly vulnerable need even more intensive guidance on how to avoid or to manage risky situations. The issue of behavioral lapse prevention will be considered later.

Combining factual information about health risks with development of risk-reduction efficacy produces good results. Because people learn and perfect effective ways of behaving under lifelike conditions, problems of transferring the new skills to everyday life are reduced. The guided mastery approach is readily adaptable in audio or videocassette format to self-protective behavior against HIV infection. Large-scale applications of self-regulative programs sacrifice the guided role-playing component. Instruction in imaginal rehearsal, however, in which people mentally practice dealing with prototypic troublesome situations, has been shown to boost perceived self-efficacy and improve actual performance in coping with threats (Bandura, 1986; Kazdin, 1978). Maibach and Flora (1993) tested the incremental benefits of cued cognitive rehearsal of self-protective strategies imbedded in videotaped modeling of how to manage potentially risky sexual activities. Cognitive rehearsal enhanced the power of symbolic modeling to strengthen a sense of personal efficacy to exercise self-protective control. The self-regulative approach, designed in a format suitable for mass distribution, has been shown to achieve some success in changing other refractory health-impairing behaviors (Sallis et al., 1986). Schinke and Orlandi (1990) are developing interactive computer formats as a vehicle for instructing youth in skills on how to manage unsafe drug and sexual activities. Participants role-play with computer characters what they would say and do in risky situations and receive instructive feedback for improving their strategies. These approaches are designed to augment the essential skill-development component in educational preventive programs that usually provide little or no opportunity to become proficient in what is being taught. The format is easily adaptable to different subcultural values, customs, and socioeconomic status.

Because of the high level of unprotected sexual activity and experimentation with drugs by adolescents, they are vulnerable to becoming a high-risk group as transmitters of the AIDS virus (Mantell & Schinke, 1990). Training materials need to be developed to assist parents and teachers on how to educate youngsters about AIDS. Winett and his colleagues devised a video prototype using modeling and cued rehearsal of self-protective skills for use in the home by parents and their teenagers (Winett et al., 1992). This home-based program increased knowledge about HIV transmission and prevention, fostered more open communication between parents and their teenagers regarding sexuality, increased family problem-solving skills, and taught teenagers strategies on

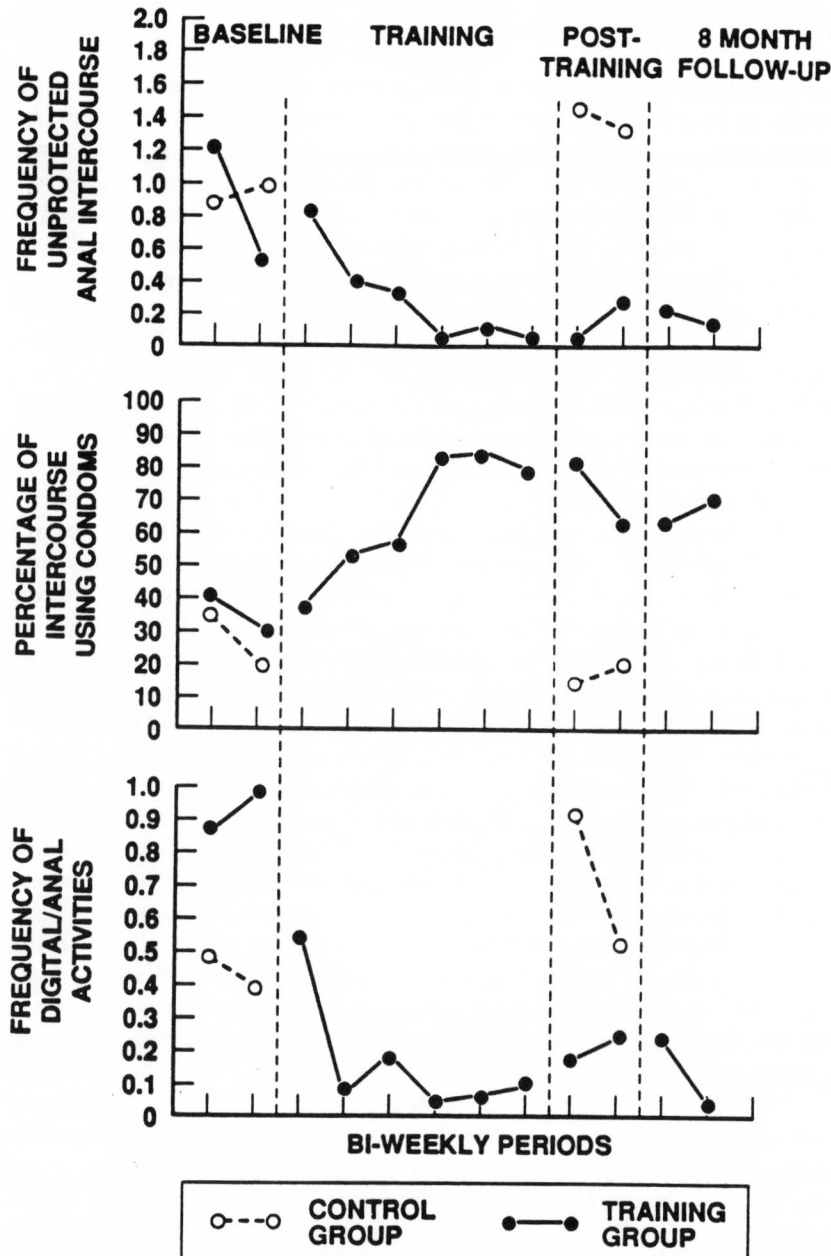

Figure 3. Frequency of unprotected anal intercourse, digital/anal activities, and proportion of condom use during intercourse by gay men who received the self-regulative program and those in a control group who did not. (Kelly, St. Lawrence, Hood, & Brasfield, 1989). Copyright 1989 by the American Psychological Association. Reprinted by permission.

how to manage common risk situations. Further efforts to increase the power of this familial approach are centered on augmenting the skill-development component. The guided mastery programs developed by Gilchrist and Schinke (1983) and Botvin and Dusenbury (1992) provide good prototypes for application in schools. Other channels of dissemination must be created, however, to reach teenagers who live in dysfunctional families and receive little guidance from school because of factional opposition to educational efforts that address self-protective behavior in an explicitly informative manner. A major segment of the teenage population can be reached by making informative audiotapes and videocassettes readily available in the settings they frequent to convey skills and peer norms for safer sexual practices. Among sexually active adolescents, those who can talk with their partners about the risks of HIV infection and perceive peer support for condom use tend to be consistent condom users (DiClemente, 1991).

Acquired immunodeficiency syndrome infection is spreading rapidly among intravenous drug users and to their sexual partners and offspring. Efforts to control this source of infection are directed mainly at curtailing the supply of drugs, instituting risk-reduction programs focused on disinfection and exchange of drug injection equipment, developing nonreusable syringes, and treating addictive conditions. These efforts must be supplemented by AIDS prevention programs designed to reduce the demand for drugs. As in other areas of habit change, informational campaigns alone will not do it. A comprehensive preventive effort must provide knowledge about the determinants, precipitants, and immediate and long-term consequences of drug use, alter the valuation of drugs, develop self-regulative and social skills to resist social pressures to use drugs, and cultivate social norms that discourage experimentation with and use of drugs. This is best achieved by school-based primary prevention programs that have proven effective in other areas of health promotion and risk reduction (Flora & Thoresen, 1988; Killen et al., 1989). Efforts at AIDS prevention are more likely to gain broad support if they are integrated into a comprehensive school-based program for health promotion rather than as a separate program.

The prototypic skills enhancement program developed by Gilchrist and Schinke (1985) has been successfully extended to the prevention and reduction of drug abuse by adolescents. This type of program informs adolescents about drug effects, provides them with interpersonal skills for managing personal and social pressures to use drugs, lowers drug use, and fosters self-conceptions as a nonuser (Gilchrist, Schinke, Trimble, & Cvetkovich, 1987). These findings are all the more interesting because they were achieved with ethnic and minority youth among whom substance abuse is prevalent. Adoption of a self-conception as a nonuser can produce major life-style changes. This is most likely to occur when the emergent new self-conception leads to severance of social ties with substance abusers and sufficient social support is provided for immersion in nonuser social networks (Stall & Biernacki, 1986).

Social Supports for Personal Change

People achieve self-directed change when they understand how personal habits threaten their well-being, are taught how to modify them, believe in their capabilities to marshall the effort and resources needed to exercise control, and have incentive to do so. However, personal change occurs within a network of social influences. Depending on their nature, social influences can aid, retard, or undermine efforts at personal change. This is especially true in the case of sexual and drug practices, which are subjected to strong social normative influences.

In social cognitive theory, normative influences regulate behavior through two regulatory systems—social sanctions and self-sanctions (Bandura, 1986). Social norms influence behavior anticipatorily by the social consequences they provide. Behavior that violates prevailing social norms brings social censure or other punishing consequences, whereas behavior that fulfills socially valued norms is approved and rewarded. People do not act like weathervanes, however, constantly shifting their behavior to conform to whatever others might want. Rather, they adopt certain standards of behavior and regulate their actions anticipatorily through self-evaluative consequences they create for themselves. Social norms convey standards of conduct. Adoption of personal standards creates a self-regulative system that operates largely through internalized self-sanctions (Bandura, 1989). People behave in ways that give them self-satisfaction, and they refrain from behaving in ways that violate their standards because it will bring self-censure. Anticipatory self-sanctions thus keep conduct in line with internal standards.

Normative consensus strengthens both its modeling and sanctioning functions. The normative influences that foster preventive measures center on the behavioral practices by which the virus is transmitted and on the cultural patterning of social relationships. Because of their proximity, immediacy, and prevalence, the interpersonal influences operating within one's immediate social network claim a stronger regulatory function than do general normative sanctions. The norms of the larger society are more distal and applied only infrequently to the behavior of any given individual because unfamiliar others are usually not around to react to it. Even when they are, if the norms of one's immediate network are at odds with those of the larger group, the reactions of outsiders carry less weight, and may be disregarded altogether. Among drug-dependent women, the more their friends use and regard condoms positively, the stronger the womens' beliefs in their efficacy to overcome interpersonal barriers to safer sex practices (Mantell et al., 1993).

The findings further suggest that efficacy beliefs both mediate the influence of peer norms and operate independently on condom use. Thus, efficacy beliefs contribute to consistent use of condoms after controlling for the effects of peer attitudes and behavioral norms.

People who are fully informed on the modes of HIV transmission and effective self-protective methods acquire the virus only if they allow it to happen to themselves. They often allow it to happen because interpersonal, sociocultural, religious, and economic factors operate as constraints on self-protective behavior. Some of those most at risk must contend with sociocultural obstacles to the use of prophylactic methods that afford protection against HIV infection. The major burden for self-protection against heterosexually transmitted diseases usually falls on women. Unlike protection against pregnancy, where women can exercise independent control through oral or implant contraceptives, use of condoms requires them to exercise control over the behavior of men. Men who possess coercive power over their partners resist the use of condoms if, in their view, it reduces their sexual pleasure, threatens their sense of manliness and authority, casts aspersions on their faithfulness, and carries the frightening implication that they may be carriers of disease. It is difficult for women, especially those of poor and minority status who are most at risk, to press the issue in the face of emotional and economic dependence, coercive threat, and subcultural prescription of compliant roles for them (Mays & Cochran, 1988). Coercive sexual experiences erode women's sense of efficacy to exercise personal control over risky sex practices (Heinrich, 1993). Women who are enmeshed in relationships of imbalanced power need to be taught how to negotiate protected sex nonconfrontationally. Women who are well equipped with condoms run the risk of being viewed as promiscuous, which creates a further impediment to self-protective action.

At the broader societal level, attitudes and social norms must be altered to increase men's sense of responsibility for the social and health consequences of their sexuality. In societies where the virus is spread heterosexually through prostitution, economic conditions that thrust women into prostitution and drug dependencies that drive them to sell sex for drugs create major obstacles to preventive efforts. In short, if AIDS prevention programs are to achieve much success they must address the sociocultural realities that impose constraints on the exercise of self-protective measures.

In the case of high-risk sexual behavior, strong involvement in a social network supportive of self-protective practices, increases knowledge of risky behaviors, beliefs in efficacy, and adoption of safer sex practices (Fisher, 1988; McKusick et al., 1990). Risk reduction through alteration of subcommunity norms is an especially important vehicle for curbing the spread of AIDS among intravenous drug users. This is because drug use is often a socially shared activity. Restricted access to drug injection equipment and the legal problems of being caught with it, promote risky shared use of drug paraphernalia. Shooting galleries involving widespread sharing of contaminated needles provide the most fertile ground for spreading the virus. Preventive efforts aimed at drug subcultures show that drug users are reachable and instructable in safer practices. Thus, provision of protective information by outreach workers about AIDS transmission, needle-exchange programs, and instruction on how to sterilize syringes can substantially reduce risky injection practices which can lower infection rates among those who continue the drug habit (Des Jarlais & Friedman, 1988a; Watters, Downing, Case, Lorvicic, Cheng, & Fergusson, 1990). Needle and syringe exchange programs do not propagate drug use, as some people have feared it might (Buning, 1991). Rather, exchange programs reduce needle sharing and curb the further spread of HIV infection among drug users. As Des Jarlais notes, most drug users now know about the modes of AIDS transmission, but many are still inadequately informed or misinformed about risk reduction techniques. For example, some dutifully wash needles in water or in other ways that do not kill the virus. Emerging subcommunity norms against needle-sharing behavior are a good predictor of reduction in risky injection practices among intravenous drug users (Des Jarlais & Friedman, 1988a). Although the subcommunity approach also serves as an excellent vehicle for enlisting drug users in treatment programs, there is not much that outreach workers can offer them because of the scarcity of treatment services.

Social influences rooted in indigenous sources generally have greater impact and sustaining power than those applied by outsiders for a limited time. A major benefit of community-mediated programs is that they can mobilize the power of formal and informal networks of influence for transmitting knowledge and cultivating beneficial patterns of behavior. A community-mediated approach is a potentially powerful vehicle for promoting both personal and social change in several ways. It provides an effective means for creating the motivational preconditions of change, for modeling requisite skills, for enlisting natural social incentives for adopting and maintaining beneficial habits, and for establishing protective practices as the normative standards of conduct. Generic principles of effective programs are readily adaptable at the subcommunity level to sociocultural differences in the populations being served. In the social diffusion of new behavior patterns, indigenous adopters usually serve as more influential exemplars and persuaders than do outsiders. Moreover, behavioral practices that create widespread health problems require group solutions that are best achieved through community-mediated efforts.

In their pioneering health-promoting programs, Farquhar and Maccoby have drawn heavily on existing community networks for transmitting knowledge and cultivating beneficial patterns of health behavior (Farquhar, Maccoby, & Solomon, 1984). This work provides a model of how to mobilize community resources to disseminate health information and to convey explicit guides on how to change refractory health habits. A socially oriented program of personal change should be applied in ways designed to create self-sustaining structures within the community for promoting behavioral practices conducive to health. Persons in the community, who serve as local organizers, are taught how to design, coordinate, and implement the programs. By teaching communities how to take charge of their own change, self-directedness is fostered at the community level as well as at the personal level.

The substantial reductions in high-risk sexual practices by gay subgroups was achieved largely through effective self-empowering organization (McKusick et al., 1990; Stall & Paul, 1989). For example, in the unprecedented social and behavioral changes brought about by the gay community in San Francisco, the members educated themselves, made safer sex practices the social norm, devised and implemented their own instructional programs to prevent HIV transmission, and established mechanisms for diffusing this knowledge. Regular updates on new research findings and available treatments were issued, social support systems were created to counteract despair and encourage meaningful life pursuits in those suffering from opportunistic infections. There was active fostering of life-style changes that might enhance immune function to prolong the lives of those infected with the virus but not yet experiencing any symptoms. There have been some attempts at self-mobilization by drug-user subgroups for self-protective change, but these have been less successful (Friedman, de Jong, & Des Jarlais, 1988). Lack of educational and financial resources, illegalities surrounding drug activities, societal restrictions of the means for safer injection practices, mistrust, and the large amount of time devoted to supporting the drug habit, impede efforts at self-organization. These conditions create a greater need for external aid in subgroup organization for risk reduction in intravenous drug users.

PREVENTION OF BEHAVIORAL LAPSES

It is not unusual for some individuals to lapse into risky practices after having adopted safer ones. A minority revert either occasionally or completely to risky drug injection behavior or unprotected sexual behavior (Des Jarlais, Abdul-Quader, & Tross, 1991; Stall, Ekstrand, Pollack, McKusick, & Coates, 1990). Development of interventions for behavioral lapses is best advanced by interactional analyses of high-risk episodes rather than by search for correlates in demographic characteristics and measures of traits disembodied from the types of situational and social influences that can override self-regulatory efforts. For example, younger individuals are more likely to engage in high-risk behavior than are their older counterparts. Such a finding is neither particularly informative nor provides any guidelines on how to maintain safer practices in problematic situations. Where each behavioral lapse carries high risk because of the relatively high prevalence of HIV infection among one's associates, individuals cannot wait for aging to protect them. While on average, younger individuals take fewer precautions than older ones, the differences within groups are usually much larger than the differences between groups. Progress in understanding human behavior and change is better achieved by clarifying the determinants of human behavior and the mechanisms through which they operate than by casting people into categories or subcategories. The research approach that is most informative and functional elucidates the high-risk episodes that arise recurrently and the modes of coping strategies that prove successful and those that are ineffectual in the interpersonal transactions.

In a retrospective analysis of high-risk episodes experienced by gay men, Kelly and his associates document the transactions that spawn lapses into behaviors that carry high risk of infection (Kelly et al., 1991). In these episodes, the individuals were unable to resist unsafe sex because of their partners' coercive pressures, misgivings and embarrassments over negotiating condom use, strong attraction and desire to please the partner, being caught up in a highly arousing intimacy without a condom, belief that condom use would reduce pleasurable sensations, revivifying pleasurable aspects of risky sex, being intoxicated, high on drugs, depressed, lonely, or distressed at the time, and conceding inefficacy to change risky practices. Those who were successful in protecting themselves against sexually transmitted infection used a variety of cognitive and behavior self-regulatory techniques to do so. They reaffirmed their personal efficacy to practice safer sex and informed their partners to that effect, they planned beforehand what they were willing to do and ensured they had condoms available, conjured up the positive outcomes of good health and the devastating consequences of AIDS, curtailed alcohol and drug use before sex, and guided the sexual activity toward the safer forms.

In managing refractory habits, effective self-regulators usually master a variety of strategies for managing risky situations and apply the strategies persistently and consistently (Bandura, 1986; Perri, 1985). A successful program of lapse prevention must equip people with cognitive and behavioral skills that enable them to exercise control over high-risk situations. Part of effective self-management is concerned with how to avoid hazardous situations that are avoidable and how to extricate oneself quickly should one venture into them. In addition to efforts aimed at lapse prevention for those who have altered their practices, there are always newcomers who need knowledge and skills on how to manage risky situations. Hence, prevention of HIV infections requires ongoing psychosocial programs that promote continuing adherence to self-protective behavior rather than a onetime campaign. Such programs need to create enduring social supports for safer practices at the level of both community norms and personal networks.

Marlatt and Gordon (1985) provide a conceptual model of the relapse process for addictive behaviors in which self-regulatory efficacy operates as an influential factor. The common precipitants in failures in self-regulation include: inability to manage negative emotional states such as stress, depression, loneliness, boredom, and restlessness; social pressures to use the substance; and interpersonal conflict. The conditions that have been identified as relapse precipitants, indeed, undermine perceived self-regulatory efficacy regarding drug use (Sitharthan, McGrath, Cairns, & Saunders, 1991). Heroin users with a low sense of efficacy cannot resist pressures to use opiates even if ill or to refrain from sharing needles that involve high risk of infection. Perceived self-efficacy predicts regular use of clean needles both directly and by intentions to do so (Kok, deVries, Mudde, & Strecher, 1991). Neither attitudes toward drug use nor social norms contributed to safer injection practices.

Some researchers have added situational precipitants that include the settings of drug use and other reminders of the effects of previous drug use (Heather & Stallard, 1989). Situational reminders activate positive outcome expectancies of the pleasurable effects of drugs experienced in the past. Such expectations create motivators for drug use that tax self-regulatory capabilities. In addition, exposure to situations in which one formerly exercised poor control over substance use can activate thoughts of past failures that weaken beliefs in one's current self-regulative efficacy (Cooney, Gillespie, Baker, & Kaplan, 1987).

Perceived self-efficacy also plays an influential role in treatment outcomes for drug addiction. The stronger the perceived self-regulative efficacy instilled by treatment the more successful are opiate users in staying off drugs (Gossop, Green, Phillips, & Bradley, 1990). Gossop and his colleagues examined a variety of predictors of drug status at short and at long follow-up periods. There were two factors that consistently emerged as significant predictors of outcome. The first was perceived self-efficacy to refrain from drug use; the second was the existence of protective factors in the form of supportive associates and involvement in those purposeful occupational activities that contribute to a satisfying early life which help individuals remain drug free. Number of coping strategies predicted short-term drug status but was unrelated to long-term status. Perceived self-efficacy accounts for variation in follow-up drug status after multiple statistical controls are applied for the effects of protective factors, time in treatment, previous history of abstinence, and coping strategies. After completing inpatient detoxification programs, individuals are often urged to seek aftercare treatment in the community for their drug problem. Perceived self-efficacy to do what is necessary to gain entry into an aftercare program predicts whether or not they enter aftercare treatment (Heller & Krauss, 1991).

Viewed from the model of triadic reciprocal causation, efforts at relapse prevention need to be extended beyond personal changes to the social environment as well. Those who have become deeply enmeshed in a subculture of substance abuse have to restructure their way of life if they are to conquer their addiction. Extending the relapse prevention model to environmental change does not minimize personal efficacy but rather factors in its influential role in shaping the very environments people experience. The environment is not simply a fixed entity that inevitably impinges upon individuals. People select, construct, and negotiate environments partly on the basis of their self-beliefs of efficacy.

One way in which severely addicted individuals restructure their lives is by staying away from detrimental social environments that are avoidable and selecting beneficial environments that promote alterative desired life-styles (McAuliffe, Albert, Cordill-London, & McGarraghy, 1991). To the extent that they are equipped to manage inducements to use drugs in risky situations that are unavoidable, by their success in self-regulation they create a different environment for themselves than if they revert to drug-related routines. It is one thing to get into a beneficial environment, but another to experience success in it. To achieve lasting changes, individuals have to develop the competencies needed to gain acceptance and satisfaction in their new lifestyle. Treatments that address these diverse facets of life produce more enduring recoveries from addiction (McAuliffe et al., 1991).

ATTITUDINAL IMPEDIMENTS TO DEVELOPMENT OF PSYCHOSOCIAL MODELS

Despite the considerable benefits of preventive measures, psychosocial research receives only a paltry 2 percent of the AIDS research budget (Siegel, Graham, & Stoto, 1990). There exist several attitudes that downgrade the priority for research into psychosocial determinants and mechanisms governing AIDS-related behavior and for further development of preventive programs for this deadly epidemic. One view, that is voiced recurrently, trivializes psychosocial approaches by regarding them as merely stopgap measures until a vaccine is discovered. This type of attitude reflects how disappointingly little has been learned from past experiences with behaviorally transmitted diseases.

The development of a generic preventive vaccine presents daunting challenges. The AIDS virus appears in differing subtypes and mutates rapidly, thus requiring new vaccines for changing viral strains. It invades immune cells and not only evades destruction by the body's defense system but turns infected T-(helper) cells into producers of more viruses, and eventually destroys the very cells that provide protective immunity. It remains latent for long periods, and it may become more virulent over time. Considering these baffling biological properties, the quest for a vaccine that will provide protective immunity against the changing forms of this virus is likely to be a prolonged, frustrating one. Because viruses merge into the host cells, the task of developing antiviral treatments that can kill the AIDS virus without destroying the host immune cells is a formidable one.

Even the more limited goal of slowing the progress of the disease or keeping it in check with antiviral drugs presents major problems of compliance with drug regimens because they produce toxicities creating severe side effects. Drugs that retard reproduction of the virus but do not eradicate it must be taken continually. Thus, in animals engrafted with human immune organs who have been infected with the HIV virus, the antiviral drug AZT reduces the virus to a very low level, but when the drug is withdrawn the infection flares (McCune, Namikawa, Shih, Rabin, & Kaneshima, 1990). Prolonged use of drugs that are beneficial in the short term by attacking nonresistant viral strains can give rise to new resistant strains and to serious physical damage that requires discontinuation of the drug. The virus usually develops resistance to given drugs or mutates in ways that outwit the drugs.

Sexually transmitted diseases, such as gonorrhea and syphilis, that have been with us for ages, have thwarted vaccine development. Discovery of effective treatments lowers the prevalence rates of a disease but does not eradicate it. With the development of a simple treatment for venereal disease, support for psychosocial control programs was curtailed, with a resultant rise in infection rates (Cutler & Arnold, 1988). The history of efforts to control diseases transmitted by behavior underscores the need for a multifaceted approach combining medical treatments with continuing psychosocial preventive programs. Contrary to the commonly voiced view, it is not that psychosocial preventive programs are of value because they provide the only means available to stem the spread of AIDS in the absence of vaccines or effective treatments. Rather, psychosocial programs constitute an integral part of a multifaceted public health strategy not only before, but even after effective treatments are found. The lessons from the past concerning behaviorally transmitted diseases should not be lost on the AIDS problem. Whether our advanced biotechnology will triumph over the AIDS virus, or the mutable virus will foil our biotechnology remains to be seen. Whatever the outcome may be, AIDS will remain with us as a continuing problem requiring ongoing psychosocial preventive programs.

Another downgrading view rests on the misbelief that psychosocial influences cannot effect much change in the transmissive risky behaviors because they serve potent drives. Amenability of behavior to change differs considerably depending on whether one seeks to eliminate certain kinds of gratifications or to alter the means of gaining those gratifications. It is much more difficult to get people to relinquish behavior that is powerfully reinforced than to adopt safer forms of the behavior that serve the same function. In the case of AIDS prevention, people who are not about to give up drugs or their preferred forms of sexuality can achieve substantial protection against HIV infection by substituting safer behaviors for risky ones. Multifaceted psychosocial programs that equip people with protective knowledge, with the means and self-beliefs to exercise effective personal control, and provide sociaı supports for their efforts at personal change, can achieve highly beneficial results. Indeed, prevention programs that incorporate many of these elements have produced substantial reductions in risky sexual and drug-injection behaviors.

IMMUNOLOGIC EFFECTS OF COPING EFFICACY

The discussion thus far has been concerned mainly with how social and self-regulative efficacy contribute to self-protective behavior. A psychosocial theory for the prevention and management of AIDS must address biological mechanisms as well as health-related behaviors. In accord with the biopsychosocial model of health and illness (Engel, 1977), psychosocial factors not only exercise control over behaviors that enhance or impair health, they also activate a wide range of biological processes that can affect susceptibility to infection. Infectious and chronic diseases are usually the product of interacting sets of determinants. The HIV virus operates in conjunction with other factors to produce the clinical manifestation of AIDS. Therefore, there is variability in whether exposure to the HIV virus will result in infection. That some people are better able than others to fight off local invasion by the virus is indicated by instances of individuals who have an ongoing sexual relationship with an infected partner but do not become infected. There is also considerable variability in the length of time before the latently infected individuals begin to develop clinical symptoms. Additionally, there is variability in the rate with which the disease progresses to the final stage of opportunistic infections and cancers as the ability of the immune system to fight infectious agents is severely impaired.

Physical cofactors account for some of the variability in immunological control of the latent virus and rate of disease development. It should be noted, however, that many of these physical cofactors that increase vulnerability to infection and disease progression, such as drug abuse, untreated venereal diseases that produce genital ulceration, and other activities that weaken health status, are largely the products of psychosocially determined behavior patterns. Not only do psychosocial influences breed many of the physical cofactors, but coping efficacy may operate as a psychosocial cofactor that influences infectability and disease progression directly through its impact on immune function. The heavy focus on the inevitability of disease development given HIV infection has retarded research on cofactors that operate as contributors to the clinical manifestations of AIDS. Such knowledge identifies cofactors over which people can exercise some control and those that are not amenable to personal change.

Perceived coping self-efficacy can affect immune function through stress and depression. Perceived self-efficacy to exercise control over stressors plays a central role in human stress reactions (Bandura, 1988a). Exposure to stressors with ability to control them has no adverse biological effects. But exposure to the same stressors without the ability to control them activates autonomic reactions, catecholamine secretion and release of endogenous opioids (Bandura, Cioffi, Taylor, & Brouillard, 1988; Bandura, Taylor, Williams, Mefford, & Barchas, 1985; Maier et al., 1985; Shavit & Martin, 1987).

Biological systems are highly interdependent. The types of biological systems activated by a weak sense of coping efficacy are intricately involved in the regulation of the immune system. Indeed, a growing body of evidence shows that exposure to stressors with weak ability to exercise control over them impairs various facets of immune function (Jemmott & Locke, 1984; Kiecolt-Glaser & Glaser, 1987; Maier et al., 1985; Shavit & Martin, 1987).

Although the stress of coping inefficacy is immunosuppressive, there is suggestive evidence that providing people with the means for managing stress may be immunoenhancing, at least for some immunologic functions (Kiecolt-Glaser et al., 1986; Kiecolt-Glaser et al., 1985). Moreover, stress aroused while gaining coping mastery over acute stressors enhances different components of the immune system (Wiedenfeld, O'Leary, Bandura, Brown, Levine, & Raska, 1990). Several studies report findings that bear on the issue of whether psychosocial interventions may help to retard disease progression. Development of skills to manage stress has been shown to increase immune function in metastatic cancer patients (Gruber, Hall, Hersh, & Dubois, 1988), and to enhance cellular and humoral immune functioning in seropositive gay men in asymptomatic stages of HIV infection (Antoni, Schneiderman, Fletcher, Goldstein, Ironson, & Laperriere, 1990). The immune system includes multiple interacting subprocesses with intricate interconnections to other biological systems, all of which complicates evaluation of level of immunity. Whether the magnitude of the immunologic changes achieved in these studies is sufficient to have significant health consequences remains to be determined.

Another path of influence of coping inefficacy on immunocompetence is through the mediating effects of depression. A sense of personal inefficacy to fulfill desired goals that affect evaluation of self-worth and to secure things that bring satisfaction to one's life create depression (Bandura, 1988b; Kanfer

& Zeiss, 1983). When the perceived self-inefficacy involves social relationships, it can induce depression both directly and indirectly by curtailing the cultivation of the very interpersonal relationships that can provide satisfactions and buffer the effects of chronic daily stressors (Holahan & Holahan, 1987a, 1987b). Depression has been shown to reduce immune function and to heighten susceptibility to disease (Ader & Cohen, 1985). The more severe the depression, the greater the reduction in immunity (Irwin, 1988).

The evidence regarding immunoregulatory interactions, suggests that a severe sense of coping inefficacy may further impair the already damaged immune system of persons infected with the HIV virus and thus exacerbate the disorder (Kiecolt-Glaser & Glaser, 1988). Apart from the common environmental stressors with which people must cope, knowledge that one has contracted the AIDS virus, the accompanying stigmatization and major social repercussions, and the reality of progressive physical deterioration and anticipated death, create major new sources of stress and despondency. Ineffectual cognitive and behavioral coping with knowledge of seropositivity and with AIDS-related problems further heightens stress and depression (Namir, Wolcott, Fawzy, & Alumbaugh, 1987).

Reactions to knowledge of seropositivity have undergone significant changes over the course of the AIDS epidemic. The early reactions of despair to the epidemic were supplanted by active pursuit of information, preventive programs, treatments, and life-style changes that might offer any hope of forestalling the onset of AIDS or prolonging the life of those in the symptomatic stage. These concerted psychosocial efforts curtailed the spread of HIV infection in gay populations. Significant progress is being made in treating the opportunistic infections that arise when immune systems are weakened by the virus. But the quest for drugs that would destroy the HIV virus or render AIDS a manageable disease is strewn with dashed hopes. As the AIDS epidemic continues to take its heavy human and emotional toll, collective enabling efforts are being replaced in many circles by a sense of despondency. The magnitude of the problem calls for increased commitment of resources to the crucial aspect of the pandemic over which we can command some control, stemming the spread of HIV infections through comprehensive preventive programs.

A multifaceted approach must address the burdensome affective dimensions of AIDS as well. Research conducted within the social cognitive framework has led to the development of self-management programs for alleviating stress and depression (Bandura, 1988b; Beck, 1976; Lewinsohn, Antonuuccio, Steinmetz, & Teri, 1984; Lewinsohn & Clarke, 1984; Rehm, 1981; Taylor & Arnow, 1988). These psychosocial approaches equip people with coping skills to manage difficult problems and to reduce their level of emotional distress. Those who do not know how to exercise control over emotional strain can be easily overwhelmed by daily confrontations with innumerable social stressors, progressive physical debilitation, bereavement experiences, and preoccupation with thoughts of their own death. Such severe chronic stressors adversely affect immunity (Kiecolt-Glaser & Glaser, 1988). The exercise of cognitive control over self-debilitating thought processes can further reduce the psychological toll of AIDS and enable patients to live out their lives as productively as they possibly can. The impact of AIDS on psychosocial functioning is, therefore, partly mediated by personal coping capabilities. Thus, some individuals who know they are infected but are still asymptomatic may sink into deep despondency, whereas others with an array of symptoms may struggle valiantly to continue a meaningful and productive life.

The conceptual model and supporting evidence reviewed in this chapter argue strongly for a multifaceted approach to the prevention and management of AIDS in which psychosocial interventions must play an influential role. With regard to prevention, equipping people with the cognitive and behavioral coping resources to exercise personal control over risky behaviors enables them to protect themselves from exposure to this most deadly of viruses. By their impact on stress, depression, and immunity, psychosocial factors can affect disease development and quality of adaptation to it. Neglect or downgrading of psychosocial models and programs will exact heavy personal tolls and impose mounting financial and social burdens on societies.

REFERENCES

Ader, R., & Cohen, N. (1985). CNS-immune system interactions: Conditioning phenomena. *The Behavioral & Brain Sciences, 8,* 379–394.

Antoni, M. H., Schneiderman, N., Fletcher, M. A., Goldstein, D. A., Ironson, G., & Laperriere, A. (1990). Psychoneuroimmunology and HIV-1. *Journal of Consulting & Clinical Psychology, 58,* 38–49.

Bandura, A. (1986). *Social foundations of thought and action: A social cognitive theory.* Englewood Cliffs, NJ: Prentice-Hall.

Bandura, A. (1988a). Self-efficacy conception of anxiety. *Anxiety Research, 1,* 77–98.

Bandura, A. (1988b). Perceived self-efficacy: Exercise of control through self-belief. In J. P. Dauwalder, M. Perrez, & V. Hobi (Eds.), *Annual series of European research in behavior therapy* (Vol. 2, pp. 27–59). Lisse (NL): Swets & Zeitlinger.

Bandura, A. (1989). Self-regulation of motivation and action through internal standards and goal systems. In L. A. Pervin (Ed.), *Goal concepts in personality and social psychology* (pp. 19–85). Hillsdale, NJ: Lawrence Erlbaum.

Bandura, A. (1991a). Self-efficacy mechanism in physiological activation and health-promoting behavior. In J. Madden, IV (Ed.), *Neurobiology of learning, emotion and affect* (pp. 229–269). New York: Raven.

Bandura, A. (1991b). Self-regulation of motivation through anticipatory and self-regulatory mechanisms. In R. A. Dienstbier (Ed.), *Perspectives on motivation: Nebraska symposium on motivation* (Vol. 38, pp. 69–164). Lincoln: University of Nebraska Press.

Bandura, A. (1992). Self-efficacy mechanism in psychobiologic functioning. In R. Schwarzer (Ed.), *Self-efficacy: Thought control of action* (pp. 355–394). Washington, DC: Hemisphere, 1992.

Bandura, A., Cioffi, D., Taylor, C. B., & Brouillard, M. E. (1988). Perceived self-efficacy in coping with cognitive stressors and opioid activation. *Journal of Personality & Social Psychology, 55,* 479–488.

Bandura, A., Taylor, C. B., Williams, S. L., Mefford, I. N., & Barchas, J. D. (1985). Catecholamine secretion as a function of perceived coping self-efficacy. *Journal of Consulting & Clinical Psychology, 53,* 406–414.

Basen-Engquist, K., Parcel, G. S. (1992). Attitudes, norms and self-efficacy: A model of adolescents' HIV-related sexual risk behavior. *Health Education Quarterly, 19,* 263–277.

Bauman, L. J., & Siegel, K. (1987). Misperception among gay men of the risk for AIDS associated with their sexual behavior. *Journal of Applied Social Psychology, 17,* 329–350.

Beck, A. T. (1976). *Cognitive therapy and the emotional disorders.* New York: International Universities Press.

Beck, K. H., & Lund, A. K. (1981). The effects of health threat seriousness and personal efficacy upon intentions and behavior. *Journal of Applied Social Psychology, 11,* 401–415.

Botvin, G. J., & Dusenbury, L. (1992). Substance abuse prevention: Implications for reducing risk of HIV infection. *Psychology of Addictive Behaviors, 6,* 70–80.

Brafford, L. J., & Beck, K. H. (1991). Development and validation of a condom self-efficacy scale for college students. *Journal of American College Health, 39,* 219–225.

Buning, E. C. (1991). Effects of Amsterdam needle and syringe exchange. *The International Journal of the Addictions, 26,* 1303–1311.

Chervin, D. D., & Martinez, A. (1987). Survey on the health of Stanford students. Report to the Board of Trustees, Stanford University, February 19, 1987.

Cooney, N. L., Gillespie, R. A., Baker, L. H., & Kaplan, R. F. (1987). Cognitive changes after alcohol cue exposure. *Journal of Consulting & Clinical Psychology, 55,* 150–155.

Cutler, J. C., & Arnold, R. C. (1988). Venereal disease control by health departments in the past: Lessons for the present. *American Journal of Public Health, 78,* 372–376.

Des Jarlais, D. C., Abdul-Quader, A., & Tross, S. (1991). The next problem: Maintenance of AIDS risk reduction among intravenous drug users. *The International Journal of the Addictions, 26,* 1279–1292.

Des Jarlais, D. C., & Friedman, S. R. (1988a). The psychology of preventing AIDS among intravenous drug users: A social learning conceptualization. *American Psychologist, 43,* 865–870.

Des Jarlais, D. C., & Friedman, S. R. (1988b). HIV infection among persons who inject illicit drugs: Problems and prospects. *Journal of Acquired Immune Deficiency Syndromes, 1,* 267–273.

DiClemente, R. J. (1991). Predictors of HIV-preventive sexual behavior in a high-risk adolescent population: The influence of perceived peer norms and sexual communication on incarcerated adolescents' consistent use of condoms. *Journal of Adolescent Health, 12,* 385–390.

Edgar, T., Freimuth, V. S., & Hammond, S. L. (1988). Communicating the AIDS risk to college students: The problem of motivating change. *Health Education Research, 3,* 59–65.

Engel, G. L. (1977). The need for a new medical model: A challenge for biomedicine. *Science, 196,* 129–136.

Farquhar, J. W., Maccoby, N., & Solomon, D. S. (1984). Community applications of behavioral medicine. In W. D. Gentry (Ed.), *Handbook of behavioral medicine* (pp. 437–478). New York: Guilford.

Fisher, J. D. (1988). Possible effects of reference group-based social influence on AIDS-risk behavior and AIDS prevention. *American Psychologist, 43,* 914–920.

Flora, J. A., & Thoresen, C. E. (1988). Reducing the risk of AIDS in adolescents. *American Psychologist, 43,* 965–970.

Friedman, S. R., de Jong, W. M., & Des Jarlais, D. C. (1988). Problems and dynamics of organizing intravenous drug users for AIDS prevention. *Health Education Research, 3,* 49–57.

Gagnon, J., & Simon, W. (1973). *Sexual conduct, the social sources of human sexuality.* Chicago: Aldine.

Gilchrist, L. D., & Schinke, S. P. (1983). Coping with contraception: Cognitive and behavioral methods with adolescents. *Cognitive Therapy & Research, 7,* 379–388.

Gilchrist, L. D., & Schinke, S. P. (Eds.). (1985). *Preventing social and health problems through life skills training.* Seattle, WA: University of Washington.

Gilchrist, L. D., Schinke, S. P., Trimble, J. E., & Cvetkovich, G. T. (1987). Skills enhancement to prevent substance abuse among American Indian adolescents. *International Journal of the Addictions, 22,* 869–879.

Gossop, M., Green, L., Phillips, G., & Bradley, B. (1990). Factors predicting outcome among opiate addicts after treatment. *British Journal of Clinical Psychology, 29,* 209–216.

Gruber, B., Hall, N. R., Hersh, S. P., & Dubois, P. (1988). Immune system and psychologic changes in metastatic cancer patients using relaxation and guided imagery: A pilot study. *Scandinavian Journal of Behaviour Therapy, 17,* 25–46.

Heather, N., & Stallard, A. (1989). Does the Marlatt model underestimate the importance of conditioned craving in the relapse process? In M. Gossop (Ed.), *Relapse and addictive behaviour* (pp. 180–208). London: Tavistock/Routledge.

Heinrich, L. B. (1993). Contraceptive self-efficacy in college women. *Journal of Adolescent Health, 14,* 110–115.

Heller, M. C., & Krauss, H. H. (1991). Perceived self-efficacy as a predictor of aftercare treatment entry by the detoxification patient. *Psychological Reports, 68,* 1047–1052.

Holahan, C. K., & Holahan, C. J. (1987a). Self-efficacy, social support, and depression in aging: A longitudinal analysis. *Journal of Gerontology, 42,* 65–68.

Holahan, C. K., & Holahan, C. J. (1987b). Life stress, hassles, and self-efficacy in aging: A replication and extension. *Journal of Applied Social Psychology, 17,* 574–592.

Irwin, M. (1988). Depression and immune function. *Stress Medicine, 4,* 95–103.

Jemmott, L. S., & Jemmott, J. B., III (1992). Increasing condom-use intentions among sexually active black adolescent women. *Nursing Research, 41,* 273–278.

Jemmott, J. B., Jemmott, L. S., & Fong, G. T. (1992). Reductions in HIV risk-associated sexual behaviors among black male adolescents: Effects of an AIDS prevention intervention. *American Journal of Public Health, 82,* 372–377.

Jemmott, J. B., III, Jemmott, L. S., Spears, H., Hewitt, N., & Cruz-Collins, M. (1991). Self-efficacy, hedonistic expectancies, and condom-use intentions among inner-city black adolescent women: A social cognitive approach to AIDS risk behavior. *Journal of Adolescent Health, 13,* 512–519.

Jemmott, J. B., III, & Locke, S. E. (1984). Psychosocial factors, immunological mediation, and human susceptibility to infectious diseases: How much do we know? *Psychological Bulletin, 95,* 78–108.

Kanfer, R., & Zeiss, A. M. (1983). Depression, interpersonal standard-setting, and judgments of self-efficacy. *Journal of Abnormal Psychology, 92,* 319–329.

Kasen, S., Vaughan, R. D., & Walter, H. J. (1992). Self-efficacy for AIDS preventive behaviors among tenth grade students. *Health Education Quarterly, 19,* 187–202.

Kazdin, A. E. (1978). Covert modeling: The therapeutic application of imagined rehearsal. In J. L. Singer & K. S. Pope (Eds.), *The power of human imagination: New methods in psychotherapy. Emotions, personality, and psychotherapy* (pp. 255–278). New York: Plenum.

Keeling, R. P. (Ed.) (1989). *AIDS on the college campus* (2nd ed.). Rockville, MD: American College Health Assoc.

Kelly, J. A., Kalichman, S. C., Kauth, M. R., Kilgore, H. G., Hood, H. V., Campos, P. E., Rao, S. M., Brasfield, T. L., & St. Lawrence, J. S. (1991). Situational factors associated with AIDS risk behavior lapses and coping strategies used by gay men who successfully avoid lapses. *American Journal of Public Health, 81,* 1335–1338.

Kelly, J. A., St. Lawrence, J. S., & Brasfield, T. L. (1991). Predictors of vulnerability to AIDS risk behavior relapse. *Journal of Consulting & Clinical Psychology, 59,* 163–166.

Kelly, J. A., St. Lawrence, J. S., Hood, H. V., & Brasfield, T. L. (1989). Behavioral intervention to reduce AIDS risk activities. *Journal of Consulting & Clinical Psychology, 57,* 60–67.

Kiecolt-Glaser, J. K., & Glaser, R. (1987). Behavioral influences on immune function: Evidence for the interplay between stress and health. In T. Field, P. M. McCabe, & N. Schneiderman (Eds.), *Stress and coping across development* (Vol. 2, pp. 189–206). Hillsdale, NJ: Lawrence Erlbaum.

Kiecolt-Glaser, J. K., & Glaser, R. (1988). Psychological influences on immunity. *American Psychologist, 43,* 892–898.

Kiecolt-Glaser, J. K., Glaser, R., Strain, E. C., Stout, J. C., Tarr, K. L., Holliday, J. E., & Speicher, C. E. (1986). Modulation of cellular immunity in medical students. *Journal of Behavioral Medicine, 9,* 521.

Kiecolt-Glaser, J. K., Glaser, R., Williger, D., Stout, J., Messick, G., Sheppard, S., Ricker, D., Romisher, S. C., Briner, W., Bonnell, G., & Donnerberg, R. (1985). Psychosocial enhancement of immunocompetence in a geriatric population. *Health Psychology, 4,* 25–41.

Killen, J. D., Robinson, T. N., Telch, M. J., Saylor, K. E., Maron, D. J., Rich, T., & Bryson, S. (1989). The Stanford adolescent heart health program. *Health Education Quarterly, 16,* 263–283.

Kok, G., deVries, H., Mudde, A. N., & Strecher, V. J. (1991). Planned health education and the role of self-efficacy: Dutch research. *Health Education Research, 6,* 231–238.

Levinson, R. A. (1986). Contraceptive self-efficacy: A perspective on teenage girls' contraceptive behavior. *Journal of Sex Research, 22,* 347–369.

Lewinsohn, P. M., Antonuuccio, D. O., Steinmetz, J. L., & Teri, L. (1984). *The coping with depression course.* Eugene, OR: Castalia.

Lewinsohn, P. M., & Clarke, G. N. (1984). Group treatment of depressed individuals: The coping with depression course. *Advances in Behaviour Research & Therapy, 6,* 99–114.

Maddux, J. E., & Rogers, R. W. (1983). Protection motivation and self-efficacy: A revised theory of fear appeals and attitude change. *Journal of Experimental Social Psychology, 19,* 469–479.

Maibach, E. W., & Flora, J. A. (1993). Symbolic modeling and cognitive rehearsal: Using video to promote AIDS prevention self-efficacy. *Communication Research, 20,* 517–545.

Maibach, E., Flora, J., & Nass, C. (1991). Changes in self-efficacy and health behavior in response to a minimal contact community health campaign. *Health Communication, 3,* 1–15.

Maier, S. F., Laudenslager, M. L., & Ryan, S. M. (1985). Stressor controllability, immune function, and endogenous opiates. In F. R. Brush & J. B. Overmier (Eds.), *Affect, conditioning, and cognition: Essays on the determinants of behavior* (pp. 183–201). Hillsdale, NJ: Lawrence Erlbaum.

Mantell, J. E., Karp, G., Majidi, K., Ramos, S. E., Glover-Walton, C., Gonzalex, V., & Brown, L. E., Jr. (1993). *Do power and powerlessness affect condom use among inner-city women?* Unpublished manuscript, Medical and Health Research Association of New York City.

Mantell, J. E., & Schinke, S. P. (1990). The crisis of AIDS for adolescents: The need for preventive risk-reduction interventions. In A. R. Roberts (Ed.), *Contemporary perspectives on crisis intervention and prevention* (pp. 185–217). Englewood Cliffs, NJ: Prentice-Hall.

Mantell, J. E., Schinke, S. P., & Akabas, S. H. (1988). Women and AIDS prevention. *Journal of Primary Prevention, 9,* 18–40.

Marlatt, A., & Gordon, J. R. (1985). *Relapse prevention: Maintenance strategies in the treatment of addictive behaviors.* New York: Guilford Press.

Mays, V. M., & Cochran, S. D. (1988). Issues in the perception of AIDS risk and risk reduction activities by Black and Hispanic/Latina women. *American Psychologist, 43,* 949–957.

McAuliffe, W. E., Albert, J., Cordill-London, G., & McGarraghy, T. K. (1991). Contributors to a social conditioning model of cocaine recovery. *International Journal of the Addictions, 25,* 1141–1177.

McCune, J. M., Namikawa, R., Shih, C., Rabin, L., & Kaneshima, H. (1990). Suppression of HIV infection in AZT-treated SCID-hu mice. *Science, 247,* 564–566.

McGuire, W. J. (1984). Public Communication as a strategy for inducing health-promoting behavioral change. *Preventive Medicine, 13,* 299–319.

McKusick, L., Coates, T. J., Morin, S. F., Pollack, L., & Hoff, C. (1990). Longitudinal predictors of reductions in unprotected anal intercourse among gay men in San Francisco: The AIDS behavioral research project. *American Journal of Public Health, 80,* 978–983.

McKusick, L., Horstman, W., & Coates, T. J. (1985). AIDS and sexual behavior reported by gay men in San Francisco. *American Journal of Public Health, 75,* 493–496.

McKusick, L., Wiley, J., Coates, T. J., & Morin, S. F. (1986, November). Predictors of AIDS behavioral risk reduction: The AIDS Behavioral Research Project. Paper presented at the New Zealand AIDS Foundation Prevention Education Workshop, Auckland, New Zealand.

Meyerowitz, B. E., & Chaiken, S. (1987). The effect of message framing on breast self-examination attitudes, intentions, and behavior. *Journal of Personality & Social Psychology, 52,* 500–510.

Namir, S., Wolcott, D. L., Fawzy, F. I., & Alumbaugh, M. J. (1987). Coping with AIDS: Psychological and health implications. *Journal of Applied Social Psychology, 17,* 309–328.

O'Leary, A. (1985). Self-efficacy and health. *Behavior Research Therapy, 23,* 437–451.

O'Leary, A., Goodhart, F., Jemmott, L. S., & Boccher-Lattimore, D. (1992). Predictors of safer sex on the college campus: A social cognitive theory analysis. *Journal of American College Health, 40,* 254–263.

Perri, M. G. (1985). Self-change strategies for the control of smoking, obesity, and problem drinking. In T. A. Wills & S. Shiffman (Eds.), *Coping and substance use.* (pp. 295–317). New York: Academic Press.

Rehm, L. P. (1981). A self-control therapy program for treatment of depression. In J. F. Clarkin & H. Glazer (Eds.), *Depression: Behavioral and directive treatment strategies* (pp. 68–110). New York: Garland Press.

Rosenthal, D., Moore, S., & Flynn, I. (1991). Adolescent self-efficacy, self-esteem, and sexual risk-taking. *Journal of Community & Applied Social Psychology, 1,* 77–88.

Rothman, A. J., Salovey, P., Antone, Ca., Keough, K., & Drake, C. (in press). The influence of message framing on health behavior. *Health Psychology.*

Sallis, J. F., Hill, R. D., Killen, J. D., Telch, M. J., Flora, J. A., Girard, J., & Taylor, C. B. (1986). Efficacy of self-help behavior modification materials in smoking cessation. *American Journal of Preventive Medicine, 2,* 342–344.

Schinke, S. P., & Orlandi, M. A. (1990). Skills-based, interactive computer interventions to prevent HIV infection among African-American and Hispanic adolescents. *Computers in Human Behavior, 6,* 235–246.

Shavit, Y., & Martin, F. C. (1987). Opiates, stress, and immunity: Animal studies. *Annals of Behavioral Medicine, 9,* 11–20.

Siegel, J. E., Graham, J. D., & Stoto, M. A. (1990). Allocating resources among AIDS research strategies. *Policy Sciences, 23,* 1–23.

Siegel, K., Mesagno, F. P., Chen, J., & Christ, G. (1989). Factors distinguishing homosexual males practicing risky and safer sex. *Social Science Medicine, 28,* 561–569.

Sitharthan, T., McGrath, D., Cairns, D., & Saunders, J. B. (1991). *An empirical investigation of situations related to opiate use.* Unpublished manuscript, Royal Prince Alfred Hospital, NSW, Australia.

Slater, M. D. (1989). Social influences and cognitive control as predictors of self-efficacy and eating behavior. *Cognitive Therapy and Research, 13,* 231–245.

Stall, R., & Biernacki, P. (1986). Spontaneous remission from the problematic use of substances: An inductive model derived from a comparative analysis of the alcohol, opiate, tobacco, and food/obesity literatures. *The International Journal of the Addictions, 21,* 1–23.

Stall, R., Ekstrand, M., Pollack, L., McKusick, L., & Coates, T. J. (1990). Relapse from safer sex: The next challenge for AIDS prevention efforts. *Journal of Acquired Immune Deficiency Syndromes, 3,* 1181–1187.

Stall, R., & Paul, J. (1989). *Changes in sexual risk for infection with the human immunodeficiency virus among gay and bisexual men in San Francisco.* (Document prepared for the World Health Organization Global Programme on AIDS). San Francisco: University of California.

Stiffman, A. R., Earls, F., Dore, P., & Cunningham, R. (1992). Changes in acquired immunodeficiency syndrome-related risk behavior after adolescence: Relationships to knowledge and experience concerning human immunodeficiency virus infection. *Pediatrics, 89,* 950–956.

Taylor, C. B., & Arnow, B. (1988). *The nature and treatment of anxiety disorders.* New York: Macmillan.

Tversky, A., & Kahneman, D. (1981). The framing of decisions and the psychology of choice. *Science, 211,* 453–458.

Watters, J. K., Downing, M., Case, P., Lorvick, J., Cheng, Y., & Fergusson, B. (1990). AIDS prevention for intravenous drug users in the community: Street-based education and risk behavior. *American Journal of Community Psychology, 18,* 587–596.

Wiedenfeld, S. A., O'Leary, A., Bandura, A., Brown, S., Levine, S., & Raska, K. (1990). Impact of perceived self-efficacy in coping with stressors on components of the immune system. *Journal of Personality and Social Psychology, 59,* 1082–1094.

Winett, R. A., Anderson, E. S., Moore, J. F., Sikkema, K. J., Hook, R., Webster, D. A., Taylor, C. D., Dalton, J. E., Ollendick, T. H., & Eisler, R. M. (1992). Family/media approach to HIV prevention: Results with a home-based, parent-teen video program. *Health Psychology, 11,* 203–206.

Zimbardo, P. G., Ebbesen, E. B., & Maslach, C. (1977). *Influencing attitudes and changing behavior.* Reading, MA: Addison-Wesley.

4

Using Information to Change Sexually Transmitted Disease-Related Behaviors

An Analysis Based on the Theory of Reasoned Action

MARTIN FISHBEIN, SUSAN E. MIDDLESTADT, and PENELOPE J. HITCHCOCK

INTRODUCTION

Given that sexually transmitted diseases (STDs) are transmitted by individuals engaging in definable physical behaviors and that many STDs are not curable, it is clear that an effective STD prevention program must include a component that focuses on changing high-risk or maintaining low-risk behaviors. Furthermore, a behavior change program is also necessary to encourage people to determine whether or not they have been exposed to a particular STD, as well as to get them to seek and use available treatments. In this chapter, we illustrate how the theory of reasoned action (Ajzen &

This is a revised chapter which appeared in J.N. Wasserheit, S.O. Aral, K.K. Holmes, and P.J. Hitchcock (Eds.), *Research issues in human behavior and sexually transmitted diseases in the AIDS era* (pp. 243–266), Washington, DC: American Society for Microbiology, 1991.

MARTIN FISHBEIN • Department of Psychology, University of Illinois, Champaign, Illinois 61820.   *SUSAN E. MIDDLESTADT* • Social Development Program, Academy for Educational Development, Washington, DC 20037.   *PENELOPE J. HITCHCOCK* • Sexually Transmitted Diseases Branch, National Institute of Allergy and Infectious Diseases, National Institutes of Health, Bethesda, Maryland 20892.

Preventing AIDS: Theories and Methods of Behavioral Interventions, edited by Ralph J. DiClemente and John L. Peterson. Plenum Press, New York, 1994.

Fishbein, 1980; Fishbein, 1980, 1967; Fishbein & Ajzen, 1975), can be used to empirically identify the determinants of any given behavior (i.e., the factors underlying it). Perhaps more important, we also try to show how, once identified, information about these determinants can be used to develop interventions that can successfully influence behaviors involved in the control and spread of STDs, including AIDS.

The theory of reasoned action is particularly useful if one is attempting to develop an intervention that includes an informational, educational, or communication component. This type of intervention has often been criticized as ineffective in producing behavior change. From the perspective of the theory of reasoned action, the problem of changing behavior is not one of converting knowledge to behavior, but instead, it is one of identifying the appropriate kinds of knowledge (or information) that must be provided and/or the structural changes that must be made if one wishes to influence the performance of a given behavior. To change or maintain a given behavior in a given population, one must first understand the determinants of that behavior in that population. The more one knows about the precise underlying factors influencing the decision to perform (or not to perform) a given behavior, the greater the probability that one can develop successful interventions to modify that behavior. Indeed, the key to successful behavioral interventions is the identification of the determinants of the specific behaviors that one wants to maintain or change.

A THEORY OF REASONED ACTION

First introduced in 1967, the theory of reasoned action (Ajzen & Fishbein, 1980; Fishbein, 1980, 1967; Fishbein & Ajzen, 1975) is a general theory of human behavior that deals with the relations among beliefs, attitudes, intentions, and behavior. Each variable in the theory has been operationally defined, and standardized procedures for assessing each of these variables have been developed. Thus, it is possible to conduct empirical tests of the hypothesized relationships among variables.

The theory of reasoned action has been used successfully to predict and explain why people have (or have not) engaged in a wide variety of behaviors including smoking (Chassin et al., 1981; Fishbein, 1980), drinking (Budd & Spencer, 1985; Schlegel, Crawford, & Sanborn, 1977), signing up for a treatment program (Fishbein, Ajzen, & McArdle, 1980), using contraceptives (Fisher, 1984; Jaccard & Davidson, 1972), dieting (Sejwacz, Ajzen, & Fishbein, 1980; Saltzer, 1978), wearing seat belts or safety helmets (Allegrante, Mortimer, & O'Rourke, 1980; Budd, North, & Spencer, 1984; Fishbein, Salazar, Rodriquez, Middlestadt, & Himelfarb, 1988), exercising regularly (Godin & Shephard, 1986), voting (Bowman & Fishbein, 1978; Schlegel, Crawford, & Sanborn, 1977; Shepherd, 1987), breast-feeding (Manstead, Proffitt, & Smart, 1983), buying various goods and services (Ryan, 1982), donating money to a university library (Middlestadt, 1990), and choosing a career (Greenstein, Miller, & Weldon, 1979).

Briefly, the theory assumes a causal chain that links beliefs to behavior. As can be seen in Figure 1, behavior is viewed as a function of the intention to perform that behavior; intention is seen as a joint function of one's overall positive or negative feeling toward performing the behavior (i.e., one's attitude toward performing the behavior), and one's overall perception of social pressure to perform or not to perform the behavior (i.e., one's subjective norm with respect to performing the behavior). Attitude and subjective norm are, in turn, viewed as a function of underlying cognitive (i.e., belief) structures. More specifically, attitudes are viewed as a function of behavioral beliefs that performing the behavior will lead to certain outcomes and one's evaluation of those outcomes. Subjective norms are viewed as a function of normative beliefs that specific referents (i.e., certain individuals or groups) think one should or should not perform the behavior and one's motivation to comply with those referents. Thus, according to the theory, behavior is ultimately determined by a cognitive structure composed of underlying behavioral and normative beliefs. In the final analysis then, changing behavior is primarily a matter of changing this cognitive structure (i.e., of changing the underlying beliefs).

THE BEHAVIORAL CRITERION

The first step in applying the theory of reasoned action is to select and identify the behavior(s) of interest. A full identification of any behavior requires

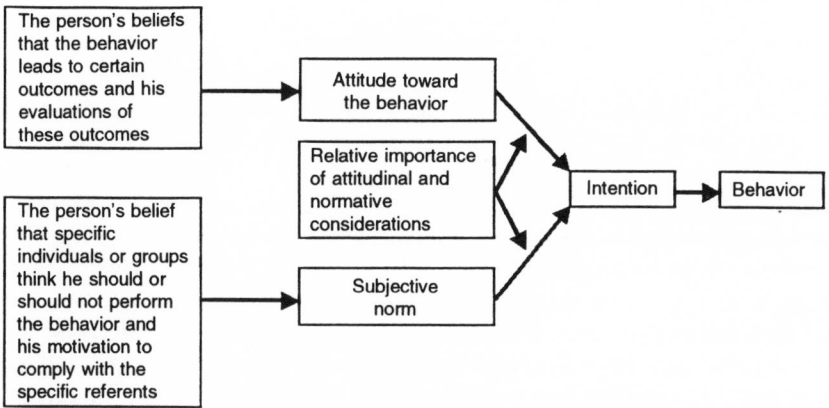

Figure 1. A theory of reasoned action: Factors determining a person's behavior. Arrows indicate the direction of influence with hypothesized relationships (From Ajzen & Fishbein, 1980).

consideration of the four elements of action, target, context, and time. That is, every action occurs with respect to some target, in a given context, and at a given point in time. Although one may arrive at more general behavioral criteria by generalizing across one or more of these elements, a change in any one of the four elements redefines the behavior of interest. For example, using a condom is a different behavior from carrying or buying a condom (a change in action); going to an STD clinic is a different behavior from going to a family doctor or going to a human immunodeficiency virus counseling and testing site (a change in target); using a condom with a spouse or long-term partner is a different behavior from using a condom with a casual partner or with a commercial sex worker (a change in context); and going to an STD clinic on a Tuesday morning is a different behavior from going to the same STD clinic on a Saturday afternoon (a change in time). It is worth noting that "using a condom *the next time* I have vaginal sex with my main partner" is a different behavior from "using a condom *every time* I have vaginal sex with my main partner" (a different type of change in time).

Since each behavior is likely to be based on its own unique set of determinants (i.e., on a cognitive structure specific to that behavior), each behavior may require a different intervention strategy. For example, the information necessary to increase condom use with one's spouse or long-term partner may be very different from that required to increase condom use with a casual date or with a commercial sex worker. Similarly, the information necessary to increase condom use for oral sex may be very different from that required to increase condom use for vaginal or anal sex. To be effective, interventions must influence the beliefs that underlie the decision to perform (or not to perform) the targeted behavior.

PREDICTING BEHAVIOR FROM INTENTIONS

The theory assumes that most socially relevant behaviors are under volitional control. Therefore, the most immediate determinant of any given behavior is the intention to perform or not to perform that behavior. This intention, however, must correspond exactly to the behavior in question (i.e., the intention must be defined in terms of the same four elements of action, target, context, and time that serve to define the behavior). There is now considerable evidence that such correspondent intentions provide very accurate predictions of most social behaviors. Thus, to change a specific behavior, one must change the intention to perform that behavior. For example, if the goal of an intervention is to increase homosexual men's use of condoms for oral sex with their long-term partners, the intervention should be designed to increase homosexual men's intentions to "always use condoms for oral sex with my long-term partner" and not to increase their intentions to "avoid AIDS," to "practice safe sex," or even their general intentions to "always use condoms when I have sex." Indeed, as we shall see below, changing intentions to reach goals (e.g., to avoid AIDS) and/or to engage in a class of behaviors (e.g., to practice safe sex) are seldom effective strategies for producing change in specific behaviors.

PREDICTING INTENTIONS FROM ATTITUDES AND SUBJECTIVE NORMS

Given that correspondent intentions are viewed as the immediate determinants of behavior, the theory is primarily concerned with identifying the factors underlying the formation and change of these correspondent intentions. According to the theory of reasoned action, a person's intention to perform (or not to perform) a given behavior is a function of two basic determinants, one personal in nature and the other reflecting social influence. The personal factor is the individual's positive or negative feelings with respect to performing the behavior in question; this factor is termed *attitude toward the behavior.* The second determinant of intention is the person's perception of the social pressure put upon him or her to perform or not to perform the behavior. Since it deals with perceptions of what others think one "should" or "ought" to do, this factor is termed *subjective norm.* Generally speaking, individuals will intend to perform a behavior when they have a positive attitude toward performing it and/or when they believe that their important others think they should perform it. Note that the attitude (and the subjective norm) specified by the theory is the individual's attitude toward (or subjective norm with respect to) his or her own performance of the behavior in question. That is, like the intention, the attitude (and the norm) must be defined in terms of the same four elements of action, target, context, and time that define the targeted behavior.

Although attitudes and subjective norms may both influence the formation of a given intention, the relative importance of these two factors is expected to vary depending on the behavior and the individual. For some behaviors (and intentions), attitudinal considerations may be more influential than normative ones, while for other behaviors, normative considerations may predominate. Similarly, the intention to perform a given behavior may be primarily under attitudinal control for some individuals (or segments of the population) and predominantly under normative control for other individuals or groups. For example, in a recent study of undergraduate males' intentions to always use a condom, it was found that, in forming this intention, those who were sexually inexperienced tended to place more weight on attitudinal considerations, while those who were sexually experienced (i.e., who had had intercourse at least once) tended to place more weight on normative considerations (M. Fishbein & S. E. Middlestadt, unpublished data).

The discussion to this point can thus be summarized by equation 1,

$$B \sim I = f[w_1 Ab + w_2 SN] \tag{1}$$

where

B is the behavior of interest (e.g., a dichotomous response to the question, "Do you always use a condom when you have vaginal intercourse with your wife?");

I is the intention to perform that behavior (e.g., the likelihood that "I intend to always use a condom when I have vaginal intercourse with my wife," measured sometime before the behavioral observation);

Ab is the attitude toward performing that behavior (e.g., positive or negative feeling toward "my always using a condom for vaginal intercourse with my wife");

SN is the subjective norm concerning this behavior (e.g., the belief that "most of my important others think I should/should not always use a condom for vaginal intercourse with my wife"); and

w_1 and w_2 are the weights (or relative importance) of the attitudinal and normative components, respectively.

Although this level of explanation provides some initial insight into why people behave the way they do, a more complete understanding of intentions requires an explanation of why people hold given attitudes or subjective norms. The theory of reasoned action also attempts to answer these questions.

THE COGNITIVE STRUCTURE UNDERLYING ATTITUDE AND SUBJECTIVE NORMS

As indicated above, the theory of reasoned action views behavior change as ultimately being a matter of changing the cognitive structure underlying that behavior. That is, one must change the evaluative implication of the behavioral beliefs underlying attitudes and/or the normative implication of the normative beliefs underlying subjective norms. Thus, to develop a successful intervention, one must first identify and examine the behavioral beliefs and outcome evaluations underlying the attitude as well as the normative beliefs and motivations to comply that determine the subjective norm.

ATTITUDE AND BEHAVIORAL BELIEFS

A person's attitude toward performing a given behavior is a function of the person's salient (i.e., "top of the mind") beliefs that performing the behavior will lead to certain outcomes and the person's evaluation of these outcomes. The more one believes that performing the behavior will lead to positive outcomes (or prevent negative outcomes), the more favorable the person's attitude. Conversely, the more one believes that performing the behavior will lead to negative consequences (or prevent positive outcomes), the more negative the attitude.

This expectancy–value relationship between attitude and behavioral beliefs is expressed mathematically in equation 2

$$Ab = f\left[\sum_{i=1}^{n} b_i e_i\right] \qquad (2)$$

where

Ab is the attitude toward one's own performance of the behavior in question (e.g., positive or negative attitude toward "my always using a condom for vaginal intercourse with my wife");

b_i is the belief that one's performance of the behavior will lead to a given outcome i (e.g., the likelihood that "my always using a condom for vaginal intercourse with my wife will reduce my sexual pleasure");

e_i is the person's evaluation of outcome i (e.g., how good or bad is "reducing my sexual pleasure");

and a behavioral crossproduct is formed for each of the n salient outcomes by multiplying the belief times the evaluation.

Finally, the n crossproducts are summed.

Note that not all of the possible outcomes of performing a behavior are seen as determinants of the attitude toward the behavior. The determinants of a given attitude in a given population are only those behavioral beliefs that are salient in the population under examination. Furthermore, one's attitude toward a behavior is determined by the evaluative implications of the total set of salient beliefs one holds; attitudes are not determined by any single belief.

SUBJECTIVE NORM AND NORMATIVE BELIEFS

A person's subjective norm with respect to a given behavior is a function of the person's normative beliefs that specific salient referents (either individuals or groups) think that he or she should or should not perform the behavior and the person's motivation to comply with those individuals or groups. Generally speaking, a person who believes that most referents with whom he or she is motivated to comply think the individual should perform the behavior, will perceive social pressure to do so. Conversely, a person who believes that most referents with whom he or she is motivated to comply think the individual should not perform the behavior, will have a subjective norm that puts perceived pressure on the person to avoid performing the behavior.

The relation between subjective norm and normative beliefs is expressed mathematically in equation 3

$$SN = f\left[\sum_{j=1}^{n} b_j m_j\right] \tag{3}$$

where

SN is the subjective norm (e.g., the person's belief that "most people who are important to me think I should/should not always use a condom when I have vaginal intercourse with my wife");

b_j is a normative belief that referent j thinks the person should/should not perform the behavior (e.g., the person's belief that "my parents think I should always use a condom when I have vaginal intercourse with my wife");

m_j is the person's motivation to comply with referent j (e.g., the belief that "generally speaking, I want to do what my parents think I should do");

and a normative belief times motivation to comply crossproduct is formed for each of n salient referents. These n normative crossproducts are then summed.

Again, note that only salient referents influence one's subjective norm. And, here too, the theory designates that subjective norms are determined by the normative implications of a set of salient normative beliefs rather than by the perceived normative pressure being exerted by any one referent.

SALIENT OUTCOMES AND REFERENTS

Just as one must determine whether a given behavior in a given population is under attitudinal or normative control, one must also identify the behavioral and normative beliefs that underlie the attitude or subjective norm. Salient outcomes and referents vary from behavior to behavior and population to population. The top-of-the-mind consequences one thinks about when one considers using a condom with a spouse or long-term partner may be very different from those that are salient when one considers using a condom with a casual or one-time partner. For example, one may think about loss of trust when one considers using a condom with a spouse but not with a casual or one-time partner. In addition, the outcomes and referents that are salient vis-à-vis either of these behaviors are quite likely to differ depending on the gender, culture, and socioeconomic status of the population of interest. Thus, in applying the theory to a new behavior or with a different population, it is imperative to conduct pilot research in a sample of the population of interest in order to identify salient outcomes and referents for that behavior in that population.

DESIGNING SUCCESSFUL BEHAVIORAL INTERVENTIONS

In this half of the chapter, we consider more directly the issues and questions involved in designing successful interventions aimed at interrupting transmission of STD pathogens or interrupting disease progression. Although one's ultimate goal may be to have an impact on a disease (e.g., reduce STD rates), and although one may believe that this can be accomplished by increasing the likelihood that a person will engage in a category of behaviors (e.g., engage in safe-sex practices), the target of an intervention should be one or more specific behaviors rather than a behavioral category or a behavioral outcome.

According to the theory of reasoned action, to be effective, an intervention must have an impact on a person's beliefs. As has been pointed out elsewhere (Fishbein & Ajzen, 1981), any given communication can be viewed as one or more belief statements. A receiver can accept or reject the information contained in the communication (i.e., the belief statements of which it is composed). If the information is accepted, this reinforces or changes the receiver's beliefs. In other words, communications essentially provide information that may lead to belief change. According to the theory of reasoned action (Fig. 1), by changing behavioral or normative beliefs, one can change corresponding attitudes and/or subjective norms, and by changing attitudes and/or subjective norms, one can change corresponding intentions. Moreover, if one changes a behavioral intention, this should influence the performance of the correspondent behavior.

Since intentions are the immediate determinants of behavior, a change in a behavioral intention should lead to a change in the correspondent behavior. In marked contrast, if one changes an intention to reach a goal, to achieve an outcome, and/or to engage in a class of behaviors, there is no guarantee that this will result in goal attainment or produce change in specific behaviors. Goal attainment often involves a number of nonbehavioral factors, many of which are beyond an individual's control. In addition, there is usually no single behavior whose performance ensures goal attainment. Instead, there are typically several behaviors, each of which increases the likelihood of reaching the goal in question. For these reasons, intentions to reach goals are often very poor determinants of actual goal attainment or of the particular behavior(s) one might perform in attempting to attain that goal.

Similarly, knowing that a person intends to engage in a category of behaviors does not mean that the person intends to perform a specific behavior within that category. Different people may define a behavioral category in different ways, and hence a person may not include a specific behavior within his or her definition of the category. In addition, a person may not know or may be incorrectly informed about the behaviors that another person would define as composing the behavioral category. For example, a commercial sex worker may have a different definition of safe sex than a doctor or a public health worker. And, even if the person knows or is told the definition of the behavioral category, there is no guarantee that an intervention that is successful in changing intentions to engage in that behavioral category will also change intentions to perform (or the actual performance of) a specific behavior within that category. Thus, if one's objective is to decrease anal sex or to increase condom use, one should focus on changing people's intentions to abstain from anal sex or their intentions to always use condoms and not on their intentions to "avoid STDs" or to "practice safe sex." To design successful behavioral interventions, it is necessary to (1) select and clearly specify an appropriate behavior to change and (2) empirically identify the beliefs underlying (i.e., the cognitive determinants of) the targeted behavior.

WHICH BEHAVIOR(S) SHOULD BE CHANGED?

From the biomedical perspective, the behavior to be changed must be one that, if altered, will result in a reduction of the spread or progression of STDs. That is, one must identify risk factors rather than risk markers. Obviously, if a valid behavioral risk factor is not identified, an intervention that is successful at modifying the behavior will not reduce or eliminate the health problem. Unfortunately, choosing and defining the behavior (or behaviors) one wishes to maintain or change is not a simple process. We often focus on outcomes (avoiding STDs, staying healthy) and behavioral categories (seeking healthcare, practicing safe sex) rather than specific behaviors. Moreover, a behavior for one person may be a goal for another. For example, although condom use is a behavior for men, it is a goal for women. Women do not use condoms; only their partners do. At best women can put a condom on their partner or they can attempt to influence the likelihood that their partners will use condoms. Thus, rather than trying to increase women's intentions to "use condoms" (a goal), a more appropriate intervention would address their intentions to engage in behaviors such as "putting a condom on my partner," "telling (or asking) my partner to use a condom," or "refusing to have sex if my partner does not use a condom."

To complicate matters even further, it is becoming increasingly clear that differences in context and target are quite important in the identification of sexual behaviors. Recall that behaviors are defined by the four elements of action, target, context, and time. Not surprisingly, our research is revealing that using a condom for oral sex is a different behavior from using a condom for vaginal or anal sex. Similarly, telling one's long-term partner to use a condom is a very different behavior from telling a casual or one-time partner to use a condom. Since "using a condom" and "telling my partner to use a condom" each refer to a number of different behaviors, they may best be viewed as behavioral categories rather than single behaviors.

Strictly speaking, variations in any one of the four elements define different behaviors. Thus, for example, "telling my *long-term* partner to always use a condom for oral sex" is a different behavior from "telling my *casual* partner to always use a condom for oral sex" or "telling my *long-term* partner to always use a condom for vaginal sex." Given practical considerations, however, it is often necessary to generalize over one or more of these elements in choosing an intervention objective. For example, one may wish to increase the likelihood of "telling *all* my partners to always use a condom for *vaginal* sex." For successful interventions, these decisions about which elements to generalize across should be based on research (both epidemiological and behavioral). That is, research is necessary in order to determine which generalizations are acceptable and to determine which types of specification are crucial.

This initial step of selecting and identifying the behavior(s) to be influenced by an intervention is a crucial one that requires substantial collaboration among behavioral scientists, medical researchers, and epidemiologists familiar with the prevention and treatment of STDs.

WHAT ARE THE DETERMINANTS OF THE SELECTED BEHAVIOR(S)?

Once a behavior has been selected and properly specified, it is necessary to identify the determinants of that behavior. As described above, the immediate determinant of any behavior is the intention to perform the behavior.

Intentions are, in turn, determined by attitudes and subjective norms, which are themselves determined by underlying cognitive structures. It is important to recognize that every behavior will have its own unique set of determinants, and thus each behavior may require a different type of intervention. For example, it is quite likely that one may have to design different interventions if the objective is to increase the frequency with which someone uses a condom for vaginal intercourse for all partners than if the goal is primarily to increase condom use for vaginal sex with casual partners. Indeed, it is conceivable that the intention to use a condom for vaginal sex with all partners is under normative control, while the intention to use a condom for vaginal sex with casual partners is under attitudinal control. Similarly, it is possible that even if these behaviors were both under attitudinal control, a key factor that might negatively influence a person's intention to use a condom for vaginal sex with all partners could be the belief that this behavior "will lead to a loss of trust between me and my partner." Yet this belief may be unimportant and/or nonsalient when one considers using a condom for vaginal sex with a casual or one-time partner.

RELATIVE IMPORTANCE OF ATTITUDINAL AND NORMATIVE FACTORS

In designing a behavioral intervention, it is necessary to determine whether the intention is primarily under attitudinal control or normative control or whether it is influenced by both types of considerations. According to the theory of reasoned action, if one wants to change or reinforce a given intention, one must change or strengthen the attitude toward performing that behavior and/or the subjective norm with respect to that behavior. Whether one should change the attitude or subjective norm, however, depends on the relative importance of these two components as determinants of that intention. If a behavior is primarily under attitudinal control, attempts to change that behavior through the use of normative pressure will not be very successful. Similarly, if the members of some group perform a given behavior because they believe that their significant others think they should perform the behavior, little will be accomplished by trying to change their attitudes toward performing that behavior.

Recall, however, that the relative weights of the two components may vary from population to population. For example, while sexually experienced male U.S. college students' intentions to "always use a condom" appear to be primarily under normative control, this same intention appears to be predominantly under attitudinal control in a sample of sexually experienced male Mexican college students (Fishbein, 1980). Thus, this step, as in all steps of the application of the theory of reasoned action, must be based on research conducted in the population that is the focus of the intervention.

SALIENT OUTCOMES AND REFERENTS

Once one has determined whether a given behavior (or intention) is attitudinally or normatively controlled, one must identify salient outcomes (e.g., costs and benefits of performing the behavior) and/or salient referents vis-à-vis the behavior. This can be done by asking a representative sample of the population of interest to report what they see as advantages and disadvantages of performing the behavior (to identify salient outcomes of performing the behavior) and to indicate people or groups who would approve or disapprove of their performing that behavior (to identify salient referents).

It is again important to recognize that salient outcomes and referents will vary as one moves from behavior to behavior and population to population. This can perhaps best be illustrated by considering some of the salient outcomes obtained in a study of condom use among commercial sex workers. More specifically, in the key participant interviews conducted as part of the Centers for Disease Control's acquired immunodeficiency syndrome (AIDS) intervention demonstration projects, commercial sex workers were asked to separately indicate what they saw as the advantages and disadvantages of using condoms for oral, anal, and vaginal sex. Not surprisingly, most of these women felt that using a condom for vaginal or anal sex would protect them from AIDS and other STDs. It is interesting that protection from AIDS was not frequently reported as an advantage of using a condom for oral sex. A unique perceived advantage of using a condom for oral sex, however, was that it meant that one did not have to get semen in one's mouth. And, not surprisingly, a unique advantage of using a condom for vaginal sex was that it would prevent pregnancy.

With respect to negative consequences, many of the professional sex workers reported that using a condom would reduce their clients' satisfaction. Breakage was seen as a major disadvantage of condom use vis-à-vis anal sex, while "it tastes bad" was frequently cited as a disadvantage of using a condom for oral sex. Even more important, the key disadvantages of using a condom differed across ethnic groups. While Hispanic sex workers were worried that using a condom could be painful and lead to injuries (e.g., it would increase friction; it would lead to urinary tract diseases; it would get stuck inside and get infected), black sex workers felt that using condoms would decrease their own sexual pleasure (e.g., it's not natural; it doesn't feel right; it's not skin-to-skin), and white sex workers worried about the mechanics of condom use (e.g., they're difficult to buy and/or to put on; they're expensive; they make the client last longer). These findings should make it clear that different populations may have very different concerns about the same behavior. More important, they provide clear evidence that different beliefs may have to be addressed and therefore that very different interventions may be necessary to change the same behavior in different populations.

WHICH ASPECTS OF THE UNDERLYING COGNITIVE STRUCTURE TO ADDRESS

Once one has identified outcomes and referents that are salient in the population of interest for the behavior of interest, one must then decide which of these behavioral or normative beliefs to target in an intervention. As described above, data must be gathered assessing two aspects for each salient outcome and two aspects for each salient referent. More specifically, with respect to each outcome, one must assess (1) the strength of the behavioral belief that performing the behavior will lead to the outcome, and (2) the evaluation of that outcome. Similarly, with respect to each salient referent, one must assess (1) the strength of the normative belief that the referent thinks the person should or should not perform the behavior, and (2) the motivation to comply with that referent. If the relative weight of the attitudinal component is high, further analyses need to be conducted on the behavioral beliefs and evaluations underlying the attitude component. If the relative weight of the normative component is high, further analyses need to be conducted on the normative beliefs and motivations to comply. These analyses should be used to identify those beliefs, outcome evaluations, and motivations to comply that discriminate between people who do and do not intend to perform the behavior in question. Once identified, these differentiating items are good aspects to address with interventions.

Consider the behavior of "telling my partner to use a condom every time I have sexual intercourse" that we examined in two groups of college women (Middlestadt & Fishbein, 1990). One of the salient outcomes of performing this behavior was that it would "protect me from STDs." Given that protection from STDs is a salient concern of these women, it would seem reasonable to develop a message directed at increasing the women's beliefs that telling their partners to use a condom would protect them from STDs. Our analyses of the underlying cognitive structure, however, indicated that while this message would be expected to be effective among sexually inexperienced college women, it is unlikely to be effective among college women who have had sexual intercourse at least once.

Among the inexperienced women, a comparison between those who do and do not intend to tell their partners to use condoms revealed a statistically significant difference in the degree to which their beliefs about STD protection contributed to their attitudes (i.e., in the behavioral belief times outcome evaluation crossproduct). Further analysis showed that this difference was due to a difference in belief strength rather than in outcome evaluation. That is, in comparison with inexperienced women who do not intend to tell their partners to use condoms, inexperienced women who intend to perform this behavior are significantly more likely to believe that telling their partners will protect them from STDs. Thus, a communication increasing the perceived likelihood of this salient outcome would make an inexperienced woman more positive toward performing the behavior, more likely to form a positive intention, and more likely to actually perform the behavior. In contrast, among the experienced women, intenders were similar to nonintenders with respect to the behavioral belief, the outcome evaluation, and the behavioral crossproduct of the two. Both intenders and nonintenders believed that it was quite likely that telling their partners to use condoms would protect them from STDs. The experienced women were thus homogeneous with respect to this belief. They all already believed the outcome would occur. There was little room for change, and addressing this belief would not be expected to successfully increase the targeted behavior.

In sum, given a targeted behavior, one can construct instruments to measure the correspondent intention, attitude, and subjective norm and then use these measures to empirically determine whether the behavior in question is under attitudinal or normative control. In contrast, one cannot simply construct instruments to measure the underlying cognitive structure. One must first empirically determine the outcomes and referents that are salient for the targeted behavior in the population of interest. Once a set of salient outcomes and referents has been identified, one can construct instruments to measure the strength of behavioral and normative beliefs as well as to measure evaluations of the salient outcomes and motivations to comply with salient referents. These measures can then be used to empirically determine those aspects of the underlying cognitive structure that would be effective ones to address in an intervention.

CONCLUSION

In this chapter, we tried to show how research based on the theory of reasoned action can be used to develop behavioral interventions. In the commercial world, interventions such as promotions and advertising campaigns are often based on extensive market research that attempts to identify the needs of consumers and/or the strategies that might be expected to influence consumer behavior. In contrast, within the health and other nonprofit domains, much less research is done. Assumptions are made about the kinds of information that should be provided to the public to achieve various goals (e.g., to reduce the spread of an STD) or to produce behavior change (e.g., to decrease the performance of behaviors that put one at risk for an STD). Educational programs, mass media communication campaigns, and other forms of health interventions are often based on intuition as to what needs to be changed and how to accomplish these changes. Rarely are the kinds of empirical and theoretical considerations discussed in this chapter taken into account. Most messages and interventions are constructed somewhat arbitrarily on the basis of what all too often turn out to be false assumptions about the determinants of the behavior one wishes to change. Indeed, more often than not, it has been assumed that providing people with information about a disease and how it is spread will lead to behavior change. However, this type of information is rarely converted into action.

One of the main reasons communications and other forms of interventions fail is that they often do not address appropriate beliefs. Messages are rarely directed at behavioral or normative beliefs about performing the behavior one is attempting to change. Instead, all too often, messages provide people with information they already have or try to convince them of something they already believe. If most members of a group already believe that performing some behavior will lead to a certain consequence or outcome (e.g., that "using a condom for anal sex will protect me from AIDS"), little will be accomplished by a persuasive communication that focuses on that information. Similarly, if most members of a group or some segment of the population are aware that their parents are strongly in favor of their telling casual partners to use condoms for vaginal intercourse, little will be accomplished by basing one's intervention on parental pressure.

It is our contention that information and education interventions can be highly effective behavior change devices. Communication of information (or knowledge) through educational or mass media channels can produce significant changes in behavior. However, the information must address the behavioral or normative beliefs underlying the behavior that one wishes to change. Given that epidemiological research has identified a behavioral risk factor, the goal of the intervention should be to change that behavior. To do this, the intervention should attempt to increase intentions to perform (or not perform) the targeted behavior. If this intention is primarily under attitudinal control, the intervention should try to change behavioral beliefs about the advantages and disadvantages of performing the behavior. If the intention is primarily under normative control, the intervention should try to change normative beliefs that specific referents think one should or should not perform the behavior. For the intervention to be successful, decisions about the specific behavioral or normative beliefs to address should not be based on intuition but must be determined empirically. We hope that medical and public health personnel concerned with STDs including AIDS will work closely with behavioral scientists to select and clearly define appropriate high-risk behaviors, to conduct the research necessary to identify the determinants of those behaviors, and to develop effective communications and other interventions that can influence these determinants.

REFERENCES

Ajzen, I., & M. Fishbein (Eds.). (1980) *Understanding attitudes and predicting social behavior.* Englewood Cliffs, NJ: Prentice-Hall.

Allegrante, J. P., Mortimer, R. G., & O'Rourke, T. W. (1980). Social-psychological factors in motorcycle safety helmet use: Implications for public policy. *Journal of Safety Research, 12,* 115–126.

Bowman, C. H., & Fishbein, M. (1978). Understanding public reactions to energy proposals: An application of the Fishbein model. *Journal of Applied Social Psychology, 8,* 319–340.

Budd, R. J., North, D., & Spencer, C. P. (1984). Understanding seat-belt use: A test of Bentler and Speckart's extension of the theory of reasoned action. *European Journal of Social Psychology, 14,* 69–78.

Budd, R. J., & Spencer, C. P. (1985). Exploring the role of personal normative beliefs in the theory of reasoned action: the problem of discriminating between alternative path models. *European Journal of Social Psychology, 15,* 299–313.

Chassin, L., Presson, C. C., Bensenburg, M., Corty, E., Olshavsky, R. W., & Sherman, S. J. (1981). Predicting adolescents' intentions to smoke cigarettes. *Journal of Health & Social Behavior, 22,* 445–455.

Fishbein, M. (1967). Attitude and the prediction of behavior, In M. Fishbein (Ed.), *Readings in attitude theory and measurement,* (pp. 477–492). New York: John Wiley.

Fishbein, M. (1980). A theory of reasoned action: Some applications and implications. In H. E. Howe & M. M. Page (Eds.), *Nebraska symposium on motivation* (pp. 65–116). Lincoln: University of Nebraska Press.

Fishbein, M. (1990). AIDS and behavior change: An analysis based on the theory of reasoned action. *Interamerican Journal of Psychology, 24,* 37–56.

Fishbein, M., & Ajzen, I. (1975). *Belief, attitude, intention and behavior: An introduction to theory and research.* Reading, MA: Addison-Wesley.

Fishbein, M., & Ajzen, I. (1981). Acceptance, yielding and impact: Cognitive processes in persuasion. In R. E. Petty, T. M. Ostrom, & T. C. Brock (Eds.), *Cognitive processes in persuasion,* (pp. 339–359). Hillsdale, NJ: Lawrence Erlbaum.

Fishbein, M., Ajzen, I., & McArdle, J. (1980). Changing the behavior of alcoholics: Effects of persuasive communication, pp. 217–242. In I. Ajzen & M. Fishbein (Eds.), *Understanding attitudes and predicting social behavior.* Englewood Cliffs, NJ: Prentice Hall.

Fishbein, M., Salazar, J. M., Rodriguez, P. R. Middlestadt, S. E., & Himelfard, T. (1988). Predicting Venezuelan students' use of seat belts: An application of the theory of reasoned action in Latin America. *Review Psicologie Sociale & Personality, 4,* 19–41.

Fisher, W. A. (1984). Predicting contraceptive behavior among university men: The role of emotions and behavioral intentions. *Journal of Applied Social Psychology, 14,* 104–123.

Godin, G., & Shephard, R. J. (1986). Psychosocial factors influencing intentions to exercise of young students from grades 7 to 9. *Research Quarterly on Exercise & Sport, 57,* 41–52.

Greenstein, M., Miller, R. N., & Weldon, D. E. (1979). Attitudinal and normative beliefs as antecedents of female occupational choice. *Personality & Social Psychology Bulletin, 5,* 356–362.

Jaccard, J. J., & Davidson, A. R. (1972). Toward an understanding of family planning behaviors: An initial investigation. *Journal of Applied Social Psychology, 2,* 228–235.

Manstead, A. S. R., Proffitt, C., & Smart, J. L. (1983). Predicting and understanding mothers' infant-feeding intentions and behaviors: Testing the theory of reasoned action. *Journal of Personality & Social Psychology, 44,* 657–671.

Middlestadt, S. E. (1990). Developing a research-based communication campaign to increase financial contributions to a University library: An application of the theory of reasoned action, In R. W. Belk (Ed.), *Advances in nonprofit marketing* (Vol. 3, pp. 51–81). Greenwich, CT: JAI Press.

Ryan, M. J. (1982). Behavioral intention formation: The interdependency of attitudinal and social influence variables. *Journal of Consumer Research, 9,* 263–278.

Saltzer, E. B. (1978). Locus of control and the intention to lose weight. *Health Education Monographs, 6,* 118–128.

Schlegel, R. P., Crawford, C. A., & Sanborn, M. D. (1977). Correspondence and mediation properties of the Fishbein model: An application to adolescent alcohol use. *Journal of Experimental Social Psychology, 13,* 421–430.

Sejwacz, R., Ajzen, I., & Fishbein, M. (1980). Predicting and understanding weight loss: Intentions, behaviors and outcomes. In I. Ajzen & M. Fishbein (Eds.), *Understanding attitudes and predicting social behavior.* pp. 101–112. Englewood Cliffs, NJ: Prentice-Hall.

Shepherd, G. J. (1987). Individual differences in the relationship between attitudinal and normative determinants of behavioral intent. *Communication Monographs, 54,* 221–231.

5

Diffusion Theory and HIV Risk Behavior Change

JAMES W. DEARING, GARY MEYER,
and EVERETT M. ROGERS

INTRODUCTION

Theories about social change are useful to the extent that they can lead to solutions for social problems. Diffusion of innovation theory has been applied to thousands of social change problems in various countries, often with successful results. But as with any social change theory, the application of diffusion theory can produce unsatisfactory results if the problem in question has certain characteristics which the theory does not adequately address. Typically, a theoretical model includes a variety of concepts which, by selective emphasis, allows change agents to fit the model to a particular problem, which may result in better descriptive, explanatory, and predictive ability, as well as a satisfactory solution to the social problem.

In certain cases, the fine-tuning of theory and problem to achieve a "best fit to application" is neither possible nor desirable. Certain models are misspecified for certain social problems. Incompatible, irrelevant, or misspecified fits between a model and a social problem lead theorists to revise existing models or to create new theoretical models. The key concepts in a social change theory may have to be revised or completely disregarded. Thus a change program may "outrun" a model, leading to modifications of the model.

JAMES W. DEARING and GARY MEYER • Department of Communication, Michigan State University, East Lansing, Michigan 48824-1212.   *EVERETT M. ROGERS* • Department of Communication and Journalism, University of New Mexico, Albuquerque, New Mexico 87131-1171.

Preventing AIDS: Theories and Methods of Behavioral Interventions, edited by Ralph J. DiClemente and John L. Peterson. Plenum Press, New York, 1994.

In the present chapter, we review certain concepts of the diffusion of innovations model as it relates to the special nature of the human immunodeficiency virus (HIV) transmission problem and to attendant programs designed to slow the further spread of HIV. We suggest that key concepts of the diffusion model may be ill-suited to apply to HIV transmission solutions unless they are reconceptualized in important ways.

Two of the present authors have been involved in scholarly research about the AIDS epidemic since 1986. Originally we investigated the agenda-setting process for the issue of AIDS, tracing how the epidemic gradually and after a four-year delay, climbed the mass media agenda in the United States, then how the AIDS issue rapidly climbed on the public agenda, and finally how federal policy-makers made the issue a high priority on the policy agenda, as evidenced by funding and other policy decisions (Rogers, Dearing, & Chang, 1991). We also compared the issue of AIDS (1) in different countries (Dearing, 1992), and (2) with other issues (Rogers & Chang, 1991). We then became interested in the special case of San Francisco, where this agenda-setting process for the issue of AIDS was much more rapid, in part because of the political influence of the gay community, which was most affected by the epidemic (Dearing & Rogers, 1992).

More recently, we have begun investigating the role of unique population groups (such as recent Asian immigrants, Native Americans, Filippino prostitutes, and youthful drug abusers) in diffusing preventive innovations (such as condoms) in San Francisco. This research led us to begin exploring the various modifications that are needed in the diffusion of innovations model when it is applied to the problem of preventing the diffusion of HIV among members of particular population groups. In the present chapter, we draw upon this research which is currently underway in San Francisco. It is our first report of some necessarily tentative conclusions.

WHAT IS DIFFUSION?

Diffusion is the process by which an innovation is communicated through certain channels over time among the members of a social system (Rogers, 1983). Diffusion consists of four main elements: (1) The innovation, an idea, practice, or object that is perceived as new by an individual or other unit of adoption; (2) communication channels, the means by which messages are exchanged; (3) time, or process; and (4) a social system, the structure and function of relations among a set of individuals or other units. Diffusion has been a popular paradigm for researchers in a number of disciplines, including (1) rural sociology, to understand why farmers decide to use new agricultural products; (2) international development and public health, to understand how disadvantaged or at-risk persons can improve or safeguard their lives; (3) marketing, for understanding customer decisions about new products and services; and (4) anthropology, where the unanticipated social consequences of adopting an innovation are often studied.

Diffusion scholars conceptualized the study of diffusion in various ways. For example, early diffusion scholars often sought to learn when in the diffusion process certain types of individuals adopt an innovation. These studies of "innovativeness" (the relative earliness in adopting a new idea), led to distinctions of adopter categories, such as innovators, early adopters, early majority, late majority, and laggards. Other scholars concentrated on distinguishing the perceived attributes of innovations that are adopted more rapidly or more slowly, such as an innovation's degree of complexity, observability, compatibility, relative advantage, and trialability.

Now, after approximately 4,500 diffusion studies have been completed, concepts such as formative design, social networks, opinion leadership, implementation and use, change agents, and the compatibility of an innovation with a targeted social system have emerged as especially important. Contemporary practitioners, consultants, and program administrators often focus on these concepts when they design and implement diffusion campaigns. Each key concept reflects one or more of the four main elements of how (1) an innovation (2) is communicated (3) over time (4) among the members of a social system.

Before considering how the importance of key diffusion concepts may differ when they are applied to HIV risk behavior change initiatives, we explore the special nature of HIV transmission and of the recommended risk behavior changes in response to this problem.

THE SPECIAL NATURE OF HIV TRANSMISSION

Communicating HIV risk behavior change messages is complicated in at least three important ways. First, HIV is transmitted primarily through sexual behavior, making communication about the problem taboo for most individuals. Taboo communication is message content which people perceive to be extremely personal (Rogers, 1983). Encouraging people to communicate taboo topics, such as how to practice safe sex by using a condom, is often unsuccessful because of embarrassment, uncertainty, and apprehension associated with the topic. Further, use of a condom often necessitates communication about it, and so its taboo nature limits its use. The communication channels for taboo topics are rather restricted.

Human immunodeficiency virus risk behavior changes are also complicated because they are preventive innovations, new ideas that an individual adopts in order to avoid the possible occurrence of some unwanted event in the future, such as contracting HIV. Adopting a preventive innovation usually involves changing and often complicating a well-established behavior. Because (1) the unwanted event may occur even if the innovation is adopted, and (2) the unwanted event may not occur even if the innovation is rejected, individual motivations to adopt preventive innovations are often weak (Rogers, 1983). For example, although policy debate, legislation, and intense mass media coverage of the innovation of automobile safety began in 1966 (Walker, 1977), through the mid-1980s large numbers of U.S. drivers were still choosing not to wear seat belts (many of them in violation of state laws). Despite seeing graphic televised crash simulations of dummies with and without seat belts, many people still knew through personal experience that not wearing a seat belt did not mean they would necessarily be seriously injured. The same logic is applied by persons who are weighing the advantages and disadvantages of adopting safe sex practices. A person considering regular condom use may reason that using condoms does not guarantee that HIV will not be contracted. Likewise, if a decision is made not to use condoms, the virus will not necessarily be contracted. Even though the probability of contracting HIV decreases as a result of a behavior change such as condom use, the lack of an "either-or" guaranteed consequence, combined with widespread public misunderstandings about probabilities and a lack of broad-based scientific literacy in the United States (Miller, 1983), means that many target audience members perceive important disincentives in the adoption of preventive innovations. Like taboo communication, the probable prevention of an occurrence that may never happen decreases the likelihood that the recommended innovation will be adopted.

Although taboo communication and the preventive nature of some innovations are important factors regarding HIV risk behavior change, the present chapter focuses on a third factor which characterizes HIV risk behavior changes: The unique nature of the population groups which are at high risk for contracting HIV. Uniqueness is an especially important factor because, while the risk of HIV is a direct result of human behavior, that behavior is typically influenced by in-group norms and social environments (Selik, Castro, & Pappaioanou, 1988). Human immunodeficiency virus spreads through a social network, an interconnected set of individuals who are linked through a pattern of interpersonal relationships (Rogers & Kincaid, 1981). Klovdahl (1985), for example, found that 40 gay men who were among the first to be diagnosed with AIDS in the United States resided in Los Angeles (and in Orange County), San Francisco, New York, and other U.S. locations, formed a social network. The social and sexual relationships among these 40 individuals determined the initial pathways in the United States of the epidemic (as diffusion theory suggests, existing social networks can also be utilized for the promotion of preventive innovations).

Population group *uniqueness* is the degree to which a set of extremely homophilous individuals is different from the larger social system of which it is a part. *Homophily* is the degree to which individuals who communicate with each other are alike. In contrast, *heterophily* is the degree to which individuals who communicate are dissimilar. What distinguishes unique population groups from other sets of people? Individuals who perceive that their values and beliefs are quite different from those of most other people may sense that they are ostracized from society. Such perceived ostracism will lead some of these individuals to become isolated from other people; they will engage in relatively little communication with others in the larger population, thus segregating themselves in an information sense. Those who feel ostracized will, through a need for socialization, seek out similar others, to engage in very frequent communication with these other like-minded persons. The distinguishing characteristic of human beings is our need to be social. Fear of social isolation drives people to act in social ways (Noelle-Neumann, 1984). So unique population group members share values and beliefs to a higher degree than do the members of other groups which may be just as highly homophilous, but which do not feel ostracized from out-group norms. It is reasonable to hypothesize that the unique population group members' reference groups, because of the high degree of interdependency among unique group members, will more closely consist of actual others in their social network than is typically the case with nonunique population group members. For example, many people normally include those whom they admire but do not personally know as members of their reference group.

So unique population groups consist of a set (1) of extremely homophilous individuals, (2) who bond together in order to cope with the ostracism and criticism that they perceive from the larger society about their values or beliefs. Because unique population groups are bound together through frequent interpersonal relationships (Rogers & Kincaid, 1981), they can act as powerful agents for or against change, by choosing either to amplify or attenuate communication messages (Renn, 1991). Dissemination efforts, unless modified in certain ways, are unlikely to be effective when directed by outsiders to unique population group members. New strategies are required for reaching and affecting behavior change among unique population group members (Bracht, 1990), partly because in sets of people that are characterized by more and more rapid communication, language and culture can be expected to change more rapidly than would otherwise occur. Typical schedules for behavior change message production can be expected to produce already outdated messages.

Besides thinking differently, unique population group members behave differently from the majority of people in a total population, the latter who are neither so ostracized from the larger society nor engage in such homophilous relationships. For example, recent immigrants, members of minority groups, and people whose social relations center around reference groups of intravenous drug users, certain homosexuals (Styles, 1979), or other tightly knit social collectivities may (1) pay more attention to specialized mass media rather than the general mass media; (2) not consider the "role-models" for a particular behavior who appear in the mass media to be credible information sources; and (3) often avoid print media altogether. In highly unique population groups, group members may shun opportunities to act as opinion leaders or change agent aides for a community-based organization, since they may risk losing status within their specific group by doing so (Motivational Educational Entertainment, 1992). The repercussions to oneself of risking one's reputation within the group can result in ostracism from the group (Cialdini, 1988). This possibility is especially a risk for the members of unique population groups.

It has been conventionally believed that the most effective community-based programs which target unique population groups communicate messages in the socioeconomic, cultural, and linguistic terms which characterize those special groups, while activating opinion leaders and social networks in the unique population group to affect behavioral change (Bowles & Robinson, 1989). Effective community-based programs commonly rely on mass communication to raise awareness and knowledge, and interpersonal and peer communication to change individuals' attitudes and behavior. In attempting to reach unique populations, mass communication is often ineffective even in raising awareness of an issue. Recent immigrants, runaway youth, substance abusers, and homeless persons may not read English, or may purposly avoid exposure to written communication messages. Thus it is quite possible for even highly targeted community-based programs to be ineffective in communicating risks, increasing knowledge, or in persuading target individuals to change their attitudes or behaviors.

RETHINKING DIFFUSION CONCEPTS FOR UNIQUE POPULATION GROUPS

Here we critically reassess certain concepts of the diffusion of innovations model, given the characteristics of unique population groups. We consider: (1) the nature of diffusion over time; (2) the role of opinion leaders in the target audience; (3) the degree of centralization of diffusion efforts; (4) characteristics of the change agent; and (5) the compatibility between an innovation and the social system.

The Process of Diffusion over Time

Most behavioral research conceptualizes but does not operationalize time as an important variable in attitudinal and behavioral change. The diffusion of an innovation model conceptualizes and operationalizes time as vital in the diffusion process. Plotting the time element is what gives diffusion its well-known cumulative, or S-shaped curve distribution. Many diffusion concepts derive from the importance given to the time element in the diffusion model. For example, the innovation–decision process through which an individual progresses from awareness of an innovation through knowledge, making a decision to adopt or not, and how feedback from others confirms that decision, is divided into time-bound stages. Time is also central to the concept of innovativeness; that is, the point at which a person or other unit of adoption, relative to other such units, decides to adopt. Similarly, rate of adoption, a systemic measure of the number of members of the system who have adopted an innovation, is determined through an analysis of time.

How does a concentration on unique population groups affect the variable of time? Because people communicate most easily and readily with others whom they believe to be most similar to themselves, we expect that communication among the members of unique population groups is (1) frequent, and (2) characterized by a high degree of trust. Communication should take less time and be relatively more effective in unique population groups. Information will travel more rapidly and face fewer obstacles. Within the group, the innovation–decision process is condensed, and the time required to adopt an innovation is reduced. Within the group, the concept of innovativeness matters less because there is less difference between early and late adopters. Both will learn of an innovation at more or less the same time because of the frequency of communication within the group, and there will be fewer reasons for potentially late adopters to delay an adoption decision (stated another way, there will be fewer reasons for potentially late adopters, and typically early adopters, to behave differently). Tracking the rate of adoption in unique population groups may also differ from less unique social systems. If perceived similarity and trust are higher, then there may be fewer cases of partially diffused innovations. Relative to less unique social systems, innovations in unique population groups will be more likely to either diffuse widely, or to fail completely. We expect that the pattern of diffusion of safe sex innovations among unique population group members may more closely approximate "critical mass" diffusion (Markus, 1990), which applies to innovations for which individuals receive great benefit if *all* social system members adopt, but much less benefit to everyone if the innovation is rejected by a considerable number of people. The special nature of critical mass diffusion is a very high degree of interdependency between early and late adopters in using the innovation. Safe sex innovations also rely on mutual adoption for shared benefit (that is, safe sex does much less good if only one partner practices it).

The rapid adoption and replacement of innovative language by urban youth is an indication of this unique population "group effect." The condensation of the time-to-adopt and time-to-reinvent complicates the task of social change agents. When urban youth reinvent their language or fashion or behavior every several months, a communication campaign which includes months of iterative formative evaluation research, careful message construction, pretesting, and field trials can be obsolete before it is developed, let alone diffused.

Opinion Leaders

Opinion leaders are highly influential members of a target group who can influence other group members to adopt an innovation. Opinion leaders, relative to other group members, have greater exposure to mass media, are more cosmopolite (that is, oriented outside of the system), have greater change agent contact and social participation, have higher socioeconomic status, and are somewhat more innovative (Rogers, 1983). Opinion leaders, due to their interpersonal influence with later adopters, play an important role in the diffusion of certain innovations (Valente, 1993). Thus opinion leaders are often sought by change agents, who seek to utilize the opinion leaders to speed the diffusion process (Kelly et al., 1991).

In the case of unique population groups, opinion leadership may play a much smaller role in the diffusion of preventive information. Why? The nature of these groups, and the impact of a shortened innovation–decision process, provide a key. Members of unique population groups are extremely homogenous and are bound together by shared norms. The scope of opinion leadership of any one individual may be curtailed because of the rapidity of communication and high degree of trust among group members. For many individuals, adoption decisions may not require interpersonal persuasion, leadership, or model behavior from a high-status person. In unique population groups, there is less difference between those persons who have certain information and those who do not. All or nearly all group members will have the same information within a short period of time.

We believe that members of unique population groups may not take an active role in the diffusion of preventive innovations because the risk of being viewed negatively by other group members is too great. Since members of unique population groups place a high value on identification with their respective groups (in part because it may be the only group that they truly feel a part of), the potential for isolation from the group may stifle both potential indigenous change agents and actual opinion leaders even if adoption of the innovation is perceived to be in the best interests of other group members.

The limited role that opinion leaders are likely to play in the diffusion of innovations within unique population groups reemphasizes the importance of change agents to the success of the diffusion effort. In unique population groups it is especially important that change agents are homophilous with the target audience, and have a high degree of safety credibility (being perceived as trustworthy) in the eyes of group members.

Decentralized Diffusion Systems

Although diffusion of innovations theory addresses both relatively centralized, as well as relatively decentralized, diffusion systems, the vast majority of diffusion initiatives have been centralized. Indeed the classical diffusion model is relatively centralized, and is characterized by the innovation being transferred from an expert source to potential adopters who are relatively less expert (Rogers, 1983). The classical model suggests that innovations are diffused from the top down, and mainly through a one-way flow of communication (although peer communication is considered to be very important in clinching adoption decisions).

Decentralized diffusion systems, on the other hand, are characterized by a high degree of shared information between source and adopter, and are based on the assumption that the members of the target group are able to manage the diffusion process themselves with little help from professional change agents (Rogers, 1983). Centralized diffusion systems are more appropriately utilized when the innovation is highly technical in nature and the target population is relatively homogeneous. Decentralized diffusion systems are most appropriate when the innovation is not represented by a high level of technology, when the users are technically competent (at least to the point of matching the technical requirements of the innovation), and when the user group is relatively heterogeneous. In this latter case, decentralized systems are likely to be more compatible with users' values and needs, creating an atmosphere for greater acceptance of the innovation.

Although unique population group members exhibit a high degree of within-group homogeneity, the high degree of heterogeneity between the various groups at high risk for HIV and the relatively low level of technology associated with preventive innovations like safe sex, suggest the use of a decentralized diffusion approach. A decentralized system enables innovation sources to more accurately identify, and more easily reach, their target audience. Dissemination attempts can be tailored to specific needs and values.

Since each high-risk group is extremely homogeneous within, only change agents with intimate knowledge of the group are able (1) to identify individuals who should be targeted in the diffusion effort, and (2) to reach them effectively. Similarly, intimate knowledge of the unique population group is necessary in order to formulate appropriate messages for the targeted individuals. This intimate knowledge means, for example, knowing the specific areas or neighborhoods in which group members live, the clubs and other entertainment outlets frequented, and the areas of concentrated employment. With intimate knowledge of the specialized group, diffusion efforts can then be designed more effectively to fit the needs and values of the homogeneous group. Consider, for example, a situation in which members of a specific group at high risk for HIV are known to frequent a particular movie theater. With this knowledge, sources may diffuse the innovation via live performances or a recorded message presented before the start of a featured movie. Within a decentralized system, sources must have intimate knowledge about group members so that the source (1) knows who the target audience is and where they can be reached; (2) shares their values, attitudes, and preferences; and (3) understands an acceptable manner in which they may be reached that is compatible with the sources' values and needs. What does a decentralized diffusion approach imply for community groups and HIV prevention organizations? If so much detailed knowledge must be known about each particular group, are lessons about HIV prevention useful from one group to another? Is generalizability less likely? Certainly the primary means of reaching the members of unique populations, that of street outreach, is highly particularistic to the social and physical circumstances of each set of target audience members.

Change Agents

A decentralized diffusion system places a great deal of emphasis on the change agent because of the intimate knowledge possessed by the change agent about both the unique population group and the innovation or information being disseminated. The successful change agent will have a high degree of homophily and credibility with members of the unique population group.

While homophilous individuals typically communicate more frequently with each other due to their commonalities, extreme homophily between individuals can actually act as a barrier to diffusion (Rogers, 1983). This barrier may occur because homophilous individuals communicate within the same networks and thus are privy to nearly identical information. Thus while much content is communicated among highly homophilous persons, the content is often of little informational value to the participants. Heterophilous individuals, on the other hand, are members of different networks and thus are likely to have knowledge others in different networks need or desire.

In the case of unique population groups at high risk for HIV, the ideal change agent would be as homophilous as possible with members of the target audience. In addition, the change agent should possess expertise (that is, knowledge) concerning strategies aimed at reducing the likelihood of acquiring HIV. In this latter sense, the change agent is quite different from target audience members. Why should the change agent/target member relationship be so characterized? First, given their relative isolation, target audience members are unlikely to trust the influence of anyone who is different from themselves. For example, the change agent working with recent immigrants from Southeast Asia should be an immigrant from Southeast Asia as well, but perhaps not quite as recent a one as the clients with whom he or she is dealing. Similarly, the change agent working with teenage prostitutes should have been a prostitute. The change agent working with intravenous drug users should have been a drug user. Second, as mentioned previously, extremely homophilous change agents are in a position to understand the target group and therefore be able to diffuse the innovation in a manner compatible with the needs and values of the target audience. Gaining access to the target group, however, is only a first step. Targeted individuals are more likely to pay attention to messages if they perceive that the change agent is an expert and can provide information that is of interest.

Credibility may be conceptualized as (1) competence credibility, and (2) safety credibility (Rogers, 1983). Competence credibility is the degree to which the source is perceived to be knowledgeable or expert about the innovation. Safety credibility is the extent to which the source is perceived as trustworthy. In many diffusion efforts, especially those characterized by a heterophilous relationship between the source and the target individual, the source possesses high competence credibility but low safety credibility. In the case of a homophilous relationship between the two parties, however, as in the case of members of unique population groups, the change agent's effectiveness rests on a high degree of safety credibility. The ideal situation, of course, is for the change agent to be perceived as having a high degree of both expertise and trustworthiness. Given the relatively closed nature of unique population groups, homophilous change agents will at least get an opportunity to demonstrate competence. Heterophilous change agents will not be given a chance to demonstrate their trustworthiness, however, because they will be rejected immediately by the unique population group.

For diffusion attempts targeting unique population groups, the recruitment of change agents who are indigenous to the group is often difficult. Potential change agents risk losing status in the unique population group if they act as proponents and sources of knowledge for preventive innovations.

Compatibility

Innovations such as condoms have long been thought to possess attributes. That is, researchers have typically conceptualized innovations as having objective characteristics. Linton (1936) took this approach in suggesting that two attributes of innovations, utility and compatibility, are most important when people are trying to decide whether or not they should adopt. So people will adopt an innovation that is (1) high in utility, and (2) highly compatible with how they already think and act.

Nearly three decades later, Katz (1963) argued that the main problem of classifying innovations was really a problem of matching the attributes of innovations with the attributes of potential adopters. Thus the problem of determining the attributes of innovations broadened. Not only did a researcher have to catalog the objective attributes of the innovation, but also those of the adopter. Katz conceptualized compatibility broadly as consisting of the four dimensions: (1) communicability (the degree to which an innovation's utility is easily explained); (2) pervasiveness (the degree to which the innovation's ramifications are readily apparent); (3) risk (the degree to which an innovation is dissimilar to what it replaces); and (4) profitability (the degree to which an innovation is perceived as more efficient or cost effective than alternatives).

Rogers (1983) lists five perceptual attributes: (1) relative advantage, the degree to which an innovation is perceived as being better than the idea it supersedes; (2) compatibility, the degree to which an innovation is perceived as consistent with the existing values, past experiences, and needs of potential adopters; (3) trialability, the degree to which an innovation may be experimented with on a limited basis; (4) observability, the degree to which the results of an innovation are visible to people; and (5) complexity, the degree to which an innovation is perceived as relatively difficult to understand and use. According to Rogers (1983), relative advantage, compatibility, trialability, and observability are positively related to adoption, while complexity is negatively related to adoption. Rogers' review suggests that of these attributes, relative advantage, compatibility, and complexity are more strongly related to adoption than are trailability or observability.

For unique population groups, *compatibility,* the degree to which an innovation is consistent with existing values, past experiences, and needs of potential adopters, is especially important. Compatibility is crucial because of the nature of a unique population group's information networks. Such groups are close-knit and tend to be characterized by one-way communication, from outside of the group, to the members inside the group. Unique population group members may, in some cases, frequently span the informational boundaries of their groups, but they will communicate relatively little to the outside about life within the group because of the constant threat of ostracism, fear, or disapproval. The special codes, language, and behavior of group members when they communicate together remain for them alone to understand. As a result, we expect unique population group members to be more selective when deciding whether or not to adopt an innovation from outside the group, and only to choose those innovations that are most consistent with their values, past experiences, and needs. We suggest that other perceived attributes, including those of effectiveness, reliability, and applicability (Dearing, Meyer, & Kazmierczak, 1993), will be relatively less effective in unique population groups.

SUGGESTIONS FOR DIFFUSION THEORY

In the present chapter we considered how the over-time nature of diffusion, the role of opinion leaders in the target audience, the degree of centralization of diffusion efforts, characteristics of change agents, and the compatibility between an innovation and the social system, may be of more or less importance when diffusion among the members of unique population groups is investigated. We suggested that because of the theoretical properties of unique population groups, where uniqueness is determined by a high degree of (1) homophily among group members, and (2) perceived ostracism from the larger society, there is reason to hypothesize that within unique population groups:

1. *The social process of diffusion occurs relatively faster than within less unique population groups.* That is, the individual's innovation-decision process is shortened.
2. *Opinion leaders play a less important role in influencing the attitudes and behaviors of others than they do within less unique population groups.* Access to unique population groups may be more important for the success of diffusion initiatives targeted to these groups than accessing certain persuasive or respected individuals within those groups.
3. *Decentralized diffusion approaches will be more effective than centralized diffusion approaches.* That is, decentralization allows for customization and reinvention, the application of intimate knowledge about each unique population group, in the design of a diffusion initiative.
4. *The selection and training of change agents is more important than within less unique population groups.* Both dimensions of credibility, expertise (competence credibility), and trustworthiness (safety credi-

bility), remain important in the perception of the target population members.

5. *The perception of compatibility between innovation and social system is more important than within less unique population groups.* The members of unique population groups are more selective when deciding whether or not to adopt an innovation such as safe sex which originates from sources outside the group.

The study of diffusion within unique population groups may point out additional modifications to the importance of various theoretical concepts. For example, a more rapid rate of diffusion, combined with less reluctance to adopt by very homogenous people, may result in a lessened distinction between adoption and implementation. Theoretically and empirically, much of the recent "action" among diffusion scholars has concerned the implementation and use of innovations, particularly in organizations, in an attempt to correct for an earlier overemphasis on the importance of adoption decisions. Perhaps the study of highly unique social systems will reverse or provide a counterbalance to this trend among scholars (we are not arguing in favor of such a paradigmatic shift, for each of the present authors also considers implementation and use to be very important diffusion stages). Also, the typical bias of change agent contact with innovators and opinion leaders may be overcome if change agents do not seek out particular-status (i.e., opinion-leading) persons, and rather "take all comers" in a democratic diffusion approach.

Lastly, we surmise that the intimate nature of sex and of the relationships which accompany it may lead to the concept of a "diffusion pair," or two persons who are intimate and thus more influential with each other. With many such relationships within unique population groups forming an intimate social network, diffusion pairs may account for a quickening of the diffusion process because of a higher degree of shared influence. With a very shared and other-dependent preventive innovation such as safe sex, the high degree of interdependency in avoiding HIV may lead to a "critical mass" curve (Markus, 1990), rather than a classical S-shaped cumulative diffusion curve (Rogers, 1983).

REFERENCES

Bowles, J., & Robinson, W. A. (1989). PHS grants for minority group HIV infection education and prevention efforts. *Public Health Reports, 104,* 552–559.

Bracht, N. (1990). Applications to special populations: Case studies. In N. Bracht (Ed.), *Health promotion at the community level* (pp. 253–256). Newbury Park, CA: Sage.

Cialdini, R. B. (1988). *Influence: Science and practice* (2nd ed.). New York: Harper Collins.

Dearing, J. W. (1992). Foreign blood and domestic politics: The issue of AIDS in Japan. In E. Fee and D. M. Fox (Eds.), *AIDS: Contemporary history* (pp. 327–345). Berkeley: University of California Press.

Dearing, J. W., Meyer, G., & Kazmierczak, J. (1993). Portraying the new: Environmental technology innovators and potential users. Paper presented at the 64th annual convention of the Western States Communication Association, Albuquerque, NM, February 14.

Dearing, J. W., & Rogers, E. M. (1992). AIDS and the media agenda. In T. Edgar, M. A. Fitzpatrick, & V. Freimuth (Eds.), *A communication perspective on AIDS* (pp. 173–194). Hillsdale, NJ: Lawrence Erlbaum Associates.

Katz, E. (1963). The characteristics of innovations and the concept of compatibility. Paper presented at the Rehovoth Conference on Comprehensive Planning of Agriculture in Developing Countries, August 19–29, Rehovoth, Israel.

Kelly, J. A., St. Lawrence, J. S., Diaz, Y. E., Stevenson, L. Y., Hauth, A. C., Brasfield, T. L., Kalichman, S. C., Smith, J. E., and Andrew, M. E. (1991). HIV risk behavior reduction following intervention with key opinion leaders of population: An experimental analysis. *American Journal of Public Health, 81,* 168–171.

Klovdahl, A. S. (1985). Social networks and the spread of infectious diseases: The AIDS example. *Social Science Medicine, 21,* 1203–1216.

Linton, R. (1936). *The study of man.* New York: Appleton-Century-Crofts.

Markus, L. (1990). Toward a "critical mass" theory of interactive media. In J. Fulk & C. Steinfield (Eds.), *Organizations and communication technology* (pp. 194–218). Newbury Park, CA: Sage.

Miller, J. D. (1983). *The American people and science policy: The role of public attitudes in the policy process.* New York: Pergamon.

Motivational Educational Entertainment Productions. (1992). *Reaching the hip-hop generation.* Philadelphia: Motivational Educational Entertainment Productions.

Noelle-Neumann, E. (1984). *The spiral of silence: Public opinion—our social skin.* Chicago: University of Chicago Press.

Renn, O. (1991). Risk communication and the social amplification of risk. In R. E. Kasperson & P. J. M. Stallen (Eds.), *Communicating risks to the public.* Dordrecht, The Netherlands: Kluwer Academic.

Rogers, E. M. (1983). *Diffusion of innovations* (3rd ed.). New York: Free Press.

Rogers, E. M., & Chang, S. (1991). Media coverage of technology issues: Ethiopian drought of 1984, AIDS, Challenger, and Chernobyl. In L. Wilkins & P. Patterson (Eds.), *Risky business: Communicating issues of science, risk and public policy* (pp. 75–96). New York: Greenwood Press.

Rogers, E. M., Dearing, J. W., & Chang, S. (1991). *AIDS in the 1980s: The agenda-setting process for a public issue.* Columbia, SC: Journalism Monographs (Vol. 126).

Rogers, E. M., & Kincaid, D. L. (1981). *Communication networks: Toward a new paradigm for research.* New York: Free Press.

Selik, R. M., Castro, K. G., & Pappaioanou, M. (1988). Racial/ethnic differences in the risk of AIDS in the United States. *American Journal of Public Health, 78,* 1539–1545.

Styles, J. (1979). Outsider/insider: Researching gay baths. *Urban Life, 8,* 135–152.

Valente, T. W. (1993). Diffusion of innovations and policy decision-making. *Journal of Communication, 32,* 30–45.

Walker, J. L. (1977). Setting the agenda in the U.S. Senate: A theory of problem selection. *British Journal of Political Science, 7,* 433–445.

6

Social Models for Changing Health-Relevant Behavior

SAMUEL R. FRIEDMAN, DON C. DES JARLAIS, and THOMAS P. WARD

INTRODUCTION

In the early days of the acquired immunodeficiency syndrome (AIDS) epidemic, public health interventions put major emphasis on education because there was an urgent need to get the news out about the dangers of a new disease and about steps that might help to combat its spread. Education, however, was clearly not all that was needed. Thus, a range of additional intervention techniques were developed, most of them focusing on individuals as their targets. These interventions were guided by theories such as: (1) the health belief model (HBM) (Becker & Joseph, 1988; Emmons et al., 1986; Montgomery et al., 1989); (2) social learning theory (Bandura, 1977; Botvin, Baker, Botvin, Filazzola, & Millman, 1984; Evans, 1976); and (3) the theory of reasoned action (Fishbein, 1980; Fishbein & Ajzen, 1975; Fishbein & Middlestadt, 1989).

These models view values, beliefs, perspectives, attitudes, and ways of thought as characteristics of individuals. The interventions based on them have been useful in helping individual gay males, drug injectors, and others to understand their risks and their alternatives, and thus have led many individuals to take actions that reduce their risks of becoming infected (Becker & Joseph, 1988; Des Jarlais & Friedman, 1992a; Friedman, Des Jarlais et al.,

SAMUEL R. FRIEDMAN • National Development and Research Institutes, 11 Beach Street, New York, New York 10013.   *DON C. DES JARLAIS* • Chemical Dependency Institute, Beth Israel Medical Center, New York, New York 10003.   *THOMAS P. WARD* • National Development and Research Institutes, 11 Beach Street, New York, New York 10013.

Preventing AIDS: Theories and Methods of Behavioral Interventions, edited by Ralph J. DiClemente and John L. Peterson. Plenum Press, New York, 1994.

in press). Individualistic models are discussed in depth in other chapters in this book.

In spite of their contributions to the fight against the spread of AIDS, however, individualistic models have serious limitations that make it necessary to develop more social theories of how to intervene against human immunodeficiency virus (HIV) spread and other threats to public health. Many persons have gone through programs based on individualistic models and still continue high-risk behaviors. Others have reduced or eliminated their risks for a while, but have subsequently returned to unprotected sex or unsafe drug-injection practices. Nevertheless, regardless of these limitations, individualistic models have not only been successful in explaining some aspects of health-relevant behavior, they can also be useful in carrying out the individual and small-group aspects of social interventions such as those discussed in this chapter (see Friedman [1993] for a more complete discussion of the strengths and limitations of individualistic models).

On a more theoretical level, it is useful to examine what individualistic models do not do, and then to adapt or construct theories that help us to understand how to intervene in matters that individualistic approaches are unable to address. In general terms, this would require using social models to understand the ways in which individual history, the properties of the social networks, groups, and subcultures to which the individual belongs, and the larger social environment interact over time, and the ways in which individuals operate within this unfolding dialectic to assert some degree of control over their own lives.

Considerable evidence exists that the experience of the AIDS epidemic among drug injectors has not conformed well with what individualistic models predict (Friedman, 1993). The epidemiology of HIV transmission highlights issues that are social rather than individualistic. For example, many studies find that, among drug injectors, racial-ethnic minorities such as African-Americans and persons of Puerto Rican descent are particularly likely to be infected with HIV; but in most cases, racial-ethnic differences in seroprevalence remain significant even when individual differences in risk behavior are statistically controlled (Friedman et al., 1987; Friedman, Sufian, & Des Jarlais, 1990; Friedman, Snyder, Shorty, Jones, Estrada, & Young, in press; Selik, Castro, & Pappaioanou, 1988; Selik, Castro, Pappaioanou, & Buehler, 1989). Moreover, rates of HIV spread after the virus first appears among drug injectors vary widely between cities even though rates of drug injection or sharing of syringes are similar (Friedman & Des Jarlais, 1991; Friedman, Des Jarlais, & Neaigus, 1992). Instead, we have suggested that differences in urban social structure and intercity differences in drug subcultures (which in turn shape the extent to which drug injectors from different neighborhoods or friendship groups inject together) probably explain these differences in transmission rates.

Moreover, the shapers of these mixing patterns are probably not individual characteristics, but social structures within the drug-injecting communities (such as shooting galleries and other multiperson injection settings) and community social dynamics (such as the extent to which neighborhood disruption by arson or gentrification leads drug injectors to move from one neighborhood to another).

Further, risk reduction among drug injectors seems to be shaped less by their personal characteristics than by the norms and behaviors of small groups of drug injectors and by their interaction with noninjecting relatives and friends. Thus, drug injectors are more likely to take steps to reduce their risk of drug-related and of sex-related HIV transmission if their drug-using friends do so, if they maintain close ties with noninjectors, and if their immediate social circles discuss AIDS (Abdul-Quader, Des Jarlais, Tross, McCoy, Morales, & Velez, 1992; Abdul-Quader, Tross, Friedman, Kouzi, & Des Jarlais, 1990; Des Jarlais et al., 1992; Friedman, 1993; Neaigus et al., 1990).

The emphasis of this chapter is not, however, on a critique of the limitations of individualistic models. Instead, the aim is to set forth ideas about theoretical frameworks that would enable us to conceptualize health-promoting interventions on a social basis. Such a perspective on health intervention models would allow us to expand our efforts to encompass: (1) changing group and subcultural norms and interests; (2) community mobilization and collective action as an approach to improving public health; and (3) removing social barriers to risk reduction. (The theoretical perspective we propose is thus somewhat different from the social ecology perspectives that have been put forward by McLeroy, Bibeau, Steckler, & Glanz [1988]; and by McBride et al., [1992], inasmuch as it focuses on social processes that can be the foci of interventions rather than on different levels of social structure that can exert influence on how individuals behave.)

As a starting point, it is useful to consider the question of how to shape the norms, values, and interests of the peer groups and other small-scale social groups that are proximate influences on behavior. In addition to the above work showing small-group influence on HIV-related risk reduction by drug injectors, research has shown that small-group pressures influence the initiation of: (1) drug injection (Casriel et al., 1990; Des Jarlais, Casriel, Friedman, & Rosenblum, 1992); (2) smoking and alcohol use among adolescents (Kandel & Logan, 1984; Moncher, Holden, & Schinke, 1991; White, 1992; White & Labouvie, 1989); and (3) risk reduction to avoid heart attack (McAlister, Puska, Salonen, Tuomilehto, & Koskela, 1982; Puska et al., 1985).

Thus, the first question to be addressed is the following: How can peer group and neighborhood subcultures change themselves, or be helped to change by outside forces, so as to reduce health risks? In addition, we discuss how existing social environments (both social policy and social structures) might either encourage high-risk behaviors or create obstacles to risk reduction, and consider theories that help to evaluate and implement some of the ways in which these policies or structures might be changed.

Thus, the focus of this discussion is quite general, aiming to present theoretical perspectives that can illuminate health-oriented interventions for a wide variety of constituencies around the world and for a wide variety of threats to health. Furthermore, we should be clear on our values: We favor the reduction of HIV transmission among gay and bisexual men and women, drug injectors, heterosexuals, and everybody else. We propose the ideas in this chapter in order both to help professionals, community and workplace activists, and others to reduce the spread of HIV, and to assist those who are trying to reduce or eliminate other threats to health and well-being. Given the limits of our own research and practical experience, many of our examples and arguments deal with AIDS among drug injectors, and we discuss these issues with considerably more background on the United States than on other countries. Nonetheless, we suggest that the need for social interventions in behalf of public health, and of theories to help guide these interventions, is worldwide.

THEORIES OF SUBCULTURAL CHANGE

There are four major theories for how to change subcultures. These are diffusion models; leadership-focused approaches; social movement theory; and models of changing the social environment. The first three, at least, form an ordered scale in terms of the degree of change in a subculture for which they are appropriate and necessary. The first three have also already been used as the basis for AIDS interventions. Since diffusion theory is considered at some length elsewhere in this volume, we discuss it only briefly below.

Diffusion Theory

The theory of cultural diffusion is a staple of anthropological and sociological models of cultural change (Ogburn, 1922; Rogers, 1982; Rogers & Shoemaker, 1971). It considers the characteristics of cultures and of innovations that make it more or less likely that a given innovation will be adopted by a culture. It also discusses the likelihood that the innovation will be used in a culture in ways that may differ considerably from the ways it was used in the culture where it originated.

From the perspective of active public-health interventions in a given subculture, diffusion theory points to several issues as salient. First, it is necessary to understand the subculture sufficiently well to be able to make reasonable predictions about what innovations might be accepted by it. Second, it may be necessary to devise an innovation that will be acceptable. Third, it is necessary to develop ways to monitor reactions to innovations that are introduced and how the subculture both uses them and itself changes as a result. Fourth, on the basis of this monitoring, it may be necessary to introduce alterations in the innovation or in the way in which it is presented.

These issues are well exemplified by what has become famous as the San Francisco model of HIV-focused outreach to drug injectors. The development of this approach has been described by Newmeyer, Feldman, Biernacki, & Watters (1989), and a process ethnography was conducted by Broadhead and Fox of how the model operated in practice (Broadhead, 1991; Broadhead & Fox, 1990; Broadhead, Fox, & Espada, 1990). On the basis of prior study of the subculture, promoting the use of bleach as a decontaminant of syringes was picked as an innovation to reduce the spread of HIV (Newmeyer, 1988). Bleach, as they saw it, met several prerequisites:

1. It would be efficacious, since a number of laboratory studies showed that it rapidly killed the free virus of HIV (Martin, McDougal, & Loskoski, 1985; Resnick, Veren, Salahuddin, Tondreau, & Markham, 1986). (Data were not then available about its efficacy in deactivating latent HIV, such as is present in proviral form inside infected white blood cells [Flynn et al., 1990]).
2. It would do no serious harm if the bleach itself were accidentally injected (Froner, Rutherford, & Rokeach, 1987; Herrmann & Heicht, 1979).
3. It would require minimal change in the rituals of drug injection; in particular, it would not seriously prolong the waiting time between obtaining the drug and injecting it.
4. Bleach is widely and easily available at low cost.

Outreach to spread this innovation was organized. At first, the project staff used only word-of-mouth education, presuming that this by itself would lead to widespread bleach use. They quickly realized, however, that having outreach workers actually distribute bleach would be an essential component in getting the innovation accepted and disseminated (Newmayer et al., 1989).

Some evidence exists that this project may have been successful in slowing the spread of HIV among San Francisco drug injectors. Bleach use has become quite widespread among drug injectors in that city. Further, although the available evidence is far from sufficient proof of causation, it is noteworthy that while seroprevalence had been rising prior to the introduction of this innovation, it subsequently leveled off at about 12% (Watters et al., 1990).

Leadership-Focused Models

Leadership-focused models are in a sense midway between diffusion theory and social-movement theory. Such models have as a central concern the question of how to get preexisting group leaders to champion an innovation, and thus combine elements of diffusion theory with elements of community organizing theory. (The term *leadership-focused model* is being proposed by us as a useful way to describe this process.) In this model, then, efforts are made to recruit influential persons to advocate health-oriented behaviors.

Several issues are problematic in this approach. First is the question of which behaviors are to be advocated. Here, the same considerations of acceptability come into play as in the diffusion model, but with greater emphasis upon how local leaders will react to the innovations. Leadership-focused approaches view the reaction of informal leadership as a decisive concern, with an important issue being how to get local leaders to be willing to spend time and, if necessary, to take risks on behalf of the innovation. The problems that leaders face in advocating an innovation, such as whether it falls outside the domain of their normal patterns of personal interaction, thus become questions that can help focus the practical discussions and problem-solving efforts of public-health theorists and practitioners.

A second issue involves the identification of local leadership. For successful health interventions, this usually means not only (or even primarily) the formal leaders of a community (Morales & Fullilove, 1992). They may sometimes have to be circumvented, if not openly opposed, since many formal leaders are often elevated above, and removed from, the daily lives of those in the surrounding community (Quimby & Friedman, 1989). Instead, it may be more important to win over the people who are influential on a given city block, or within a given friendship group or extended family, or a particular network of drug injectors. In order to identify appropriate individuals, a detailed understanding of social relationships at the local level is helpful. Such an understanding is best achieved by devoting a substantial period of time to direct observation of the target group and intimate association with it. During this period, careful attention should be paid to differentiated network and influence patterns that might affect how men and women can most easily be won over.

A third issue is how to select and recruit local leaders to work with the project. Ethnographic, snowball sampling, and sociometric techniques can provide data about interaction patterns, and about which persons are most likely to be able to persuade others to accept the innovation.

A fourth issue is the relationship between the local leaders and the rest of the intervention project. Local leaders need to be trained about the substantive issues so that they can answer questions and, indeed, so they can defend themselves against criticism for advocating it. Often, the project is asking local influentials to put their prestige and influence on the line in working for the project. They will be more willing to do this to the extent that (1) they see the importance of the health issue and the efficacy of the intervention; and (2) see ways to increase their own standing by being the advocates of the "necessary" changes. Moreover, since local influentials are usually intelligent people with a good understanding of their community and subculture, they will usually see ways to "improve upon" the intervention model. The project needs to be alert to the variety of ways in which this process can take place in practice, and will be aided in doing so to the extent that it is able to conduct extensive field ethnography. In many cases, the local leaders will indeed find ways to improve upon the model, and these improvements may be transferable to other local leaders or even to other projects.

On other occasions, however, the particular needs of the local leader might weaken or distort the behavioral changes that are recommended in ways that weaken or obviate their efficacy. In such cases, detailed understanding of the community will help the project and the local leader to determine whether there are ways whereby a health-enhancing message can in fact be delivered. Moreover, if a large proportion of local leaders prove to be unable or unwilling to work effectively toward risk reduction, then it may be necessary to use community organizing or other techniques discussed below.

Leadership-focused models have been applied in a number of areas of health intervention. Among the more famous are: (1) the interventions around coronary health in North Karelia, Finland (McAlister et al., 1982; Puska et al., 1985); (2) the Chicago model for AIDS intervention with drug injectors (Wiebel, 1988, 1990, 1991; Wiebel, Fritz, & Chene, 1989); and (3) the AIDS interventions among gay men by Kelly and colleagues (Kelly et al., 1991; Kelly et al., 1992). Here, we will briefly describe how the model has been applied by Kelly et al. (Kelly et al., 1991; Kelly et al. 1992) as a way to exemplify the leadership-focused approach and to show its success in promoting risk reduction.

Kelly and his collaborators set up interventions in three cities: Biloxi and Hattiesburg, Mississippi, and Monroe, Louisiana. In each of these cities, there were preexisting gay bars that were well-established community institutions with stable clienteles. This provided a framework for a fairly straightforward technique of identifying local leaders, training them, and contracting with them about what they would do after their training. Opinion leaders were identified by a multistep process: First, bartenders were asked to unobtrusively observe and record interaction patterns among their patrons for one week, and to nominate those who socialized with others and those who were most often seen being greeted positively by others. Their nominee lists were compared, and those who were named at least twice (and who could be found) were asked to take part in the program. In Biloxi, at least, these nominees were also asked to name one friend each whom they considered to be highly popular among gay men but who had not yet been nominated (Kelly et al., 1991; Kelly et al., 1992).

Training consisted of four weekly 90-minute group sessions that covered (1) epidemiology, risk behaviors, and reduction techniques; (2) characteristics of effective health-promotion messages; (3) modeling and role-playing of scenarios; and (4) after a week in which trainees each tried out their new skills with four gay male friends, discussion of what happened and how to improve upon their efforts.

Trainees contracted to have a total of at least 14 conversations with peers, and their efforts were monitored during a 17-day posttraining period. During this period, they reported having an average of 6.1 conversations, although it is highly likely that they engaged in further conversations thereafter (Kelly et al., 1992).

Using a quasi-experimental design, Kelly et al. found that significant declines occurred in unprotected anal intercourse, and significant increases occurred in condom use. Indeed, the data suggest that the intervention led to substantial changes in the social norms of the gay men attending these bars (Kelly et al., 1992).

Kelly and his collaborators do not report any significant difficulty in getting cooperation from the owners of the bars or from the local leaders whom they contacted. They also do not report on any problems from the police or from neighborhood residents. This is probably because gay communities in the United States are well aware of the dangers of AIDS, and because the gay patrons of these bars have considerable organizational resources and stability. In many cases, however, conditions will not be so conducive as to enable interventions of this type to proceed so easily. To the extent that hierarchies of influence change rapidly, or that social networks are short-lived (such that social relationships are transient rather than long-rooted), or that there is serious resistance to change among influential segments of a subculture or scene, leadership-focused approaches might be less effective. In such cases, social movements or projects aimed at changing the larger social environment might be most efficacious.

Social Movement Theory

Cultures also change as a result of social movements on the part of their members (Ash, 1972; Davies, 1962; Gamson, 1975; Geschwender, 1964; Gurr, 1969; McAdam, 1982; McCarthy & Zald, 1973; Oberschall 1973; Piven & Cloward, 1979; Rudé, 1980; Tilly, 1978). Examples of social movements include Solidarnosc in Poland in 1980 and 1981, the black lung strikes in West Virginia in the late 1960s, the civil rights movement in the United States, and women's and gay rights movements in many countries. Usually, these movements develop out of the efforts of indigenous persons and local leaders, but outside intervention may on occasion stimulate or support such efforts. Community organizing efforts, for example, are often part of social-movement activities in specific localities. Social movements differ from diffusion and leadership-focused models in that they usually involve immediate challenges to the influence of some local informal leaders (and, often, to public policies or authorities as well). Although some local leaders are a major force in the making of social movements (Rudé, 1980), others usually oppose them. Thus, for public-health interventions, the social-movement approach becomes necessary primarily in circumstances where either or both of the following circumstances are true:

1. An extreme degree of local popular involvement is necessary in order to implement the changes required to prevent disease.
2. Opposition is likely. Such opposition may be on the level of small groups (e.g., sex partners who resist condom use), local informal leaders (e.g., the rare needle seller or shooting gallery operator who opposes syringe exchanges or bleach use), or from political or economic elites (e.g., resistance to making experimental drugs available to people with AIDS, or to occupational safety and health measures in many countries.)

For purposes of public-health interventions, several issues are salient: the first is to investigate whether some people within the target group have already begun to mobilize around the relevant issues; and, if so, whether the kind of mobilization they have initiated is likely to develop in ways that further or impede public health. For example, in the early 1980s in New York, gay men were beginning to mobilize against AIDS, and drug users in Rotterdam and other Dutch cities were setting up their own *junkiebonden* (drug users' unions) to pursue issues of concern to them, including health-related ones.

Second, if mobilization is not occurring, it is necessary to consider why not. Here, it may simply be the case that no one is sufficiently informed, in which case mobilization may be relatively easy to organize. More normally, however, there are obstacles to mobilization. The obstacles to and facilitators of mobilization are a major concern of social movement theory (Ash, 1972; Davies, 1962; Gamson, 1975; Geschwender, 1964; Gurr, 1969; McAdam, 1982; McCarthy & Zald, 1973; Oberschall, 1973; Piven & Cloward, 1979; Rudé, 1980; Tilly, 1978), and include issues such as (1) the extent to which the target population has mobilization resources—particularly including the strength of preexisting social networks and organization, but also including mundane matters, such as access to meeting places and money; (2) the extent to which (a) police action or (b) stigmatization (or even victimization) by civil society prevents organization through repressing the target population; and (3) the extent to which preexisting influentials will oppose or support mobilization.

Third, if it is possible to work with a preexisting social movement in the population, then issues similar to those that affect working with local influentials in a leadership-focused model become relevant. These include educating the leaders about the public health and biological issues they will be faced with, and working with them to develop ways in which their specific political and prestige needs can be made to coincide with effectively changing local norms and interests in ways that encourage healthier behaviors. This may involve working with people who may be more experienced than are local influentials (and who may be even less trusting of authority, including that of public-health agencies and scientists).

Fourth, if it is necessary to organize the group, this will involve locating potential group leaders (some of whom will already be local influentials) and training them not only in the public-health issues as such, but also in the organizational and political skills they will need to mobilize and lead the target population. This will include helping them figure out which local influentials to recruit to the cause and which have to be circumvented or opposed.

Specific techniques for public-health interventions by social-movement organizations include the publishing of newsletters and leaflets that provide health information and convey strategic and tactical suggestions about how to implement risk reduction. Such publications may also include other materials of whatever sort is necessary to attract readers and supporters to the movement. Moreover, once groups are established, even if they first came into existence through the initiative of public-health agencies, they will usually be somewhat autonomous, and may need to take actions that some public-health agencies would be unable to sponsor or support. For example, AIDS-related projects that have been set up by autonomous groups have included underground needle exchanges and the provision of extralegal experimental AIDS medicines. Similarly, some of the *junkiebonden* in the Netherlands in the early 1980s set up their own mechanisms for the distribution of non-prescription methadone at a time when they perceived the established drug-treatment facilities as prescribing dosages too low to block the craving for heroin.

The best example of a public-health social movement may be the mobilization that has occurred among gay men and lesbians to combat AIDS. This has been described elsewhere by others with more direct knowledge of the topic (Adam, 1987; Altman, 1986, 1991; Gamson, 1989; Patton, 1985, 1990), so here we will only present a brief interpretive sketch. First, however, it is worth briefly considering the issue of how to *evaluate* the impacts of social movements. Clearly, randomized experimental designs are not appropriate, since social movements are "naturally occurring" social phenomena outside the ability of researchers to create or prevent. Thus, their study has to rely on research designs used in studying natural–historic processes rather than controlled designs. (Some related issues—such as the efficacy of different community organizing techniques in promoting social movements and/or behavior change—can to some extent be studied using controlled designs, although such projects are expensive.)

When AIDS became visible, gays were able to respond relatively quickly. This was done, in part, by making use of the mobilization resources that had already been assembled through a succession of previous social-movement activities (Adam, 1987; Altman, 1986, 1991; Patton, 1985). In particular, there were many organizationally experienced people with widespread social networks; ongoing community institutions such as newspapers, informal gathering spots, and formal meeting places; and individuals and organizations that had money to donate for action against AIDS. Thus, in many cities around the world, groups formed to pressure the medical and public-health establishments into committing substantial resources for AIDS research (Shilts, 1987). These groups also organized immediate practical assistance for the sick in terms of social support, running errands, providing legal services, and the like. Other groups later formed, such as those of people with AIDS and groups dedicated to disseminating news about possible medications that orthodox medicine was not making available (and later, to make these available themselves, regardless of regulations). Groups like STOP AIDS held numerous small-group workshops that aimed at developing peer support for safer sex, and also at helping the gay community come to some definition and agreement on what changes in sex practices were appropriate (Bye, 1990). The gay press provided a forum for heated debates over safer sex, and also over the politics of AIDS prevention activities in the context of the entire gamut of interests of gay communities.

Later, when a sizable number of gay and lesbian activists became convinced that standard interest-group pressures were not sufficient to get governments and drug companies to respond in the ways they wanted, direct action groups like ACT UP formed. These have held demonstrations around many issues, including access to experimental medicine and increasing resources for AIDS research and prevention activities. ACT UP has also been involved in establishing underground syringe exchanges for drug injectors in localities like New York, where until recently laws and/or public-health officials prevented official exchanges from being set up.

The effect of this community mobilization was impressive. High-risk anal sex without condoms decreased considerably among gay men with ties to the mobilized gay communities and seroconversion rates were greatly reduced (Coutinho, van Griensven, & Moss, 1989). In gay communities with less organization and less mobilization, such as among African-American gays and bisexuals in San Francisco in 1990, norms supporting condom use were weaker and high-risk sex was more widespread (Peterson et al., 1992). Although there has been considerable attention paid to issues of: (1) relapse to high-risk behavior among some gay men (de Wit et al., 1992); (2) how to socialize young gays to safer sex as soon as they become sexually active (Stall et al., 1992); and (3) how to reach homosexually active African-American men (Peterson et al., 1992), nonetheless, the collective achievement of this gay and lesbian mobilization is one of the most effective health behavior interventions on record (Altman, 1991; Patton, 1990).

CHANGING THE SOCIAL ENVIRONMENT

Risk behaviors and peer groups are situated in larger social contexts. People who live in communities where despair and rampant violence are widespread are more likely to prioritize other issues than avoiding heart disease, cancer, or AIDS. Further, some social locations require behaviors that risk one's health; examples include, working in carcinogenic jobs when the alternative is poverty; taking amphetamines to stay awake while driving a truck or being a medical intern—or marijuana, tobacco, or alcohol use to be able to tolerate a boring job; and sex without a condom if this is what it takes to prevent violence or desertion by one's husband or boyfriend. Furthermore, some of the most large-scale patterns of social relationships in society seem to create a broad variety of inimical health effects through a variety of mechanisms. As one example of this, there is considerable evidence that racial stratification produces a wide range of deleterious health effects (Geschwender, 1978; Willis, 1987).

Where social environments predispose people to behave in unsafe ways, efforts to change these environments are an essential part of public-health activity. These attempts at change include changing public policies or large-scale social structures that make change difficult or impossible, or that directly facilitate the spread of infectious agents. Changing policies or social structures involves considerations that are deeply intertwined with issues of political values and interests. Thus, research on these issues is inherently controversial. It is often difficult to get such research funded. For example, in terms of research on a policy level, the Federal government was for years unwilling to fund research on the efficacy of syringe exchanges; and research on the sexual behavior of the American people was also denied funding for political reasons. Similarly, given the American aversion to seeing the United States as a class-divided society, official statistics present health and illness data by race and gender, and sometimes by income, but almost never by social class (Krieger, 1991; Turshen, 1989). Furthermore, the sociology of knowledge suggests that, on many issues, it may be impossible to get scholars to agree on appropriate evaluation criteria or models on some of these issues (Kuhn, 1962; Mannheim, 1936; Ossowski, 1963). Thus, in this section of the chapter, we will first present examples of policy and structural issues that are relevant to the HIV epidemic; then discuss three modes of trying to bring about change in these areas; and then consider what research issues need to be studied (although we have no illusions that definitive studies could ever be designed that would bring about scientific agreement on many of these issues).

Issues

Social Policy Issues

The HIV epidemic has raised many policy issues, some of them quite controversial. Examples include the distribution of condoms in schools; the content of AIDS education in the schools; and syringe-exchange programs and/or changes in the laws that outlaw the possession of syringes by drug injectors. The degree to which these programs are controversial varies, both geographically and over time. Within the United States, for example, syringe exchanges are still prohibited in many areas, controversial but at least tolerated in others, yet legally sanctioned (and not particularly controversial) in others. In much of Australia and the Netherlands, on the other hand, needle exchanges were implemented with minimal opposition, and indeed many public-health personnel in these countries have expressed amazement that syringe exchange could be so vehemently opposed in other places (Des Jarlais & Friedman, 1992b).

Social Structural Issues

Social structural issues are also important in the HIV epidemic. Racial stratification affects the extent to which people engage in drug injection, and also the extent to which drug injectors, noninjecting heterosexuals, and non-injecting gay men become HIV-infected and, indeed, become diagnosed with AIDS (Friedman, 1993; Friedman, Stepherson, Woods, Des Jarlais, & Ward, 1992; Selik, Castro, & Pappaioanou, 1988; Selik, Castro, Pappaioanou, & Buehler, 1989).

The social structuring of gender also creates difficulties for HIV prevention. Sexual stratification in the economy, politics, and everyday life means that women are less able to protect themselves by insisting on condom usage (Chavkin, 1990; Paone, Chavkin, Willets, Friedmann, & Des Jarlais, 1992; Patton, 1985, 1990; Sotheran, 1991). The stigmatization and repression of homosexuality (that may be a product of sexual stratification between men and women [Worth, 1989]) has made it difficult to get resources for AIDS programs and also has made it particularly difficult to implement effective prevention work targeting closeted gay men.

As another example, in the United States at least, discussion of issues of sexuality is extremely circumscribed. Spouses and other partners find it extremely difficult to talk candidly about sex, and this makes it very hard to deal with condom use or other safer sex approaches. Furthermore, the extent to which sexual discussion is circumscribed probably provides fertile ground for moralistic approaches to HIV that make it difficult to implement needed harm-reduction programs. The reasons for the inability to discuss sexuality are unclear. They may be rooted in value systems, but they are very widespread in persons from different ethnic and racial groups and both among recent immigrants and persons whose families have been here for many generations. They may be rooted in patterns of sexual stratification, or in patterns of alienation that include alienation from human sexuality as just one aspect of alienation from the realities of social life.

MODES OF ACTION

In general, the question is: Which modes of action will be most effective in changing a policy or social structure? Three salient modes of action will be discussed. The first is to conduct research about the benefits and disadvantages of different policies and structures, which is usually done in terms of consequences of a direct sort (e.g., in regard to syringe exchange: Does it lead to increases or decreases in the numbers of drug injectors? In high-risk behaviors? In HIV seroconversions?). Such research can also consider the differing consequences for different groups of people (e.g., on the fortunes of politicians who advocate or resist change, or on strategies for maintaining or opposing general social stability in a country).

A second approach is political interest-group activity based upon pluralist political theories. Many groups have lobbied federal or state executive or legislative officials about AIDS prevention and other HIV-related issues. Sometimes, such efforts have led to change, or at least have prevented negative outcomes. For example, when the United States Congress passed legislation to end funding of bleach-distribution programs for drug injectors, concerned organizations and individuals active in the field succeeded in getting this reversed (Des Jarlais & Bailey, 1990). Here again, though, the efficacy of this strategy will vary depending on the degree to which there are powerful opponents and/or the degree to which the policy may have other meanings or implications beyond those which are openly discussed.

A third approach is direct action. Examples of this include establishing underground syringe exchanges and then fighting for the public legitimation of their de facto existence; civil-disobedience actions, such as distributing syringes to drug injectors in ways that might provoke authorities into making arrests that would then lead to showcase trials; or distributing free condoms at school entrances. Unofficial syringe exchanges initiated policy changes in Australia, and the widespread underground exchanges in San Francisco and the surrounding areas of California created a supportive political atmosphere in which public authorities have refrained from arresting syringe-exchange staff. Direct action has also been used to attack structures of racial and sexual stratification through sit-ins, mass demonstrations, strikes, and other tactics.

THEORY AND RESEARCH NEEDS ABOUT SOCIAL CHANGE

In developing a theory-based understanding of how to change social policies and structures, several issues become salient. First, social policies exist for historically understandable reasons (although it is possible that a given policy is vestigial in that the reasons that brought it into being have ceased to be relevant and no others have as yet replaced them). Understanding these reasons is useful both because it may indicate that a specific policy change would entail other related problems that would still have to be addressed, and because it can provide insight into the bases on which opposition might arise.

Similarly, social structures usually have long histories, and are deeply entrenched and institutionalized. Thus, although structural racism may seem to be irrational, obsolete, and inefficient (Becker, 1957), it remains deeply imbedded in the entire history and institutional framework of our society. Many financial and real-estate companies make profits from the dynamics of racially segregated neighborhoods; and work forces that are divided by racial antagonisms are easier to control and to pay low wages (Geschwender, 1978). It has been suggested that many whites continue to derive compensatory emotional comfort from feeling superior to nonwhite groupings (Sennett & Cobb, 1972). Efforts to change racial stratification or other social structures have to take account of the ways in which they are institutionalized, and must develop ways to win over, neutralize, or defeat opponents of change.

Third, the people in a given geographic area have different interests, different values, and to some extent as a result of this, different beliefs (Mannheim, 1936; Ossowski, 1963). This means that proposals for change may be opposed by different groups for different reasons. On the other hand, it may be beneficial to the leaders of some groups to obscure the real differences among these reasons.

The battles around syringe exchange provide an example of how different supporters of the same position may be motivated by quite different considerations. Opponents of syringe exchange have included not only top-level Federal executive-branch officials and law-enforcement officials, but also African-American clergy and politicians. The focus of statements by the Federal and law-enforcement officials was their priority on the "War on Drugs," and their view of syringe exchange as undermining this campaign by "sending the wrong message." Leaders of the African-American community in New York, on the other hand, focused on their fears that syringe exchange might be funded at the expense of drug abuse treatment and prevention programs. That is, they saw it as a strategy whereby white officials might avoid dealing with the needs of their local neighborhoods. Individuals in neighborhoods in which there are large quantities of drug sales and drug injection, on the other hand, seem (at least on the basis of anecdotal evidence and of what we have learned in conversations with syringe-exchange operators) to vary widely in how they view these efforts (J. Rivera-Beckman, personal communication, August 23, 1992). In many neighborhoods, they have been quite supportive of underground syringe-exchange efforts because they see them as a way to reduce the spread of HIV among their drug-injecting neighbors and relatives. Other individuals may oppose exchanges because they find drug users so abhorrent that their death from AIDS is not a major concern. Still others may see the value in preventing deaths from AIDS, but may be led by their own experiences with drug injectors to believe that interventions based on harm-reduction principles will not work. Research is clearly needed on what causes individuals and leaders to take one approach rather than another; and about how positions that block needed public-health interventions can be changed.

Fourth, different modes of action operate through different mechanisms and through changing the positions of different people. Research is usually aimed at decision makers and, through dissemination in the mass media, the "general public." Lobbying usually focuses on these same groups and perhaps on specialized constituencies or interest groups. Direct action may have a similar focus, but also aims to change the sociopolitical environment by forcing authorities to make publicly visible choices about issues under circumstances chosen by the activists. There is a clear need for research to be conducted on the processes of social advocacy and/or social transformation by which research, lobbying, and direct action operate; on the conditions that make each approach more or less likely to succeed; and on the ways in which combinations of these approaches can be merged most successfully.

Fifth, we need to develop theories of society as a totality that will enable us to understand why certain social structures or policies are particularly resistant to change; if and why there are institutional interests and groups that benefit from the social conditions which lead to other persons having to undergo serious health risks; which social groupings may be most likely to join efforts for social change; and which actions such groups can take to produce change with the least damage.

Examples of efforts to change the social conditions that lead to ill health and to high-risk behaviors include but are not limited to: the occupational safety and health field; environmentalist activities; efforts to abolish racism and poverty; efforts to make medical care easily accessible to all.

CONCLUSIONS

Health behavior is a socially situated phenomenon. It is shaped by a range of forces. Some of these inhere primarily in the individual, others in small groups, still others in communities or subcultures, and some are characteristics of national or world social orders. From another perspective, of course, these distinctions are obfuscatory, since the dialectic among these different levels of organization means that all interact with each other. Thus, "individuals" in New York in the 1990s are shaped and defined by, and in turn, help to shape and define, the small groups, subcultures, communities, and societies in which they live.

Theories of health behavior, then, need to be equally far-ranging, and able to synthesize all these levels of analysis in their synchronic and historical interactions. Although action need not always wait on theoretical development, adequate theories make it much easier not only to understand the world but to change it.

By these standards, all models of health behavior, including those discussed in this chapter, are just bare beginnings. We are far from knowing how to combine the different modes and levels of analysis. In practice, however, this dilemma may be less crippling than it would first appear. In designing interventions, the models presented here can fruitfully coexist with each other and with individualistic interventions, to the mutual benefit of all. Projects to educate and increase the skills of individuals can provide a resource that can be used by diffusionist or mobilization-oriented projects, and these projects aimed at subcultural change often use the techniques of individual intervention as tactics.

Nonetheless, the distinction between individualistic and more sociological theories of health behavior is extremely important. In part, this is because of American society's ideological domination by a narrow individualism. The presuppositions of funding agencies are primarily individualistic, and their methodological preconceptions and biases toward the classic experimental design with random assignment can make it even more difficult to get community- or subculturally-focused interventions funded. The limited development to date of supraindividual theories of health behaviors aggravates this problem.

Finally, then, we suggest that insights are offered by looking at health behaviors as imbedded within and, in part, as constitutive of, small groups and subcultures. By studying the ways in which subcultural change occurs, in its interactions with other forces at all levels of analysis, we can begin to develop a sociological theory of health behaviors. The particular typology of ways in which subcultures change that is offered here emphasizes four kinds of processes: diffusion, working with preexisting leaders, mobilization, and change of the larger social environment. This typology is doubtless incomplete, but it also clearly enables us to expand our scope to encompass social as well as individual shapers of behavior change.

REFERENCES

Abdul-Quader, A. S., Tross, S., Friedman, S. R., Kouzi, A. C., & Des Jarlais, D. C. (1990). Street-recruited intravenous drug users and sexual risk reduction in New York City. *AIDS, 4*, 1075–1079.
Abdul-Quader, A. S., Des Jarlais, D. C., Tross, S., McCoy, E., Morales, G., & Velez, I. (1992). Outreach to injecting drug users and female sexual partners of drug users on the Lower East Side of New York City. *British Journal of Addiction, 87*, 681–688.
Adam, B. (1987). *The rise of a gay and lesbian movement.* Boston: Twayne.
Altman, D. (1986). *AIDS in the mind of America.* Garden City, NY: Doubleday.
Altman, D. (1991). The primacy of politics: Organizing around AIDS. *AIDS, 5,* (suppl 2):S231–S238.
Ash, R. (1972). *Social movements in America.* Chicago: Markham.
Bandura, A. (1977). *Social learning theory.* Englewood, NJ: Prentice-Hall.
Becker, G. S. (1957). *The economics of discrimination.* Chicago: University of Chicago Press.
Becker, M. H., & Joseph, J. K. (1988). AIDS and behavioral change to reduce risk: A review. *American Journal of Public Health, 78*, 394–410.
Botvin, G. J., Baker, E., Botvin, E. M., Filazzola, B. S., & Millman, R. (1984). Prevention of alcohol misuse through development of personal and social competence. *Journal of Studies on Alcohol, 45*, 550–552.
Broadhead, R. S. (1991). Social constructions of bleach in combating AIDS among injection drug users. *Journal of Drug Issues, 21*, 711–734.
Broadhead, R. S., & Fox, K. J. (1990). Takin' it to the streets: AIDS outreach as ethnography. *Journal of Contemporary Ethnography, 19*, 322–348.
Broadhead, R. S., Fox, K. J., & Espada, F. (1990). AIDS outreach workers. *Society, 27*, 66–70.
Bye, L. L. (1990). Moving beyond counseling and knowledge-enhancing interventions: A plea for community-level AIDS prevention strategies. In D. G. Ostrow (Ed.), *Behavioral aspects of AIDS* (pp. 157–170). New York: Plenum Medical Book Company.

Casriel, C., Des Jarlais, D. C., Rodriguez, R., Friedman, S. R., Stepherson, B., & Khuri, E. (1990). Working with heroin sniffers: Clinical issues in preventing drug injection. *Journal of Substance Abuse Treatment, 7,* 1–10.

Chavkin, W. (1990). Drug addiction and pregnancy: Policy crossroads. *American Journal of Public Health, 80,* 483–486.

Coutinho, R. A., van Griensven, G. J. P., & Moss, A. (1989). Effects of preventive efforts among homosexual men. *AIDS, 3,* (Suppl. 1):S53–S56.

Davies, J. C. (1962). Toward a theory of revolution. *American Sociological Review, 27,* 5–19.

Des Jarlais, D. C., & Bailey, W. (1990). Almost banning bleach. Paper presented at the 118th Annual Meeting of the American Public Health Association, Boston.

Des Jarlais, D. C., Casriel, C., Friedman, S. R., & Rosenblum, A. (1992). AIDS and the transition to illicit drug injection: Results of a randomized trial prevention program. *British Journal of Addiction, 87,* 493–498.

Des Jarlais, D. C., & Friedman, S. R. (1992a). AIDS prevention programs for intravenous drug users. In G. P. Wormser (Ed.), *AIDS and other manifestations of HIV infection* (2nd ed. pp. 645–658). New York: Raven Press.

Des Jarlais, D. C., & Friedman, S. R. (1992b). The AIDS epidemic and legal access to sterile equipment for injecting illicit drugs. *Annals of the American Academy of Political & Social Science, 521,* 42–65.

Des Jarlais, D. C., Friedman, S. R., Choopanya, K., Vanichseni, S., & Ward, T. P. (1992). International epidemiology of HIV and AIDS among injecting drug users. *AIDS, 6,* 1053–1068.

de Wit, J. F. B., de Vroome, E. M. M., Sandfort, T. G. M., van Griensven, G. J. P., Coutinho, R. A., & Tielman, R. A. P. (1992). Safe sexual practices not reliably maintained by homosexual men. *American Journal of Public Health, 82,* 615–616.

Emmons, C. A., Joseph, J. G., Kessler, R. C., Wortman, C. B., Montgomery, S. B., & Ostrow, D. G. (1986). Psychosocial predictors of reported behavior change in homosexual men at risk for AIDS. *Health Education Quarterly, 13,* 331–345.

Evans, R. J. (1976). Smoking in children: Developing a social psychological theory of deterrence. *Preventive Medicine, 5,* 122–127.

Fishbein, M. (1980). A theory of reasoned action. Some applications and implications. In H. E. Howe & M. M. Page (Eds.), *Nebraska Symposium on Motivation, 1979* (pp. 65–116). Lincoln: University of Nebraska Press.

Fishbein, M., & Ajzen, I. (1975). *Belief, attitude, intention, and behavior: An introduction to theory and research.* Reading, MA: Addison-Wesley.

Fishbein, M., & Middlestadt, S. E. (1989). Using the theory of reasoned action as a framework for understanding and changing AIDS-related behaviors. In V. M. Mays, G. W. Albee, & S. F. Schneider (Eds.), *Primary prevention of AIDS: Psychological approaches* (pp. 93–110). Newbury Park, CA: Sage.

Flynn, N., Jain, S., Keddie, E., Carlson, J., Jennings, M., & Haverkos, H. (1990). Bleach is not enough: Giving IV drug users a choice of disinfectants when they share needles and syringes. Paper presented at the Sixth International Conference on AIDS, San Francisco, CA [abstract S.C. 761].

Friedman, S. R. (1993). AIDS as a sociohistorical phenomenon. In G. L. Albrecht & R. S. Zimmerman (Eds.), *Advances in medical sociology, vol. 3: The social and behavioral aspects of AIDS* (pp. 19–36). Greenwich, CT: JAI Press.

Friedman, S. R., & Des Jarlais, D. C. (1991). HIV among drug injectors: The epidemic and the response. *AIDS Care, 3,* 239–250.

Friedman, S. R., Des Jarlais, D. C., & Neaigus, A. (1992). AIDS among drug injectors: The first decade. In V. deVita Jr., S. Hellman, & S. A. Rosenberg (Eds.), *AIDS: Etiology, diagnosis, treatment, and prevention. (3rd ed.* pp. 453–461). Philadelphia: J. B. Lippincott.

Friedman, S. R., Des Jarlais, D. C., Ward, T. P., Jose, B., Neaigus, A., & Goldstein, M. (in press). Drug injectors and heterosexual AIDS. In L. Sherr (Ed.), *Heterosexual AIDS.* Reading, UK: Harwood Academic Publishers.

Friedman, S. R., Snyder, F. R., Shorty, V., Jones, A., Estrada, A. L., & Young, P. A. (in press). Racial differences in HIV risk behaviors among drug injectors: Multicity data. In *Proceedings of the Second National AIDS Demonstration Research Conference.* Rockville, MD: National Institute on Drug Abuse.

Friedman, S. R., Sotheran, J. L., Abdul-Quader, A., Primm, B. J., Des Jarlais, D. C., Kleinman, P., Mauge, C., Goldsmith, D. S., El-Sadr, W., & Maslansky, R. (1987). The AIDS epidemic among Blacks and Hispanics. *The Milbank Quarterly, 65,* 455–499.

Friedman, S. R., Stepherson, B., Woods, J., Des Jarlais, D. C., & Ward, T. P. (1992). Society, drug injectors, and AIDS. *Journal of Health Care for the Poor & Underserved, 3,* 73–89.

Friedman, S. R., Sufian, M., & Des Jarlais, D. C. (1990). The AIDS epidemic among Latino intravenous drug users. In R. Glick and J. Moore (Eds.), *Drug Abuse in Hispanic Communities* (pp. 45–54). New Brunswick, NJ: Rutgers University Press.

Froner, G. A., Rutherford, G. W., & Rokeach, M. (1987). Injection of sodium hypochlorite by intravenous drug users. *Journal of the American Medical Association, 258,* 325.

Gamson, J. (1989). Silence, death, and the invisible enemy: AIDS activism and social movement "newness." *Social Problems, 36,* 351–367.

Gamson, W. (1975). *The strategy of social protest.* Homewood, IL: Dorsey Press.

Geschwender, J. A. (1964). Social structure and the Negro revolt. *Social Forces, 43,* 250–256.

Geschwender, J. A. (1978). *Racial stratification in America.* Dubuque, IA: Wm. C. Brown.

Gurr, T. R. (1969). *Why men rebel.* Princeton, NJ: Princeton University Press.

Herrmann, J. W., & Heicht, R. C. (1979). Complications in therapeutic use of sodium hypochlorite. *Journal of Endodontology, 5,* 160.

Kandel, D. B., & Logan, J. (1984). Patterns of drug use from adolescence to young adulthood. *American Journal of Public Health, 74,* 660–666.

Kelly, J. A., St. Lawrence, J. S., Diaz, Y. E., Stevenson, L. Y., Hauth, A. C., Brasfeld, T. L., Kalichman, S. C., Smith, J. E., & Andrew, M. E. (1991). HIV risk behavior reduction following intervention with key opinion leaders of population: An experimental analysis. *American Journal of Public Health, 81,* 168–171.

Kelly, J. A., St. Lawrence, J. S., Stevenson, L. Y., Hauth, A. C., Kalichman, S. C., Diaz, Y. E., Brasfeld, T. L., Koob, J. J., & Morgan, M. G. (1992). Community AIDS/HIV risk reduction: The effects of endorsements by popular people in three cities. *American Journal of Public Health, 82,* 1483–1489.

Krieger, N. (1991). The making of public health data: Political considerations and implications. Paper presented at the 119th Annual Meeting of the American Public Health Association, Washington, DC, November 10–14 [session 2065].

Kuhn, T. (1962). *The structure of scientific revolutions.* Chicago: University of Chicago Press.

Mannheim, K. (1936). *Ideology and utopia,* Trans. New York: Harcourt, Brace.

Martin, L. S., McDougal, J. S., & Loskoski, S. L. (1985). Disinfection and inactivation of the human T-lymphotropic virus type III/lymphadenopathy-associated virus. *Journal of Infectious Diseases, 152,* 400–403.

McAdam, D. (1982). *Political process and the development of Black insurgency, 1930–1979.* Chicago: University of Chicago Press.

McAlister, A., Puska, P., Salonen, J. T., Tuomilehto, J., & Koskela, K. (1982). Theory and action for health promotion: Illustrations from the North Karelia Project. *American Journal of Public Health, 72,* 43–50.

McBride, C., Curry, S. J., Anderman, C., Cheadle, A., Wagner, E., & Pearson, D. (1992). *Testing a social ecology model to explain adolescent risk-taking behavior.* Paper presented at the 120th Annual Meeting of the American Public Health Association, Washington, DC [session 2002].

McCarthy, J., & Zald, M. (1973). *The trend of social movements in America.* Morristown, NJ: General Learning Press.

McLeroy, K. R., Bibeau, D., Steckler, A., & Glanz, K. (1988). An ecological perspective on health promotion programs. *Health Education Quarterly, 15,* 351–377.

Moncher, M. S., Holden, G. W., & Schinke, S. P. (1991). Review of current etiological constructs. *International Journal of the Addictions, 26,* 337–414.

Montgomery, S. B., Joseph, J. G., Becker, M. H., Ostrow, D. G., Kessler, R. C., & Kirscht, J. P. (1989). The health belief model in understanding compliance with preventive recommendations for AIDS: How useful? *AIDS Education & Prevention, 1,* 303–323.

Morales, E. S., & Fullilove, M. T. (1992). "Many are called . . .": Participation by minority leaders in an AIDS intervention in San Francisco. *Ethnicity & Disease, 2,* 389–401.

Neaigus, A., Friedman, S. R., Sufian, M., Stepherson, B., Goldsmith, D. S., & Mota, P. (1990). *Effects of peer culture, race, and gender on IV drug use risk reduction.* Paper presented at the 118th Annual Meeting of the American Public Health Association, New York City, October.

Newmeyer, J. A. (1988). Why bleach? Development of a strategy to combat HIV contagion among San Francisco intravenous drug users. In R. J. Battjes & R. W. Pickens (Eds.), *Needle sharing among intravenous drug users: National and international perspectives* (pp. 151–159). Washington, DC: U.S. Government Printing Office, NIDA Research Monograph 80.

Newmeyer, J. A., Feldman, H. W., Biernacki, P., & Watters, J. K. (1989). Preventing AIDS contagion among intravenous drug users. *Medical Anthropology, 10,* 167–175.

Oberschall, A. (1973). *Social conflict and social movements.* Englewood Cliffs, NJ: Prentice-Hall.

Ogburn, W. F. (1922). *Social change.* New York: Huebsch.

Ossowski, S. (1963). *Class structure in the social consciousness,* Trans. New York: Free Press.

Paone, D., Chavkin, W., Willets, I., Friedmann, P., & Des Jarlais, D. C. (1992). The impact of sexual abuse: Implications for drug treatment. *Journal of Women's Health, 1,* 149–153.

Patton, C. (1985). *Sex and germs: The politics of AIDS.* Boston: South End Press.

Patton, C. (1990). *Inventing AIDS.* New York: Routledge.

Peterson, J. L., Coates, T. J., Catania, J. A., Middleton, L., Hilliard, B., & Hearst, N. (1992). High-risk sexual behavior and condom use among gay and bisexual African-American men. *American Journal of Public Health, 82,* 1490–1494.

Piven, F. F., & Cloward, R. (1979). *Poor people's movements.* New York: Vintage.

Puska, P., Nissinen, A., Tuomilehto, J., Salonen, J. Y., Koskela, K., McAlister, A., Kottke, T. E., Macoby, N., & Farquhar, S. W. (1985). Strategy to prevent coronary heart disease: Conclusions from ten years of the North Karelia project. *Annual Review of Public Health, 6,* 147–193.

Quimby, E., & Friedman, S. R. (1989). Dynamics of Black mobilization against AIDS in New York City. *Social Problems, 36,* 403–415.

Resnick, L., Veren, K., Salahuddin, S. Z., Tondreau, S., & Markham, P. D. (1986). Stability and inactivation of HTLV-III/LAV under clinical and laboratory environments. *Journal of the American Medical Association, 255,* 1887–1891.

Rogers, E. M. (1982). *Diffusion of innovations. Third edition.* New York: The Free Press.

Rogers, E. M., & Shoemaker, F. F. (1971). *Communication of innovation: A cross-cultural approach.* (2nd ed.). New York: The Free Press.

Rudé, G. F. E. (1980). *Ideology and popular protest.* New York: Pantheon Press.

Selik, R. M., Castro, K. G., & Pappaioanou, M. (1988). Racial/ethnic differences in the risk of AIDS in the United States. *American Journal of Public Health, 78*, 1539–1545.

Selik, R. M., Castro, K. G., Pappaioanou, M., & Buehler, J. W. (1989). Birthplace and the risk of AIDS among Hispanics in the United States. *American Journal of Public Health, 79*, 836–839.

Sennett, R., & Cobb, J. (1972). *The hidden injuries of class.* New York: Vintage.

Shilts, R. (1987). *And the band played on: Politics, people and the AIDS epidemic.* New York: St. Martin's Press.

Sotheran, J. L. (1991). *HIV risk and social relationships among IV drug users.* Paper presented at the Annual Workshop on Psychosocial Factors in Population Change, Washington, DC, March 19–20.

Stall, R., Burrett, D., Bye, L. L., Catania, J. A., Frutchey, C., Henne, J., Lemp, G., & Paul, J. (1992). A comparison of younger and older gay men's HIV risk-taking behaviors: The communications technologies 1989 cross-sectional survey. *Journal of the Acquired Immune Deficiency Syndrome, 5*, 682–687.

Tilly, C. (1978). *From mobilization to revolution.* Reading, PA: Addison-Wesley.

Turshen, M. (1989). *The politics of public health.* New Brunswick, NJ: Rutgers University Press.

Watters, J. K., Cheng, Y., Segal, M., Lorvick, J., Case, P., & Carlson, J. (1990). *Epidemiology and prevention of HIV in intravenous drug users in San Francisco, 1986–1989.* Paper presented at the 6th International Conference on AIDS, San Francisco, CA [abstract F.C.106].

White, H. R. (1992). Early problem behavior and later drug problems. *Journal of Research in Crime and Delinquency, 29*, 412–429.

White, H. R., & Labouvie, E. W. (1989). Towards the assessment of adolescent problem drinking. *Journal of Studies on Alcohol, 50*, 30–37.

Wiebel, W. (1988). Combining ethnographic and epidemiologic methods for targeted AIDS interventions: The Chicago Model. In R. J. Battjes & R. W. Pickens (Eds.), *Needle sharing among intravenous drug abusers: National and international perspectives* (pp. 137–150). Washington, DC: U.S. Government Printing Office, NIDA Research Monograph 80.

Wiebel, W. (1990). Identifying and gaining access to hidden populations. In E. Y. Lambert (Ed.), *The collection and interpretation of data from hidden populations* (pp. 4–11). Washington, DC: U.S. Government Printing Office, NIDA Research Monograph 98.

Wiebel, W. (1991). Factors influencing personal decisions to use heroin. In D. Forster & J. Salloway (Eds.), *The socio-cultural matrix of alcohol and drug use: A sourcebook of patterns* (pp. 367–391). Lewiston, NY: Edwin Mellen Press.

Wiebel, W., Fritz, R., & Chene, D. (1989). Description of intervention procedures utilized by the AIDS Outreach Intervention Projects—University of Illinois at Chicago, School of Public Health. *Proceedings of the Community Epidemiology Work Group: Chicago-June 1989* (Vol. 3, pp. 68–79). Rockville, MD: National Institute on Drug Abuse.

Willis, D. P. (1987). Currents of health policy: Impact on Black Americans. *Milbank Quarterly, 65* (Supplements 1 & 2).

Worth, D. (1989). Sexual decision-making and AIDS: Why condom promotion among vulnerable women is likely to fail. *Studies in Family Planning, 20*, 297–307.

7

School-Based Interventions to Prevent Unprotected Sex and HIV among Adolescents

DOUGLAS KIRBY and RALPH J. DiCLEMENTE

INTRODUCTION

At present, acquired immunodeficiency syndrome (AIDS) remains a relatively uncommon diagnosis among adolescents; those between 13 and 19 years of age account for less than 1% of diagnosed cases of AIDS in the United States (Centers for Disease Control and Prevention, 1993). Recent data indicate, however, that the rate of AIDS among adolescents has increased markedly over the course of the epidemic (Hein, 1992), with African-American adolescents disproportionately represented among AIDS cases (Bowler, Sheon, D'Angelo, & Vermund, 1993; DiClemente, 1992a; 1993).

AIDS case surveillance data is not, however, a useful marker for evaluating the threat human immunodeficiency virus (HIV) poses for adolescents. Given the long latency period between infection with HIV to clinical endpoints (i.e., symptoms of disease), many adolescents infected as teenagers will not experience HIV-associated symptoms until well into their twenties. Thus, relatively few of the reported AIDS cases have occurred among adolescents, but more than 20% have occurred among individuals in their twenties, many of whom were probably infected as adolescents (Centers for Disease Control, 1991b).

A more precise measure of the impact of HIV in the adolescent population is HIV seroprevalence. At present, there are no representative population-

DOUGLAS KIRBY • ETR Associates, P.O. Box 1830, Santa Cruz, California 95061-1830.   *RALPH J. DiCLEMENTE* • School of Public Health, Department of Health Behavior and School of Medicine, Departments of Medicine and Pediatrics, and Center for AIDS Research, University of Alabama, Birmingham, Alabama 35249.

Preventing AIDS: Theories and Methods of Behavioral Interventions, edited by Ralph J. DiClemente and John L. Peterson. Plenum Press, New York, 1994.

based studies for estimating HIV seroprevalence. A recent review of HIV seroepidemiologic surveys among adolescents in selected populations indicates that HIV infection is not uncommon, with rates varying widely by ethnicity and gender (DiClemente, 1992a). For example, among youths younger than 20 applying to the military, the prevalence of HIV infection per 1000 whites, blacks, and Hispanics was .17, 1.00, and .29 respectively (Burke et al., 1990). Among military personnel under 20, the prevalence of HIV infection per 1000 soldiers was 0.5 (Kelley et al., 1990). Among Job Corps entrants aged 16 to 21, the prevalence per 1000 entrants for whites, blacks, and Hispanics respectively was 1.2, 5.3, and 2.6 (Centers for Disease Control, 1990).

While representative HIV seroprevalence surveys are limited, survey data well describe the prevalence of adolescents' HIV-associated risk behaviors. In 1990, of all students in grades 9 to 12, 54% reported ever having had sexual intercourse; this percentage increased with each grade (Centers for Disease Control, 1992a). In a different national survey of females, 26% reported having had sex by age 15; 75% before they turned 20 (Centers for Disease Control, 1991a). In a nationally representative sample of males the figures are higher, with 86% having sex prior to age 20 (Sonenstein, Pleck, & Ku, 1989). Among high school students sexually active at the time of their survey, only 49% of the males and 40% of the females reported using a condom during their last intercourse (Centers for Disease Control, 1992a).

Most adolescents do not have large numbers of sexual partners, but when most adolescents initiate intercourse at early ages and most of them fail to use condoms during every act of intercourse, their exposure to STD and HIV accumulates over time. Thus, by age 21, about one out of four teens becomes infected with an STD (Department of Health and Human Services, 1990) and about 2.5 million adolescents are infected with an STD annually (Centers for Disease Control, 1989).

Thus, these data demonstrate the need for the urgent development and rapid implementation of HIV prevention programs that effectively reduce unprotected sex.

THE ROLE OF SCHOOLS IN HIV PREVENTION

School-based HIV prevention programs have an important role to play in preventing HIV infection by encouraging the adoption and maintenance of HIV-preventive behaviors and enhancing adolescents' tolerance toward persons infected with HIV or living with AIDS (DiClemente, 1989). Schools are an obvious intervention site for the implementation of HIV prevention efforts as they are the one institution in our society regularly attended by most young people; nearly 95% of all children and youth are in elementary or secondary schools (Iverson & Kolbe, 1983). Moreover, virtually all youth are in schools before they initiate risk-taking behaviors that may expose them to HIV infection.

For almost a century, school-based programs have attempted to reduce unprotected sexual activity and sexually transmitted disease (Imber, 1982). As the threat of HIV became more prominent in our society, schools responded dramatically and many schools developed programs which focused primarily upon HIV. In earlier years other programs attempted to reduce sexual intercourse outside of marriage, unintended pregnancy, and sexually transmitted diseases other than HIV. These efforts targeted similar risk behaviors related to the transmission of HIV—the onset of sexual intercourse, the frequency of intercourse, the number of sexual partners, and the use of condoms. Understanding the evolution of sex education efforts provides a historical context with which to examine current and proposed HIV prevention efforts. Moreover, many health professionals believe that HIV prevention programs will be most effective if they are taught as part of more comprehensive sex education programs that attempt to teach skills and change norms.

THE GENERATIONS OF SEX AND HIV EDUCATION CURRICULA: HOW EFFECTIVE?

Many sexuality education programs are concerned with a wide range of sexual issues and do not focus primarily upon reducing unprotected intercourse. Since the mid-1970s, however, when concern about teenage pregnancy increased, many programs have focused more upon the behaviors that cause pregnancy. Since the mid-1980s when this country became more concerned about the threat of AIDS, there have also been many programs that focused upon the behaviors leading to HIV transmission.

Although the hundreds of curricula that have been developed contain activities or elements reflecting a wide variety of approaches, these curricula fall loosely into five groups. Because some of these groups evolved out of other groups, to some extent they can be perceived as "generations." Notably, these generations somewhat parallel the generations of curricula to reduce smoking, alcohol, and illegal drug use.

The first generation of sex education curricula focused primarily upon increasing knowledge and emphasizing the risk and consequences of pregnancy. They were based upon the premise that if youth had greater knowledge about sexual intercourse, pregnancy, methods of birth control, the probability of pregnancy, and the consequences of childbearing, then they would rationally choose to avoid unprotected intercourse. This generation of curricula paralleled the first smoking and substance abuse curricula which described different drugs and emphasized the consequences of substance use (e.g., the long-term impact of smoking and its relationship to cancer).

The next generation of sex education curricula included considerable knowledge content, but did not give as much emphasis to "the endless pursuit of the fallopian tubes." Instead, they devoted much more emphasis to values clarification and skills, especially decision-making and communication skills. The values clarification exercises were designed to help the students become more clear about their basic values as well as their values about sexual behavior. Teachers gave students dilemmas to solve and discuss, but commonly did not emphasize that particular values were right or wrong. These curricula emphasized generic skills, such as the basic steps involved in making a decision and the basic components in communicating with one's partner (e.g., "I" messages, paraphrasing, and careful listening). When these skills and values were applied to sexual issues, curricula often spelled out the pros and cons of engaging in sexual intercourse and the pros and cons of using contraception, but did not consistently and clearly emphasize that the students should not engage in unprotected sexual activity. Proponents of this approach believed that if students' values became more clear and their decision-making skills improved, then they would become more likely to decide to avoid risk-taking behavior, and, if their communication skills improved, then they would be more likely to communicate effectively those decisions to their partners.

Numerous studies have measured the impact of these first two generations of programs upon the knowledge of students and the findings from these studies are nearly unanimous—instruction did increase knowledge of sexuality (Kirby, 1984). There have been similar findings for STD education programs (Yarber, 1986). It has been increasingly recognized, however, that knowledge about sexual issues such as contraception is very weakly related to behavior and that increasing knowledge may not produce much reduction in risk-taking behavior (Whitley & Schofield, 1985–1986).

A smaller number of studies examined the impact of these sex education programs upon values and attitudes. Those studies indicate that when specific values were not given prominent emphasis in the course, there was little evidence that the courses had any measurable impact upon the students' values. When several more liberal courses taught during the 1970s focused upon increasing the students' acceptance of the sexual practices of other students, however, there was some change in that direction (Hoch, 1971; Parcel & Luttman, 1980, 1981). Finally, during the early 1980s, when several courses focused upon increasing the clarity of students' values, they succeeded in making them slightly more clear (Kirby, 1984).

Whether or not these sex education courses measurably affected students' skills depended both upon how the skills were taught and how they were measured. One curriculum used an intensive cognitive–behavioral approach that focused upon teaching and practicing communication skills in the classroom through modeling, role-playing, and rehearsal. When the evaluators measured these skills with vignettes and videotapes, they found a measurable impact (Schinke, Blythe, & Gilchrest, 1981). In contrast, a different study used questionnaires to evaluate the impact of a variety of exemplary sex education programs upon skills as they were practiced in everyday life and not in the classroom. That study did not find a measurable impact (Kirby, 1984).

Five major studies have examined the impact of sex education upon the initiation of intercourse and the subsequent frequency of sexual intercourse. Four of these studies were based upon surveys of large random samples of teenagers or young adults in this country and included questions both about participation in sex education programs and personal sexual experience. Thus, those studies measured the impact of a cross section of sex education programs existing at that time. Two of these studies found that for older teens, participation in sex education was not associated with subsequently initiating intercourse, but for younger teens (e.g., 14 or 15 years old), participation in sex education was associated with subsequent initiation of intercourse (Dawson, 1986; Marsiglio & Mott, 1986). The third study found no statistical relationship between sex education and sexual experience (Zelnik & Kim, 1982), and finally the fourth found that sex education was associated with delayed initiation of intercourse (Furstenberg, Moore, & Peterson, 1985). The fifth study examined the impact of 14 specific sex education programs and had smaller sample sizes in each of the programs (Kirby, 1984). That study found that none of the programs increased or decreased sexual experience.

Four of these five studies examined the impact of sex education upon the use of birth control; the first three also relied upon national surveys of youth. Their results were also mixed. The study with the most positive results found that having taken pregnancy and contraceptive education was positively related to use of birth control during first intercourse and to use of birth control ever. However, pregnancy and contraceptive education were not related to current use of contraception. Similarly, a second survey found weak relationships between having had sex education and use of contraception both during first intercourse and during any sexual activity, but these relationships were statistically significant only for blacks. A third study focused upon current use of birth control and found inconsistent results which depended upon how sex education was defined. Finally, in the study of 14 sex education courses it was possible to measure the impact of 11 of the courses upon contraceptive use; none of these courses had a measurable impact upon use of contraception.

Three of these studies examined the relationship between sex education and pregnancy; none found a measurable and significant impact of sex education upon pregnancy.

Although the results of these evaluations produced somewhat inconsistent results, they clearly demonstrated that these first two generations of sex education programs did not dramatically reduce sexual risk-taking behavior or measurably reduce teenage pregnancy; at best they may have slightly increased the use of birth control among selected groups.

The third generation of programs did not evolve out of the first two generations, but instead developed in reaction to the first two generations of sex education programs. Concerned that the first two generations of programs were "value free," a different group of educators developed the third generation of programs. They generated a moralistic and ideological fervor and consistently emphasized the message that youth should not engage in intercourse until marriage. To avoid any possibility of a "double-message," these programs commonly did not discuss contraception or only emphasized the risks associated with contraception.

Abstinence programs such as *Teen Aid* and *Sex Respect* have been evaluated and the evaluation results indicate that the programs did affect a wide variety of attitudes regarding premarital intercourse (Donahue, 1987; Weed & Olsen, 1988, 1992). In all cases, attitudes became significantly less accepting of premarital intercourse in the short term. These effects may have been partially produced by response biases, however, and the studies either did not measure long-term effects or, alternatively, they measured long-term effects and found that the effects had greatly diminished. Only a few studies have examined the impact upon behavior of abstinence programs and the methods employed in all of them have been quite limited. Two of the studies failed to find a positive impact upon behavior (Christopher & Roosa, 1990; Roosa & Christopher, 1990). A third study found that *Sex Respect, Teen Aid,* and *Values and Choices* (evaluated as a group and not individually) did not delay the initiation of intercourse among middle-school youth or among high-school youth, but did delay the onset of intercourse among high-school students with values unfavorable to abstinence before the program (Weed, Olsen, DeGaston, & Prigmore, 1992).

The fourth generation of programs designed to change adolescent sexual behavior are the HIV education programs. Many of these developed quite independently of the previous three generations of sex education programs and, at least initially, they did not build upon the successes and failures of sex education programs.

These programs typically had a variety of goals, including: increasing recognition of HIV transmission routes; reducing misinformation and misconceptions about HIV infection and transmission; reducing unnecessary fears associated with the disease; encouraging young people to delay premature sexual intercourse; supporting safer sex by encouraging teenagers who are sexually active to use condoms every time they have any kind of intercourse or to practice only those sexual behaviors that do not place one at risk of HIV infection; encouraging youth to avoid drug use; and helping students develop compassion for people infected with HIV.

Many of the HIV education curricula developed during the first few years relied heavily upon didactic presentations and group discussions of information about HIV. Partially because of the short length of most HIV program units, rarely were there serious attempts to improve skills or to change norms. Thus, like the early sex education programs, they either explicitly or implicitly assumed that correcting youths' myths about HIV and AIDS would, as a logical consequence, result in adolescents changing their behavior.

Recognizing that most youth knew few people who were infected with HIV and that consequently most youth would deny any personal vulnerability, some curricula also focused upon personalizing the information by having a person living with HIV or AIDS, especially a young person, speak to students.

Early evaluations of these programs indicated that many of them were successful at increasing adolescents' HIV knowledge. Some made youth more sensitive to the rights of people infected with HIV or living with AIDS. And some reduced unnecessary fear about getting HIV from improbable sources such as blood donations and mosquito bites (Ashworth, DuRaut, Newman, & Gaillard, 1992; DiClemente, Boyer, & Mills, 1987; Farley, Pomputius, Sabella, Helgerson, & Hadler, 1991; Huszti, Clopton, & Mason, 1989; Miller & Downer, 1987; Rickert, Gottleib, & Jay, 1990). Few studies rigorously measured the impact of these programs upon sexual behaviors.

Although the impact of individual programs upon behavior was not well evaluated, national surveys provide some evidence that school-based programs may have had some impact. First, numerous studies have indicated that teenagers are remarkably knowledgeable about the transmission of HIV (DiClemente, 1990; Hingson & Strunin, 1992). Second, a national survey of teenage males conducted in 1988 indicated that there were large increases in the use of condoms among males; specifically, use more than doubled from 21 to 58% between 1979 and 1988 (Sonenstein et al., 1989). Although these data suggest that school-based programs might have contributed to greater knowledge and greater use of condoms, it is not possible to determine whether this increase was due to school-based AIDS education programs, the innumerable other AIDS education programs in communities and the media, or other factors. Third, two other studies examined the impact of AIDS education upon condom use. One of these (Anderson et al., 1990) failed to find a significant direct relationship between AIDS instruction and condom use, but there may have been an indirect relationship through knowledge. In contrast, the second study (Ku, Sonenstein, & Pleck, 1992) found that among adolescent males (the only gender studied), instruction on AIDS, contraception, and resistance skills were all significantly and independently associated with greater condom use.

There is now emerging a fifth group of sex education and AIDS education programs and evaluation studies. This generation differs from the previous generations in several ways: the curricula are based upon theoretical approaches that have been demonstrated to be effective in other health areas; they build upon the successes and failures of previous programs; and the behavioral effects of each program are far more rigorously evaluated.

Thus far, there is only one curriculum that is school based, that covers condoms and other methods of contraception, that has been well evaluated with a rigorous research design, that has demonstrated a clear impact upon behavior, and that has been published (Kirby, Barth, Leland, & Fetro, 1991). That curriculum is *Reducing the Risk* (Barth, 1989). Evaluations of other curricula are currently under way, however, show promising results, and will shortly be published.

The *Reducing the Risk* curriculum is based upon social learning theory, cognitive-behavior theory, and social-influence theory. It clearly emphasizes the value that students should avoid unprotected intercourse by abstaining from intercourse or using contraception. The curriculum incorporates many active learning or experiential activities, especially role-playing. These role-playing activities are designed to reinforce the norm against unprotected sex, teach skills to avoid unprotected sex, and increase students' self-efficacy in those skills. Other experiential activities, designed to increase both comfort and self-efficacy, include discussions of lines that youth give for having sex and responses to them, visits to a family planning clinic, and reviews of condoms at a drug store.

Reducing the Risk did not have a significant impact upon all the students who had already had sex. However, it did significantly increase the use of contraception among some groups of sexually experienced students (e.g. females and lower risk youth) and it did significantly prevent unprotected sexual behavior among those who had not had intercourse prior to the program, mostly by delaying the onset of sexual intercourse and partially by increasing the use of contraception among those who initiated sex after the program (Kirby et al., 1991).

There are 11 studies of specific school-based sex and AIDS education programs that measured impact upon behavior and have been published, or are available as government or agency reports (Kirby & Coyle, 1994). These programs include *AIDS Prevention for Adolescents in School* (*APAS*) (Walter & Vaughn, 1993); *Life Skills and Opportunities Curriculum* (*LSO*) (Baldwin-Grossman & Sipe, 1992); the Mathtech programs (Kirby, 1984); the *McMaster Teen Program* (Thomas et al., 1992); *Postponing Sexual Involvement* (*PSI*) (Howard & McCabe, 1990); *Reducing the Risk* (*RTR*) (Kirby et al., 1991);

the Schinke, Blythe, and Gilchrest curriculum (hereafter referred to as the Schinke curriculum) (Schinke et al., 1981); *Sex Respect* (Weed et al., 1992); *Teen Aid* (Weed et al., 1992); *Teen Talk* (Eisen, Zellman, & McAlister, 1990); and *Values and Choices* (Weed et al., 1992).

About half of these programs effectively reduced unprotected intercourse, either by delaying the onset of intercourse, increasing the use of condoms, or reducing the number of sexual partners; the other half did not. There are several common elements among the five effective programs that may be linked to their success. These programs:

- Used social learning theories as a foundation for program development (e.g., social-learning theory, cognitive–behavioral theory, social-influence theory).
- Included a narrow focus on reducing sexual risk-taking behaviors that may lead to HIV/STD infection and/or unintended pregnancy; relatively little time was spent addressing other sexuality issues, such as gender roles, dating, and parenthood.
- Used active learning methods of instruction. Students were actively involved in generating, obtaining, and/or sharing the information and they were involved in other experiential activities designed to personalize the information (e.g., games, videos, simulation activities, reviews of condoms in drug stores).
- Included activities that address the social and/or media influences and pressures to have sex. This took several forms. Some programs addressed media influences; others discussed "lines" that are typically used to get someone to have sex; whereas others discussed social barriers to using protection. In all programs, strategies for responding to these pressures were identified, discussed, and/or practiced.
- Focused upon and reinforced clear and appropriate values against unprotected sex (i.e., postponing sex, avoiding unprotected intercourse, using condoms, and avoiding high-risk partners). Critically, these values and norms were tailored for the age and sexual experience of the target population. The values or norms were reinforced throughout each curriculum in a variety of ways. All of the programs provided basic, accurate information about the risks of unprotected intercourse and methods of avoiding unprotected intercourse. A few programs provided accurate information on the rates of certain behaviors and/or acceptability of those behaviors to emphasize that "not everyone is doing it," as is often assumed by teens. In some programs students were guided through decision-making processes to reach appropriate conclusions about risk-taking behaviors. Students also identified "pressure lines" and then shared and modeled personal approaches for responding

to these lines. Finally, students participated in role-playing activities to further reinforce these norms.

- Provided modeling and practice of communication or negotiation skills. All of the effective programs devoted some time to skill development (i.e., communication, negotiation, and refusal skills). Typically, the programs provided information about the skills, modeled effective use of the skills, and then provided some type of skill rehearsal and practice (e.g., verbal role-playing and/or written practice). There was, however, significant variation in the quality and amount of time devoted to skill practice.

Despite these commonalities, there is very little evidence regarding which of these factors contributes most to the overall success of the programs.

There appear to be several characteristics that distinguish the effective programs from the ineffective ones. First, the ineffective curricula tend to be more comprehensive and less focused; that is, they cover a broader array of topics and discuss many values and skills, but they fail to emphasize those particular facts, values, norms, and skills necessary to avoid sex or unprotected sex.

Second, the less effective curricula tend to use a decision-making model in which the decision-making steps are taught; the model is applied to important decisions; and students are implicitly instructed to make their own decision. This approach is in contrast to the methods used in the effective curricula, which present a clear stand and emphasize clear behavioral values and norms.

The fact that all five of the effective programs focused upon specific behavioral values and norms, in combination with the fact that none of the ineffective programs did so, strongly suggests that this focus may be an especially important characteristic of effective programs.

SCHOOL-BASED PROGRAMS TO IMPROVE ACCESS TO CONTRACEPTIVES

As the problems of unintended teenage pregnancy and AIDS have gained greater prominence in our society, some schools have developed programs to directly improve access to contraceptives. The first such efforts were school-based clinics. These are health clinics located on school campuses that provide youths with a wide range of medical and counseling services including primary health care, physical examinations, laboratory tests, diagnosis and treatment of illness and minor injuries, immunizations, gynecological exams, birth control information and referral, pregnancy testing and counseling, nutrition education, weight reduction programs, and counseling for substance abuse. Some of them prescribe and dispense contraceptives. The first clinics opened in 1970; the first clinics to prescribe or dispense contraceptives did so in 1973. By 1993, more than four hundred clinics had been opened in high schools and middle schools throughout the country (Center for Population Option, 1993). According to a 1991 study of these clinics, more than 60% provided counseling, referral, or follow-up for family planning methods, about 28% wrote prescriptions for birth control pills, and fewer than 20% dispensed any type of contraceptive on site (Waszak & Neidell, 1991).

There has been relatively little research on the clinics' impact on student sexual behaviors, in part because most of the growth in school-based clinics has occurred in the last few years. A few studies, however, provide mixed evidence for the impact of clinics.

The most widely quoted findings are those based upon the St. Paul clinics. They reported substantial percentages of students using the clinics for reproductive health services and large decreases in birth rates (Edwards, Steinman, Arnold, & Hakanson, 1980). Subsequent analyses of improved birth rate data indicate, however, that the clinics did not significantly reduce birth rates (Kirby et al., 1993).

Additional evidence for the effectiveness of school-linked services was found in a study examining an experimental pregnancy prevention program that combined classroom presentations and small-group discussions in two inner-city Baltimore schools with reproductive health services provided to the students at a nearby clinic. Data indicated that after the program was implemented students in the program schools initiated intercourse later and were more likely to use contraception if they did have intercourse (Zabin, Hirsch, Smith, Street, & Hardy, 1986).

A more recent study of the impact of school-based clinics revealed that the clinics studied did not increase sexual activity and had varying effects upon contraceptive use (Kirby & Waszak, 1991). In one site where the clinic school focused upon high risk youth, emphasized pregnancy prevention, and dispensed birth control pills, there was a significantly greater use of birth control pills among females than in the comparison school. Unfortunately, there was not a significantly greater use of condoms. In two other sites which dispensed both condoms and oral contraceptives, there were no significant differences in the student use of condoms between the clinic schools and their comparison schools.

Because of the increasing threat of AIDS in some communities, schools are dispensing condoms even if they do not have school-based clinics. In the few short years since the idea of school condom availability has been seriously contemplated, more than three hundred schools throughout the country have decided to make condoms available and many more schools are currently considering condom availability programs (ETR, 1993). Furthermore, this idea has broad support; 68% of American adults have voiced support for condom availability in high schools (Roper Organization, 1991).

Supporters of school condom availability view it as a promising method of reducing unprotected sex. First, they believe that it may increase students' perceptions that other youth in school use condoms when they have intercourse, and that using condoms is the proper thing to do if having sex. Second, they believe that making condoms available in school may reduce barriers to availability such as discomfort, cost, and ease of access.

Unpublished data indicate that in some schools making condoms available, relatively small numbers of condoms are given to students and could not significantly affect schoolwide rates of condom use, while in other schools large numbers of condoms are, in fact, distributed to students and may reduce instances of unprotected intercourse. For example, a Santa Monica high school with approximately 2,700 students distributes 2,600 to 3,000 condoms per month (Rosenfield, personal communication, February 18, 1993). In six Baltimore schools with school-based clinics, between 100 and 600 condoms were distributed monthly to the students through the school-based health clinics (Rosenthal, personal communication, February 18, 1993). In Florida a school clinic distributed about 1,500 condoms per month to the 1,300 students in its school (Martin, personal communication, February 16, 1993). Given that many of the students in these schools have either never had sex or do not have intercourse each month, the condoms distributed through these schools have the potential for significantly reducing the amount of unprotected intercourse.

COMPREHENSIVE SCHOOL-BASED PROGRAMS

These research findings suggest that educational approaches with the characteristics described above and school condom availability may significantly reduce unprotected intercourse. Neither of these approaches alone, however, represents a complete solution to the problems of unprotected intercourse; many students in schools with these programs continue to engage in unprotected intercourse. More generally, no single approach is likely to produce a dramatic impact. Multiple components in a single school though may have either an additive or synergistic effect.

Few studies have evaluated such programs, but a San Francisco high school implemented a variety of components and was evaluated (Kirby & Waszak, 1991). In particular, it introduced a widely recognized educational component called the Wedge, which included both information about HIV/ AIDS and presentations in each class by a young person with AIDS. There were also after-school group sessions that dealt with sexual issues and a variety of schoolwide activities that heightened student consciousness about AIDS. Finally, the school opened a school-based clinic that did not dispense condoms, but did emphasize condom use and did provide students with a prescription that enabled them to get condoms anonymously and free of charge at a nearby community health clinic. Of course, all of this took place in a community where AIDS became very prominent and where there were many media and community activities that influenced a reduction in unprotected sexual activity. Over a two-year period there was a substantial increase in the percentage of males in the school who used condoms the last time they had sex. Although it is impossible to distinguish the impact of the school activities from community activities, it seems likely that the school activities contributed to the change.

PROGRAMMATIC RECOMMENDATIONS

As the tragedies of the AIDS epidemic continue to accumulate, it is very important to design, implement, and evaluate potentially effective programs. There are innumerable suggestions in the HIV prevention literature for improving the effectiveness of HIV prevention programs; for example, developing curricula that are developmentally appropriate; reaching youth early before risk-taking behaviors are initiated and become established; accepting teenagers' sexual behavior; discussing contraception in a straightforward manner; providing explicit education about safe sex; giving more emphasis to the risks of unprotected intercourse; providing complete information about HIV testing; involving parents in the instruction; providing counseling; and providing free condoms. Some of these changes may or may not improve the effectiveness of HIV prevention programs. Because it is costly in both dollars and time to implement all of these ideas, there needs to be some more compelling rationale for implementing particular approaches.

There are a few potentially effective approaches to determine which of these and other ideas may be most effective. First, program designers can address the reasons that adolescents provide for having unprotected sex. In numerous studies (Kirby & Waszak, 1991; Whitley & Schofield, 1985–1986), youth have most frequently cited two reasons for having sex without using birth control. First, they did not expect to have intercourse ("It just happened"). To counter this, effective programs must reduce the frequency of unexpected sex either by reducing the frequency of intercourse or increasing the expectedness of and the planning for intercourse. The second most important reason is that they didn't think pregnancy would occur—they felt invulnerable. Teens' perception of invulnerability to the risk of harmful outcomes has been well documented (Gruber & Chambers, 1987; Weinstein, 1984).

A very real problem for AIDS education is that for most teenagers the probability of having sex with someone infected with the HIV virus is quite small, and the probability of their actually contracting the HIV virus from that person is smaller still. Because teenagers, like adults, have difficulty making decisions when probabilities are very small, they are less likely to change their behavior, even when they have been given accurate information. This is especially likely given that many young people *overestimate* the number of cases of AIDS in this country and *overestimate* the chances of getting AIDS from a single unprotected act of heterosexual intercourse (Freimuth, Edgar, & Hammond, 1987). Thus, exposure to more correct estimates may logically reduce their concern, not increase it. In addition, numerous studies in psychology and health education have demonstrated that people are less likely to avoid a risk when the negative consequences are remote—both unlikely and in the distant future (U.S. General Accounting Office, 1988).

This problem may be partially overcome by providing more certain and more immediate positive rewards for avoiding unprotected sex. These rewards probably need to be symbolic in the form of social approval for avoiding risks. This, of course, requires changing peer norms. Reducing both the frequency of unplanned intercourse and perceptions of invulnerability is a challenging task; nevertheless these goals should provide new direction for AIDS education programs.

Another potentially effective means for determining which programmatic ideas may be effective is to employ a risk-factor approach which attempts to identify the factors associated with risk-taking behavior and, more importantly, those factors which reinforce health-promoting behaviors. The history of implementing risk-factor approaches indicates that this approach has been effective in other adolescent risk-taking areas. For example, neither smoking education nor drug education were effective when they emphasized knowledge, but when programs focused upon those factors that were both related to the smoking and drug behaviors and amenable to change, programs became substantially more effective.

One important risk factor which is related to condom use and is amenable to change is perceived referent-group norms (Fisher, 1988; Fisher & Fisher, 1992; Fisher & Misovich, 1990; Fisher, Misovich, Fisher, 1992). Adolescents are strongly affected by their perception of peer norms regarding consistent condom use (DiClemente & Fisher, under review; DiClemente, 1991, 1992b; Walter et al., 1992). In one recent study, DiClemente & Fisher (under review) tested the relative explanatory ability of a social influence model compared with a behavioral–demographic model. The findings indicate that social influence factors (perceived peer norms regarding condom use and communicating with sex partners about AIDS) significantly increased the power of the model to classify a school-based sample of sexually active adolescents into their self-reported condom use categories by 76%. Furthermore, adolescents who perceived peer norms as supporting condom use were more than four times as likely to be consistent condom users. This suggests that modifying adolescents' perceptions of peer norms in a proprevention direction can be a crucial factor in helping establish safer sex behavior as normative.

The importance of changing peer norms is also supported by the review of effective and ineffective programs which demonstrated that in contrast to the ineffective programs, all the effective programs emphasized clear values and attempted to change norms.

There are a variety of ways to change peer norms. One way is to use respected peers to support HIV prevention norms to students. Though largely untested with respect to modifying HIV risk behaviors, the importance of peer support in changing other risky behavior has been reported in the adolescent substance prevention literature (Botvin, 1986; Hansen & Graham, 1991; Klepp, Halper, & Perry, 1986; Perry & Grant, 1988; Robinson, Killen, Taylor et al., 1987; Telch, Miller, Killen, Cooke, 1990). While peer-assisted interventions have been used effectively to prevent and, with less efficacy, to modify adolescents' substance use (e.g., cigarettes, alcohol, marijuana), these strategies have not been adequately applied or evaluated with respect to changing adolescents' HIV-related sexual risk behaviors.

Another way to improve peer norms is to provide accurate information to the students on the rates of certain behaviors and/or acceptability of those behaviors. Typically these data demonstrate that "not everyone is doing it," as is often assumed by teens, and that most youth believe that condoms should be used during intercourse. Yet another way to improve norms is to guide students in small groups through group decision-making processes to reach appropriate conclusions about risk-taking behaviors. Finally, identifying "pressure lines" and sharing responses and both modeling and practicing role-plays can also reinforce norms. At the very least, these activities may give students the support or "permission" they need to feel comfortable using the strategies outside the classroom.

Another risk factor that is related to unprotected intercourse is perceived self-efficacy in avoiding sex or using condoms. It seems likely that actual ability to avoid sex or use condoms would also be related to these behaviors, but because of the difficulty of measuring these abilities, these relationships have not been empirically examined. The review of effective and ineffective curricula indicated that curricula which modeled refusal and assertiveness skills and then provided sufficient practice through role-playing in these skills were more likely to be effective than the curricula which did not do so (Kirby & Coyle, 1994).

Many past HIV/AIDS education programs have lasted for only four hours. Although well-crafted four-hour programs may have some impact upon behavior, four hours is not sufficient time in which to substantially change norms, skills, and perceived self-efficacy in those skills. Thus, effective HIV education programs need to be longer. One way to increase their length and potential effectiveness is to embed them within longer, more comprehensive sexuality education programs.

Integrating pregnancy prevention, STD prevention, and HIV pregnancy has an additional advantage. At least two studies have demonstrated that the majority of students who use condoms do so primarily to prevent pregnancy and not to prevent HIV transmission. Thus, by emphasizing both pregnancy prevention and HIV prevention, curricula may have a greater impact than if only one of the goals is emphasized.

A caveat is in order at this point. This integration can also diminish the effectiveness of the HIV program if the sexuality education program is too broad and too unfocused. The review of the studies above indicated that it is important to maintain a clear focus and a clear message. This can be done in a sexuality education program, such as *Reducing the Risk,* that emphasizes the avoidance of unprotected intercourse.

In the past, people and institutions concerned with HIV transmission have not joined forces with those concerned with pregnancy prevention. This has had at least three negative consequences; (1) it prevented HIV educators from quickly learning from the mistakes made and lessons learned in sex education; (2) it constrained HIV education to a small number of hours of instruction; and (3) it prevented using pregnancy prevention to reinforce condom use. It is past time to more fully integrate the two areas of instruction so that curricula can more adequately change norms, skills, and self-efficacy.

RESEARCH RECOMMENDATIONS

To achieve progress in the field of school-based behavioral interventions more quickly and with greater confidence, more rigorous standards must be applied to the evaluation of HIV prevention programs. Limitations in the design of programmatic evaluations have reduced the ability to identify and adequately assess the effectiveness of interventions to modify risk behaviors. Below are several critical issues which directly affect the ability to detect programmatic effect and the quality of the research data.

Statistical Power

One major limitation which decreases the ability to detect programmatic effect is sample size. Selection of the appropriate sample size needs to be determined prior to the evaluation, using power analytic methods. These calculations should recognize the analyses of subsamples that must be conducted. For example, when examining behavior, samples typically must be divided into youth who are sexually inexperienced at the beginning of the study, youth who are sexually experienced at that time, and youth who initiated intercourse during the study. In a study by Siegel, DiClemente, Durbin, Krasnovsky, and Saliba (under review), the authors found that the magnitude of changes in behavior were comparable to the significant changes in knowledge and attitudes toward persons living with AIDS, but the changes in behavior were not statistically significant, in large part, because the sample of sexually active adolescents represented only about one-quarter of the total sample. This problem occurs frequently and limits our understanding of program impact upon behavior.

Randomization

Individual students, classrooms, or entire schools should be randomly assigned to the intervention and control conditions. If programs are schoolwide and may affect all students, then entire schools should be randomized to intervention and control conditions, and then either schools should be used as the unit of analysis or multilevel statistics should be used. It is not proper to use students as the unit of analysis when schools are randomly assigned to treatment and control groups.

Long-Term Follow-Up

Too many studies follow students for only three months after the pretest or after the intervention. This is an insufficient amount of time in which to measure possible degradation in program effect. It is also insufficient time in which to measure actual behavioral change. For example, in most studies much more than three months is needed for a sufficient proportion of the control group to initiate intercourse and for the difference in the program and control group proportions to be statistically significant. In the evaluation of *Reducing the Risk,* significant effects in sexual initiation appeared at 18 months that were not yet significant at 6 months. Thus, the appropriate follow-up period should be determined prior to the evaluation, and study participants tracked for sufficient periods of time.

Selection of Appropriate Outcome Measures

In general, the objective of most HIV prevention programs should be to reduce and/or eliminate risk behaviors. If the goal of the program directly targets reduction in risk behaviors, then these behaviors need to be assessed. Adequate assessment requires use of measurement instruments which are culturally, linguistically, and developmentally appropriate for the target population. Moreover, efforts must be taken to insure that social desirability biases are minimized when inquiring about sensitive behaviors such as sexual intercourse and drug use.

CONCLUSION

This is a historic time in the history of research to reduce unprotected intercourse among adolescents. First, there now exists strong evidence that some theory-based and school-based interventions, such as the *Reducing the Risk* curriculum, do reduce unprotected intercourse among at least some groups of youth. This is very encouraging. Second, there are emerging enough good studies of individual prevention programs so that researchers can assess which curricula and approaches are most effective with different groups of youth. Clearly there is much yet to be learned and much to be done, but we now have more evaluation research on which to base our thinking.

Past research indicates that HIV education programs, in combination with other sources of information, especially the media, have significantly increased adolescents' knowledge about HIV and reduced the prevalence of commonly held myths and misconceptions about disease transmission. This important role should not be minimized as there is evidence to indicate that reducing misconceptions about casual contact among adolescents results in increased tolerance toward those individuals infected with HIV or who have AIDS (Siegel et al., under review). And, of course, this greater knowledge has undoubtedly caused many youth to use condoms or otherwise avoid unprotected intercourse with some partners.

While surveys indicate that most adolescents now know the basic facts about the transmission of HIV (Anderson & Christenson, 1991; DiClemente, 1990; Hingson & Strunin, 1992) there is a growing belief that knowledge about HIV is no longer related to risk-taking behavior (DiClemente, 1990, 1992; Stevenson & DeBord, 1988) or only weakly related to risk-taking behaviors (Anderson et al., 1990) and that HIV prevention programs are not likely to produce greater reductions in risk-taking behavior unless they do substantially more than increase knowledge (DiClemente et al., 1987; Greico, 1987).

Research also supports additional conclusions. Even though some youth, particularly youth at higher risk of becoming HIV infected, drop out of school, and even though some conservative communities constrain the development of potentially effective HIV prevention programs, schools are nevertheless a promising institution through which to reach youth. There are programs in many classrooms which reach youth before they drop out of school and which effectively reduce unprotected intercourse.

These programs do have programmatically and statistically significant effects upon behavior. They share several common characteristics: (1) they have a theoretical grounding in one or more variations of social-learning theory; (2) they focus narrowly on reducing sexual risk-taking behaviors; (3) they use active learning methods of instruction to convey information on the risks of unprotected sex and how to avoid those risks; (4) they include experiential activities on social influences and pressures; (5) they reinforce individual values and group norms against unprotected sex; and (6) they model and provide at least a minimum of practice in social skills to avoid unprotected intercourse. Because of the demonstrated success of these programs, they should be implemented more broadly throughout the country.

Programs which do all of these things adequately must last more than four hours; thus, many programs either need to be lengthened or integrated into sexuality education programs that are also focused upon reducing unprotected intercourse.

Finally, there is limited evidence indicating that programs which reinforce classroom instruction with schoolwide activities, with access to condoms or with reproductive health counseling and services may have a greater impact.

Despite the successes of these programs, there do not currently exist any evaluated programs which reduce unprotected intercourse to an acceptable level. Thus, there remains a great need both for the development of more effective programs and for rigorous research on the behavioral impact of these programs, particularly in ethnically diverse communities. Only by systematically monitoring programmatic developments and outcome evaluations and providing for timely feedback of information to program planners, can school-based HIV prevention programs achieve their ultimate objective, the reduction of risk behaviors associated with HIV transmission.

REFERENCES

Anderson, J. E., Kann, L., Holtzman, D., Arday, S., Truman, B., & Kolbe, L. (1990). HIV/AIDS knowledge and sexual behavior among high school students. *Family Planning Perspectives, 22,* 252–255.

Anderson, M. D., & Christenson, G. M. (1991). Ethnic breakdown of AIDS related knowledge and attitudes from the National Adolescent Student Health Survey. *Journal of Health Education, 22,* 30–34.

Ashworth, C. S., DuRant, R. H., Newman, C., & Gaillard, G. (1992). An evaluation of a school-based AIDS/HIV education program for high school students. *Journal of Adolescent Health, 13,* 582–588.

Baldwin-Grossman, J., & Sipe, C. (1992). *Life skills and opportunities curriculum—Summer training and education program. Report on long-term impacts.* Philadelphia, PA: Public/ Private Ventures.

Barth, R. (1989). *Reducing the risk: Building skills to prevent pregnancy.* Santa Cruz, CA: Network Publications.

Botvin, G. (1986). Substance abuse prevention research: Recent developments and future directions. *Journal of School Health, 56,* 369–373.

Bowler, S., Sheon, A. R., D'Angelo, L. J., & Vermund, S. H. (1993). HIV and AIDS among adolescents in the United States: increasing risk in the 1990s. *Journal of Adolescence, 15,* 345–371.

Burke, D. S., Brundage, J. F., Goldenbaum, M., Gardner, L. I., Peterson, M., Visintine, R., Redfield, R. R., & the Walter Reed Retro Virus Research Group (1990). Human immunodeficiency virus infections in teenagers. *Journal of the American Medical Association, 263:* 2074–2077.

Centers for Disease Control & Prevention. (1991a). Premarital sexual experience among adolescent women, United States, 1970–1988. *Morbidity and Mortality Weekly Report, 39,* 929.

Centers for Disease Control & Prevention. (1991b, June). *HIV/AIDS Surveillance Report.* Atlanta, GA: Author.

Centers for Disease Control & Prevention. (1992). Sexual behavior among high school students— United States, 1990. *Morbidity and Mortality Weekly Report, 40,* 885–888.

Centers for Disease Control & Prevention. (1993). *HIV/AIDS Surveillance Report,* April 5. Atlanta, GA: Author.

Centers for Disease Control & Prevention. (1990). *National HIV Seroprevalence Surveys: Summary of Results.* Atlanta, GA: Author.

Centers for Disease Control & Prevention. (1989). *Annual Report.* Atlanta, GA: Author.

Center for Population Options (1993). *Links.* Spring/Summer.

Christopher, S., & Roosa, M. (1990). An evaluation of an adolescent pregnancy prevention program: Is "Just Say No" enough? *Family Relations, 39:* 68–72.

Dawson, D. (1986). The effects of sex education on adolescent behavior. *Family Planning Perspectives, 18,* 162–170.

Department of Health & Human Services. (1990). *Healthy People 2000: National Health Promotion and Disease Prevention.* Washington, DC: Author.

DiClemente, R. J. (1989). Prevention of human immunodeficiency virus infection among adolescents: The interplay of health education and public policy in the development and implementation of school-based AIDS educations programs. *Journal of AIDS Education & Prevention, 1,* 70–78.

DiClemente, R. J. (1990). The emergence of adolescents as a risk group for human immunodeficiency virus infection. *Journal of Adolescent Research, 5,* 7–17.

DiClemente, R. J. (1991). Predictors of HIV-preventive sexual behavior in a high-risk adolescent population: The influence of perceived peer norms and sexual communication on incarcerated adolescents' consistent use of condoms. *Journal of Adolescent Health, 12,* 385–390.

DiClemente, R. J. (1992a). Epidemiology of AIDS, HIV seroprevalence and HIV incidence among adolescents. *Journal of School Health, 62,* 325–330.

DiClemente, R. J. (1992b). Psychosocial determinants of condom use among adolescents. In R. J. DiClemente (Ed.), *Adolescents and AIDS: A generation in jeopardy* (pp. 34–51). Newbury Park, CA: Sage.

DiClemente, R. J. (1993). Confronting the challenge of AIDS among adolescents: Directions for future research. *Journal of Adolescent Research, 8,* 156–166.

DiClemente, R. J., Boyer, C. B., & Mills, S. (1987). Prevention of AIDS among adolescents: Strategies for the development of comprehensive risk-reduction health education programs. *Health Education Research, 2,* 287–291.

DiClemente, R. J., & Fisher, J. D. (under review). Factors associated with consistent condom use among adolescents in an HIV epicenter: Test of a social influence model.

Donahue, M. (1987). *Technical report of the national demonstration project field test of human sexuality: Values and choices.* Minneapolis, MN: Search Institute.

Edwards, L., Steinman, M., Arnold, K., & Hakanson, E. (1980). Adolescent pregnancy prevention services in high school clinics, *Family Planning Perspectives,* 12:6–14.

Eisen, M., Zellman, G. L., & McAlister, A. L. (1990). Evaluating the impact of a theory-based sexuality and contraceptive education program. *Family Planning Perspectives, 22,* 262.

ETR (1993). Working papers.

Farley, T. A., Pomputius, P. F., Sabella, W., Helgerson, S. D., & Hadler, J. L. (1991). Evaluation of the effect of school-based education on adolescents' AIDS knowledge and attitudes. *Connecticut Medicine, 55,* 15–18.

Fisher, J. (1988). Possible effects of reference group-based social influence on AIDS-risk behavior and AIDS prevention. *American Psychologist, 43,* 914–920.

Fisher, J. D., & Fisher, W. A. (1992). Changing AIDS risk behavior. *Psychological Bulletin, 111,* 455–474.

Fisher, J. D., & Misovich, S. J. (1990). Social influence and AIDS-Preventive Behavior. In J. Edwards, R. S. Tindale, & L. Heath, (Eds.), *Social influence processes and prevention* (pp. 39–70). New York: Plenum Press.

Fisher, J. D., Misovich, S. J., & Fisher, W. A. (1992). Impact of perceived social norms on adolescents' AIDS-risk behavior and prevention. In R. J. DiClemente (Ed.), *Adolescents and AIDS: A generation in jeopardy* (pp. 117–138). Newbury Park, CA: Sage.

Freimuth, V., Edgar, T., & Hammond, S. (1987). College students' awareness and interpretation of the AIDS risk. *Science, Technology & Human Values, 12.*

Furstenberg, F., Moore, K., & Peterson, J. (1985). Sex education and sexual experience among adolescents. *American Journal of Public Health, 75,* 1331–1332.

Greico, A. (1987). Cutting the risks for STDs. *Medical Aspects of Human Sexuality, 21,* 70–84.

Gruber, E., & Chambers, C. V. (1987). Cognitive development and adolescent contraception: Integrating theory and practice. *Adolescence, 22,* 661–670.

Hansen, W. B., & Graham, J. W. (1991). Preventing alcohol, marijuana and cigarette use among adolescents: Peer pressure resistance training versus establishing conservative norms. *Preventive Medicine, 20,* 414–430.

Hein, K. (1992). Adolescents at risk for HIV infection. In R. J. DiClemente (Ed.), *Adolescents and AIDS: A generation in jeopardy* (pp. 3–16). Newbury Park, CA: Sage.

Hingson, R., & Strunin, L. (1992). Monitoring adolescent's response to the AIDS epidemic: Changes in knowledge, attitudes, beliefs and behaviors. In R. J. DiClemente (Ed.), *Adolescents and AIDS: A generation in jeopardy* (pp. 17–33). Newbury Park, CA: Sage.

Hoch, L. (1971). Attitude change as a result of sex education. *Journal of Research in Science Teaching, 8,* 363–367.

Howard, M., & McCabe, J. (1990). Helping teenagers postpone sexual involvement. *Family Planning Perspectives, 22,* 21–26.

Huszti, H. C., Clopton, J. R., & Mason, P. G. (1989). Effects of an AIDS educational program on adolescents' knowledge and attitudes. *Pediatrics, 84,* 986–991.

Imber, M. (1982). Toward a theory of curriculum reform: An analysis of the first campaign for sex education. *Curriculum Inquiry.* 12:4, 339–362.

Iverson, D. C., & Kolbe, L. J. (1983). Evaluation of the national disease prevention and health promotion strategy: Establishing a role for the schools. *Journal of School Health, 53,* 294–302.

Kelley, P. W., Miller, R. N., Pomerantz, R., Wann, F., Brundage, J. F., & Burke, D. S. (1990). Human immunodeficiency virus seropositivity among members of the active duty US Army. *American Journal of Public Health.* 80:405–410.

Kirby, D. (1984). *Sexuality education: An evaluation of programs and their effects.* Santa Cruz, CA: Network Publications.

Kirby, D., Barth, R. P., Leland, N., & Fetro, J. V. (1991). Reducing the risk: Impact of a new curriculum on sexual risk-taking. *Family Planning Perspectives, 23,* 253–262.

Kirby, D., & Coyle, K. (1994). Changing risk-taking behavior: Preliminary conclusions from research. In J. Drolet & K. Clark, (Eds.), *The sexuality education challenge.* Santa Cruz, CA: ETR Publications.

Kirby, D., Resnick, M. D., Downes, B., Kocher, T., Gunderson, P., Potthoff, S., Zelterman, D., & Blum, R. W. (1993). The effects of school-based health clinics in St. Paul on school-wide birth rates. *Family Planning Perspectives, 25,* 12–16.

Kirby, D., & Waszak, C. (1991). Six school-based clinics: Their reproductive health services and impact on sexual behavior. *Family Planning Perspectives, 23,* 6–16.

Klepp, K. I., Halper, A., & Perry, C. L. (1986). The efficacy of peer leaders in drug abuse prevention. *Journal of School Health, 56,* 407–411.

Ku, L. C., Sonenstein, F. L., & Pleck, J. H. (1992). The association of AIDS education and sex education with sexual behavior and condom use among teenage men. *Family Planning Perspectives, 24,* 100–106.

Marsiglio, W., & Mott, F. (1986). The impact of sex education on sexual activity, contraceptive use and premarital pregnancy among American teenagers. *Family Planning Perspectives, 18,* 151–162.

Miller, L., & Downer, A. (1988). AIDS: What you and your friends need to know—A lesson plan for adolescents. *Journal of School Health, 58,* 137–141.

Parcel, G., & Luttman, D. (1980). Effects of sex education on sexual attitudes. *Journal of Current Adolescent Medicine, 2,* 38–46.

Parcel, G., & Luttman, D. (1981). Evaluation of a sex education course for young adolescents. *Family Relations, 30,* 55–60.

Perry, C. L., & Grant, M. (1988). Comparing peer-led to teacher-led youth alcohol education in four countries. *Alcohol Health Research World, 12,* 322–326.

Rickert, V., Gottleib, A., & Jay, M. (1990). A comparison of three clinic-based AIDS education programs on female adolescents' knowledge, attitudes, and behavior. *Journal of Adolescent Health, 11,* 298–303.

Robinson, T. N., Killen, J. D., Taylor, B., Kelch, M., Bryson, S. W., Saylor, K. E., Maron, D. J., Maccoby, N., & Farguhar, J. W. (1987). Perspectives on adolescent substance abuse. *Journal of the American Medical Association, 258,* 2072–2076.

Roosa, M., & Christopher, S. (1990). Evaluation of an abstinence-only adolescent pregnancy prevention program: A replication. *Family Relations, 39,* 363–367.

The Roper Organization, Inc. (1991). *AIDS: Public Attitudes and Education Needs.* New York: Author.

Schinke, S., Blythe, B., & Gilchrest, L. (1981). Cognitive-behavioral prevention of adolescent pregnancy. *Journal of Counseling Psychology, 28,* 451–454.

Siegel, D., DiClemente, R. J., Durbin, M., Krasnovsky, F., & Saliba, P. (under review). Change in junior high school students' AIDS related knowledge, misconceptions, attitudes, and HIV-preventive behaviors: Effects of a school-based intervention.

Sonenstein, F. L., Pleck, J. H., & Ku, L. C. (1989). Sexual activity, condom use and AIDS awareness among adolescent males. *Family Planning Perspectives, 21,* 152–158.

Stevenson, M. R., & DeBord, K. (1988). *AIDS awareness: Will knowledge of the facts change behavior?* Paper presented at the meetings of the Society for the Scientific Study of Sex, Chicago, IL.

Telch, M. J., Miller, L. M., Killen, J. D., Cooke, S., & Maccoby, M. (1990). Social influences approach to smoking prevention: The effects of videotape delivery with and without same-age peer leader participation. *Addictive Behavior, 15,* 21–28.

Thomas, B., Mitchell, A., Devlin, M., Goldsmith, C., Singer, J., & Watters, D. (1992). Small group sex education at school: The McMaster teen program. In B. Miller, J. Card, R. Paikoff, & J. Peterson, (Eds.), *Preventing adolescent pregnancy* (pp. 28–52). Newbury Park, CA: Sage.

U.S. General Accounting Office. (1988). *AIDS education: Reaching populations at higher risk.* Washington, DC: Author.

Walter, H. J., & Vaughn, R. D. (1993). AIDS risk reduction among a multi-ethnic sample of urban high school students. *Journal of the American Medical Association 270*(6), 725–730.

Walter, H. J., Vaughn, R. D., Gladis, M. M., Ragin, D. F., Kasen, S., & Cohall, A. T. (1992). Factors associated with AIDS risk behavior among high school students in an AIDS epicenter. *American Journal of Public Health, 82,* 528–532.

Waszak, C., & Neidell, S. (1991). *School-based and school-linked clinics: Update 1991.* Washington DC Center for Population Options.

Weed, S., & Olsen, J. (1988). *Evaluation of the sex respect program: Results for the 1987–88 school year.* Salt Lake City, UT: The Institute for Research and Evaluation.

Weed, S. E., Olsen, J. A., DeGaston, J., & Prigmore, J. (1992). *Predicting and Changing Teen Sexual Activity Rates: A Comparison of Three Title XX Programs* (Report to the Office of Adolescent Pregnancy Programs). Washington, DC: DHHS.

Weinstein, N. D. (1984). Why it won't happen to me: Perceptions of risk factors and susceptibility. *Health Psychology, 3,* 431–457.

Whitley, B. E. Jr., & Schofield, J. W. (1985–1986). Meta-analysis of research on adolescent contraceptive use. *Population & Environment, 8,* 173–203.

Yarber, W. (1986). *Pilot testing and evaluation of the CDC-sponsored STD curriculum.* Bloomington: Indiana University, Center for Health and Safety Studies.

Zabin, L. S., Hirsh, M. B., Smith, E. A., Street, R., & Hardy, J. B. (1986). Evaluation of a pregnancy prevention program for urban teenagers. *Family Planning Perspectives, 18,* 119–126.

Zelnik, M., & Kim, Y. (1982). Sex education and its association with teenage sexual activity, pregnancy, and contraceptive use. *Family Planning Perspectives, 16,* 117–126.

8

Interventions for Adolescents in Community Settings

JOHN B. JEMMOTT III and
LORETTA SWEET JEMMOTT

INTRODUCTION

Although in the United States the largest number of reported cases of acquired immunodeficiency syndrome (AIDS) have involved white men who engaged in same-gender sexual activities, a confluence of evidence suggests that inner-city African-American adolescents are at risk for infection with human immunodeficiency virus (HIV). It may be possible to reduce the risk of AIDS among inner-city African-American adolescents by identifying the key HIV risk-associated behaviors in this population, the intervention-sensitive conceptual variables that determine those behaviors, and the most effective behavior-change intervention strategies. In this chapter, we will summarize and review critically the literature on interventions to reduce the risk of HIV infection among adolescents in community settings.

HIV RISK-ASSOCIATED SEXUAL BEHAVIOR AMONG AFRICAN AMERICANS

In this section, we review the literature on the extent to which the sexual practices of African-American adolescents contribute to risk of HIV infection.

JOHN B. JEMMOTT III • Department of Psychology, Princeton University, Princeton, New Jersey 08544.   *LORETTA SWEET JEMMOTT* • College of Nursing, Rutgers, The State University of New Jersey, Newark, New Jersey 07112.

Preventing AIDS: Theories and Methods of Behavioral Interventions, edited by Ralph J. DiClemente and John L. Peterson. Plenum Press, New York, 1994.

Epidemiological studies have identified behaviors that increase risk of sexually transmitted infection (Hatcher et al., 1990), and these behaviors are risky with respect to HIV infection. In general, HIV risk-associated sexual behaviors are those sexual activities that involve the exchange of semen, vaginal secretions, or blood. This would include sexual (vaginal) or anal intercourse that is unprotected (i.e., intercourse without the use of a latex condom), sexual involvement with many partners, and sexual involvement with partners who engage in high-risk behaviors such as injection drug use. Of course, the only way to eliminate the possibility of sexually transmitted HIV infection is to practice abstinence. However, avoiding these high-risk sexual behaviors should substantially decrease the chances of HIV infection.

In general, there are scant data on the prevalence of sexual behaviors other than coitus and contraceptive usage among blacks. Data on black adolescent men are particularly limited. This is problematic because adolescent men are often initiators of sexual activity with their female partners and because the latex condom, the best currently available method of preventing sexually transmitted HIV infection, must be worn by men. Indeed, unprotected coitus is perhaps the most common HIV risk-associated behavior among heterosexuals. Studies suggest that substantial numbers of African-American adolescents engage in unprotected coitus.

Failure to Use Condoms during Coitus

More than two-thirds of American adolescents have had sexual intercourse by the time they are 19 years of age (Centers for Disease Control, 1991; Sonenstein, Pleck, & Ku, 1989). National surveys of adolescents consistently have indicated that a greater proportion of African Americans than whites or Latinos report having had sexual intercourse (Centers for Disease Control, 1991; Hofferth & Hayes, 1987; Pratt, Mosher, Backrach, & Horn, 1984; Sonenstein et al., 1989; Taylor Kagay, & Leichenko, 1986). In part, the greater reports of sexual experience among African-American adolescents may be attributed to socioeconomic background. On average, rates of poverty and low socioeconomic background, which are associated with early sexual experience, are greater among African-American adolescents than among white adolescents. However, some studies have found greater reports of sexual intercourse among African-American adolescents even when socioeconomic background was controlled statistically (Hofferth, Kahn, & Baldwin, 1987).

Although the use of latex condoms can substantially reduce the risk of sexually transmitted disease (STD) (Centers for Disease Control, 1988; Stone, Grimes, & Magder, 1986), it seems clear that many sexually active adolescents do not use condoms consistently (Hingson, Strunin, Berlin, & Heeren, 1990; Jemmott & Jemmott, 1990; Keller et al., 1991; Sonenstein et al., 1989). Statistics on STD and unintended pregnancy document the consequences of unprotected sexual intercourse among adolescents. In general, rates of syphilis, gonorrhea, and hospitalization for pelvic inflammatory disease have been highest among adolescents and have declined exponentially with age (Bell & Holmes, 1984). But inner-city African-American adolescents are particularly at risk: STDs are two to three times more common among low-income people who reside in urban areas than among people of higher income or those who live in suburban or rural areas (Cates, 1987; Hatcher et al., 1990; Jones et al., 1986; Pratt et al., 1984). In addition, the adolescent pregnancy rate is nearly twice as high among African-American adolescents as among white adolescents. The juxtaposition of elevated pregnancy rates and the potential for perinatally transmitted HIV infection (Centers for Disease Control, 1993) also suggests the urgency of intervening with African-American adolescents.

More direct evidence of the high prevalence of unprotected coitus among African-American adolescents comes from national surveys of contraceptive utilization (Mosher & Pratt, 1990; Sonenstein et al., 1989). In general, the first contraceptive methods that adolescents use are male methods, including not only the condom, but also the method that is especially risky from the perspective of HIV infection, withdrawal before ejaculation. As adolescents grow older and more sexually experienced, their use of female methods, particularly the contraceptive pill, becomes more common (Jemmott & Jemmott, 1990; Pleck, 1989). Thus, as adolescents grow older, their risk of pregnancy declines, but their risk of sexually transmitted infection may increase. Failure to use condoms is especially likely among younger adolescents (Pratt et al., 1984; Taylor et al., 1986; Zelnik, Kantner, & Ford, 1981). Inasmuch as younger adolescents who are having sexual intercourse for the first time are particularly unlikely to use condoms or any other contraception (Zelnik et al., 1981), and African-American adolescents are likely to have sexual experience at a younger age, it is not surprising that African-Americans are less likely than are whites to use condoms or any contraception at first coitus.

It has been suggested that awareness of the AIDS epidemic may be having an ameliorative impact on condom use. Sonenstein et al. (1989) found that 58% of sexually active 17- to 19-year-old black and white male adolescents living in metropolitan areas in 1988 reported using condoms the last time they had coitus. This represents a substantial increase from 1979 levels, when only 21% of 17- to 19-year-old black and white male adolescents living in metropolitan areas reported condom use at last coitus.

Noncoital Sexual Behaviors

Research on sexual behavior, for the most part, has focused on coitus with the aim of understanding fertility. Consequently, little is known about the dynamics of noncoital sexual behaviors such as anal intercourse and oral sex. This is unfortunate because the behavior associated with the most well-documented risk for sexual transmission of HIV is noncoital: namely, unprotected receptive anal intercourse. Although anal intercourse is chiefly associated with homosexual men, there is growing recognition that it is a fairly common practice among heterosexuals (Reinisch, Sanders, & Ziemba-Davis, 1988). Indeed, of all men who have engaged in anal intercourse, a greater percentage may have had such experience with women than with other men. Much better data are available on the noncoital sexual behaviors of white middle-class, well-educated individuals than on the noncoital sexual behaviors of other populations, but the available evidence suggests that these behaviors may be somewhat less common among blacks than among whites. Drawing on data from seven studies, Reinisch et al. (1988) estimated that 39% (range = 20%–43%) of white middle-class women had ever participated in anal intercourse. In contrast, a study of black college students at an east coast university revealed a relatively low incidence of anal intercourse among black women. Only 10% of black women reported ever experiencing anal intercourse (Thomas, Gilliam, & Iwrey, 1989). In a similar vein, Jemmott and Jemmott (1991) found that only 16% of black female undergraduates at a university in an inner-city area of New Jersey reported ever experiencing anal intercourse. One of the few studies to compare noncoital sexual behaviors in blacks and whites was Wyatt, Peters, and Guthrie's (1988a, 1988b) study of women ages 18 to 36 years in the Los Angeles area. The study revealed that 21% of black women, as compared with 43% of a matched sample of white women, reported having ever experienced anal intercourse.

As in the case of anal intercourse, evidence suggests tentatively that although oral sex is common among both blacks and whites, it may be less common among blacks. For instance, studying college students, Belcastro (1985) found that reports of ever engaging in heterosexual oral sex were lower among black men and women than among their white counterparts. About 48% of the black women, as compared with 81% of the white women, reported having engaged in fellatio. In addition, 34% of black women, as compared with 50% of white women, reported having engaged in cunnilingus with a man. Among male students, blacks (50%) were less likely to report having engaged in cunnilingus than were whites (72%), although they were only nonsignificantly less likely to report experiencing heterosexual fellatio. Wyatt et al. (1988a, 1988b) also found evidence of less oral sex among blacks: 87% of white women and 70% of black women reported ever engaging in cunnilingus with a man, and 93% of white women, but only 65% of black women reported ever engaging in fellatio.

In summary, these data suggest that although black adolescents may engage in a range of HIV risk-associated sexual behaviors, the chief sexual risk behavior is the failure to use condoms during sexual intercourse. The key to risk of exposure to HIV and other sexually transmitted diseases is not simply frequency of sexual intercourse or frequency of condom use, but the frequency of unprotected coitus. Thus, the high rate of sexual intercourse among inner-city black adolescents must be viewed in light of their relatively low rates of condom use. A high rate of sexual intercourse would be less worrisome if condoms were used each time. A low rate of condom use would be less worrisome if the person had sexual intercourse only rarely. It is the combination—high rates of intercourse coupled with low rates of condom use—that is potentially deadly. It is the combination that heightens risk of exposure to HIV.

To be sure, adolescents currently represent less than 1% of all reported AIDS cases in the United States (Centers for Disease Control, 1993). But this statistic may underestimate the potential for HIV infection among adolescents. Young adults in their twenties constitute 20% of all AIDS cases, and because several years typically elapse between the time a person is infected with HIV and the appearance of clinical signs sufficient to warrant a diagnosis of AIDS, many of these young adults were infected during adolescence. The prevalence of injection drug use in the inner city also heightens the risk of HIV infection for African-American adolescent residents. Although the adolescents themselves may not use injection drugs—indeed some data (Turner, Miller, & Moses, 1989) indicate that injection drug use among adolescents is rare—they may have unprotected sex with injection drug users or with individuals who have had unprotected sex with such potentially infected persons. The fact that increasing percentages of adolescents are reporting use of condoms is encouraging. It raises the prospect that condom use is malleable and may be subject to influence by HIV risk-reduction interventions.

INTERVENTIONS TO REDUCE HIV RISK-ASSOCIATED BEHAVIOR AMONG INNER-CITY AFRICAN-AMERICAN ADOLESCENTS

Although relatively few studies have tested HIV risk-reduction interventions on black adolescents, studies on white gay men and black adult men undergoing treatment of STDs suggest that HIV risk-reduction interventions may increase self-reported procurement and use of condoms and decrease self-reported number of sexual partners (e.g., Coates, McKusick, Kuno, & Stites, 1989; Kelly, St. Lawrence, Hood, & Brasfield, 1989; Kelly et al., 1991; Solomon & DeJong, 1989; Valdiserri, Lyter et al., 1989). These studies raise the possibility that similar effects might occur among black adolescents.

One of the earliest studies to report the impact of an HIV risk-reduction intervention was the Lanier and McCarthy (1989) study on a predominantly

African-American sample of adolescents in juvenile corrections facilities in Alabama. Juvenile delinquents are at elevated risk for early sexual activity, sexually transmitted disease, and injection drug use, which makes them an important population for HIV risk-reduction efforts. The AIDS intervention used by Lanier and McCarthy consisted of one hour of instruction on each of five days. It was designed to increase AIDS knowledge and emphasized abstinence as the preferred means of AIDS prevention, though the article did not provide further details of the intervention's content. The evaluation involved a posttest-only design in which adolescents at some institutions received the full five-day intervention, adolescents at other institutions received three days of the intervention, and those at other institutions received no intervention. Analyses centered on responses to an anonymous questionnaire administered several weeks after implementation of the intervention. Although the effects of the intervention on the behavior were not examined, the adolescents who received the five days of intervention, as compared with other adolescents, scored higher in AIDS knowledge, believed more strongly that AIDS is a significant problem, believed more strongly that they themselves had a high risk of infection, and expressed a greater willingness to inform potential sexual partners if they tested positive for AIDS.

An experiment by Schinke, Gordon, and Weston (1990) tested the efficacy of an intervention designed to reduce the risk of HIV infection associated with drug use and unsafe sex among 60 black and Hispanic adolescents enrolled in an urban job-training program. The intervention involved the use of a self-instructional guide written in comic book format. It included rap lyrics presented by cartoon characters drawn to mirror participants' age and ethnic–racial background. The characters provided information about AIDS risk behaviors, myths, and prevention strategies. To enhance decision-making skills, the guide introduced participants to the steps involved in cognitive problem solving. In a game format, the youths made hypothetical decisions about drug use and AIDS risks.

The adolescents were assigned randomly to one of three conditions: (1) a self-instructional guide plus group instruction condition in which they received the self-instructional guide and met with intervention leaders for three one-hour sessions on the rationale for the guide and how it should be used; (2) a guide-only condition in which they received the guide but no group sessions; or (3) a control condition in which they received neither the guide nor the group sessions. Data were collected before the intervention and one month after it. Although the pattern of means across several dependent measures suggested positive effects of the self-instructional interventions, there were few significant differences. Analyses of covariance revealed no between-condition differences in AIDS knowledge, fear of AIDS, approval of casual drug use, or intentions to use condoms, controlling for preintervention beliefs.

There was a significant effect on participants' disapproval of injection drug use, which seemed to indicate that participants who received the self-instructional guide plus small group intervention, as compared with the control subjects, decreased their permissiveness toward intravenous drug use.

Rickert, Gottlieb, and Jay (1990) conducted a study to test the effects of HIV risk-reduction interventions on black and white female adolescents who attended an adolescent medicine clinic in a metropolitan area in central Arkansas. The adolescents were assigned randomly to one of three conditions: (1) a control condition in which they were given the opportunity to ask questions about AIDS and were given a booklet on AIDS; (2) an education condition in which they were given the booklet and a brief AIDS lecture based on Centers for Disease Control (CDC) guidelines; or (3) an enhanced education condition in which they received the booklet and the lecture and viewed a humorous videotape explaining the purpose of condoms and demonstrating their use. Immediately after the intervention, adolescents in all conditions completed questionnaire measures and were given a coupon that they could redeem for free condoms at an on-site pharmacy. Although there were no significant differences between groups in attitudes toward practicing preventive behaviors, attitudes toward persons with AIDS, or perceived seriousness of AIDS, adolescents in the education and enhanced education conditions scored significantly higher in AIDS knowledge than did those in the control condition. Considering the whole sample, there were no significant between-condition differences in the proportion of adolescents who redeemed coupons for free condoms. In the subsample of adolescents who had reported previously purchasing condoms, however, those who received enhanced education were more likely to redeem the coupons than were those in the other two conditions.

SOCIAL PSYCHOLOGICAL APPROACH TO HIV RISK-REDUCTION INTERVENTIONS

In collaboration with our colleagues and students, we have been conducting a series of studies designed to elucidate the modifiable social psychological factors that underlie behaviors that create risk of sexually transmitted HIV infection in inner-city African Americans and to develop theory-based, culturally sensitive, developmentally appropriate interventions to reduce these behaviors (Jemmott & Jemmott, 1991, 1992; Jemmott, Jemmott, & Fong, 1992, 1993; Jemmott, Jemmott, & Hacker, 1992; Jemmott, Jemmott, Spears, Hewitt, & Cruz-Collins, 1992). Our research has drawn upon Bandura's social cognitive theory (1986) and the theory of planned behavior (Ajzen, 1985, 1991; Madden, Ellen, & Ajzen, 1992), an extension of the more widely known theory of reasoned action (Ajzen & Fishbein, 1980; Fishbein & Ajzen, 1975).

According to the theory of planned behavior, specific behavioral intentions are the determinants of behaviors. Consider, for instance, condom use: Based on the theory, it might be predicted that adolescents' use of condoms is a function of their intentions to use condoms. The theory further holds that a behavioral intention is determined by both attitudes toward the specific behavior and subjective norms regarding the behavior. Thus, people intend to perform a behavior when they evaluate that behavior positively and when they believe significant others think they should perform it.

A valuable feature of the theory of planned behavior is that it directs attention to why people hold certain attitudes and subjective norms. Attitudes toward behavior are seen as reflecting behavioral beliefs about the consequences of performing the behavior. By targeting beliefs about sexual behavior, interventions may be able to change attitudes toward those behaviors. In the case of unprotected sexual intercourse, perhaps the most obvious is the belief that it increases the risks of pregnancy and STD, including HIV infection. Another key consideration is what has been termed "hedonistic beliefs" (Jemmott et al., 1992; Jemmott & Jones, 1993) or beliefs about the consequences of sexual activities for sexual enjoyment (Catania et al., 1989; Hingson et al., 1990; Jemmott & Jemmott, 1992; Valdiserri, Arena, Proctor, & Bonati, 1989).

Subjective norms are seen as reflecting normative beliefs about what specific reference persons or groups think should be done regarding the behavior. People may modulate their risk-associated behavior as a function of their beliefs about how significant others would view it (Fishbein & Middlestadt, 1989). Quite apart from people's beliefs about other consequences of the behavior—as might be reflected in hedonistic beliefs, for example—if people believe that significant others disapprove of a risk behavior, they may be less likely to engage in that behavior than if they believe that others approve of the behavior. In the case of adolescents' sexual behavior, the key referents would certainly include girlfriends/boyfriends. Other significant referents who may affect adolescents' risky sexual behavior include friends or peers and family members (Fox & Inazu, 1980; Furstenberg, 1971; Handelsman, Cabral, & Weisfeld, 1987; Hofferth & Hayes, 1987; Milan & Kilmann, 1987; Morrison, 1985; Nathanson & Becker, 1986). In social cognitive theory terms (Bandura, 1986), salient behavioral beliefs and normative beliefs can be seen as types of outcome expectancies (Jemmott & Jones, 1993).

A fundamental assumption of the theory of reasoned action is that its predictive power is greatest for behaviors that are fully under the volitional control of individuals. In contradistinction, Ajzen (1985, 1991) proposed the theory of planned behavior to account for behaviors that are subject to forces that are *beyond* individuals' control. For instance, performance of the behavior might depend on another person's actions or the behavior might be performed in the context of strong emotions. Individuals use condoms, not by themselves, but in concert with their sexual partners. This would seem to lend credence to the notion that perceived behavioral control is important to condom use. Thus, individuals' perceptions of their ability to negotiate condom use are critical to reducing unprotected sexual intercourse. Perceived behavioral control reflects past experience as well as anticipated impediments, obstacles, resources, and opportunities. It has an affinity with the social cognitive theory construct of perceived self-efficacy (Bandura, 1982, 1986, 1989; O'Leary, 1985). If people believe that they have little control over performing a behavior because of a lack of requisite skills or resources, their intentions to perform the behavior may be low, even if they have favorable attitudes or perceive supportive subjective norms regarding it.

The theory of planned behavior does not include many variables that traditionally have been studied in attempts to understand preventive health behavior. Thus, for instance, low socioeconomic background, low parental education, residing in a female-headed household, and residing in households with a large number of children are not in the theory but have been linked to heightened sexual activity (Brown, 1985; Fox & Inazu, 1980; Hofferth & Hayes, 1987; Hogan, Astone, & Kitagawa, 1985; Hogan & Kitagawa, 1985; Zelnik et al., 1981). The theory of planned behavior holds that those variables that are external to the model would affect specific behavioral intentions and behaviors by influencing attitudes toward those behaviors, subjective norms regarding them, or perceptions of control over them. In other words, the effects on intentions and behaviors of other variables are seen as mediated by their effects on the attitudinal component, the normative component, the perceived control component, or all three. In this way, the theory can accommodate variables that are external to it (Ajzen, 1991; Fishbein & Middlestadt, 1989).

Intervening with African-American Male Adolescents

Our initial intervention study was a field experiment designed to test the effectiveness of an HIV risk-reduction intervention on African-American male adolescents (Jemmott, Jemmott, & Fong, 1992). The study also addressed an important practical question regarding the implementation of HIV interventions with inner-city African-American male adolescents. It might be hypothesized that a black male educator would be a good role-model for African-American male adolescents. Hence, the second issue the study addressed was whether intervention effects would be enhanced if the facilitator was a black man as opposed to a black woman. The participants were 157 African-American male adolescents from Philadelphia who volunteered for a "Risk-Reduction Project" designed to reduce important risks faced by African-

American youth, including unemployment, pregnancy, and AIDS. They were recruited from a local medical center, community-based organizations, and a local high school, and assigned randomly to an HIV risk-reduction condition or a control condition on career opportunities and to a small group of about six boys led by a specially trained male or female black facilitator. Few participants reported *ever* sharing needles (4%), *ever* having receptive anal intercourse (2%), having sexual relationships with males exclusively (2%), or having sexual relationships with both males and females (1%). Their chief HIV risk was from sexual relationships with women. Although the mean age of the sample was only 14.6 years, about 83% of the adolescents reported having had coitus at least once. About 21% of respondents who had coitus in the past three months reported that they *never* used condoms during those experiences, and only 30% reported *always* using condoms.

Adolescents in the HIV risk-reduction condition received a five-hour intervention involving videotapes, games, and exercises aimed at increasing AIDS-related knowledge, weakening problematic beliefs and attitudes toward HIV risk-associated sexual behavior, and increasing skill at negotiating safer sex. One video, *The Subject is AIDS,* narrated by a black woman in conjunction with a multiethnic cast, presented factual information about AIDS. Another video, *Condom Sense,* addressed negative attitudes toward the use of condoms, hedonistic beliefs, and normative beliefs. It disputed the idea that sexual intercourse is substantially less pleasurable when a condom is used. One black male character tries to convince a basketball buddy that his girl friend's request that they use condoms during sex is reasonable. The intervention also addressed perceived behavioral control, including confidence in technical skills in the use of condoms, and negotiation skills to convince partners that condoms should be used or that abstinence should be practiced. A condom exercise focused on familiarity with condoms and the steps involved in the correct use of them. Participants engaged in role-playing situations depicting potential problems in trying to implement safer-sex practices, including abstinence.

To control for Hawthorne effects, to reduce the likelihood that effects of the HIV risk-reduction intervention could be attributed to nonspecific features, including group interaction and special attention, adolescents randomly assigned to the control condition also received a five-hour intervention. Structurally similar to the HIV risk-reduction intervention, it involved culturally and developmentally appropriate videotapes, exercises, and games, but regarding career opportunities. This control intervention was designed to be both enjoyable and valuable. Although career opportunity subjects did not learn about AIDS, given the high unemployment among inner-city black adolescents, the goal was to provide information that would be valuable to them as they planned their future.

Adolescents in both conditions completed questionnaires before, immediately after the intervention, and three months after the intervention. Analyses of covariance, controlling for preintervention measures, revealed that adolescents who received the HIV risk-reduction intervention subsequently had greater AIDS knowledge, less favorable attitudes toward risky sexual behavior, and reduced intentions for such behavior compared with adolescents in the control condition. Responses to debriefing questions on the postintervention questionnaire indicated that participants in the two conditions were equally involved in their respective activities and felt that they had a valuable and enjoyable experience. Of the original participants, 150 (96%) completed follow-up questionnaires three months after the intervention. Adolescents in the HIV risk-reduction condition reported less risky sexual behavior in the three months postintervention than did those in the control condition. For instance, they reported having coitus less frequently and with fewer women, they reported using condoms more consistently during coitus, and fewer of them reported engaging in heterosexual anal intercourse. Moreover, the AIDS-intervention participants still had greater AIDS knowledge and weaker intentions for risky behavior in the next three months than did the other participants. The study revealed scant evidence that the use of black male facilitators would enhance intervention effects on black male adolescents. Although analyses on the postintervention questionnaire revealed a Condition times Gender of Facilitator interaction such that the HIV risk-reduction intervention caused a greater increase in AIDS knowledge among participants who had a male facilitator than among those who had a female facilitator, this interaction was not evident on other postintervention measures or at the three-month follow-up. In addition, the effects of the HIV risk-reduction intervention on attitudes and sexual behavior measured at the three-month follow-up were significantly *stronger* with female facilitators than with male facilitators.

Intervening with Young Inner-City African-American Adolescents

Jemmott, Jemmott, and Fong (1993) recently conducted an HIV risk-reduction study that focused on male and female African-American adolescents. The study was designed not only to test the HIV risk-reduction intervention, but to pursue further, practical questions about how interventions are implemented with inner-city African-American adolescents. The study was designed to test whether intervention effects varied depending on whether the facilitator was African American or white, whether the gender of the facilitator and the gender of the adolescent were matched or different, whether the adolescents in the small group were homogeneous or heterogeneous on gender, and theoretically and practically important combinations of these factors. The participants were 506 seventh and eighth graders (mean age, 13.1 years) recruited from the public junior high schools and elementary schools of Trenton, New Jersey for a study designed to discover ways to reduce important health risks that African-American youth face. About 55% of respondents reported having experienced coitus at least once, and about 31% of all respondents reported having coitus in the past three months. About 25% of those reporting coitus in the past three months indicated that they never used condoms during those experiences, whereas 30% indicated they always used condoms during those experiences.

The adolescents were assigned randomly to either an HIV risk-reduction condition or a control condition and to a small group that was either homogeneous or heterogeneous in gender and that was led by a specially trained male or female facilitator who was African American or white. Adolescents in the HIV risk-reduction condition received a five-hour intervention designed to influence variables theoretically important to behavior change and to be meaningful and culturally and developmentally appropriate for young inner-city African-American adolescents. From a theoretical perspective, the intervention was designed (1) to increase self-efficacy regarding the ability to implement condom use, including confidence that they could get their partner to use one; (2) to address hedonistic beliefs to allay participants' fears regarding adverse consequences of condoms on sexual enjoyment; and (3) to increase general knowledge of AIDS and STDs and specific beliefs regarding the use of condoms to prevent sexually transmitted HIV infection. The intervention included information about risks associated with injection drug use and specific sexual activities. The value of abstinence as the safest sex practice was discussed. Videotapes, games, and exercises were used to facilitate learning and active participation.

As in our previous intervention study, participants in the control condition also received an intervention. Instead of an intervention on career opportunities, however, this control group received an intervention targeting behaviors (e.g., dietary and exercise habits and cigarette smoking) that affect the risk of certain health problems other than AIDS. These health problems, including cardiovascular disease, hypertension, and certain cancers, are leading causes of morbidity and mortality among African Americans (Gillum, 1982; Ibrahim, Chobanian, Horan, & Roccella, 1985; Page & Asire, 1985). Structurally similar to the HIV risk-reduction intervention, the general health promotion intervention also lasted five hours and used culturally and developmentally appropriate videotapes, exercises, and games to reinforce learning and to encourage active participation.

After the interventions, the participants completed the postintervention questionnaires. Adolescents in the HIV risk-reduction condition subsequently expressed stronger intentions to use condoms; had more favorable beliefs about the effects of condoms on sexual enjoyment and about the ability of condoms to prevent pregnancy, STD, and AIDS; had greater perceived self-efficacy to use condoms; and had greater knowledge about AIDS than did those in the control condition, controlling for preintervention measures of the particular dependent measure. Responses to debriefing questions indicated that participants in the HIV risk-reduction and general health promotion conditions did not differ in ratings of how much they talked during the interventions, liked the intervention activities, or learned from the activities.

Of the original participants, 489 (97%) took part in the three-month follow-up and 469 (93%) took part in the six-month follow-up. The effects of the HIV risk-reduction intervention on the motivational variables were sustained over the six-month time interval. At both follow-ups, participants in the HIV risk-reduction intervention scored higher on intentions to use condoms, AIDS knowledge, hedonistic beliefs, and perceived self-efficacy to use condoms than did the participants in the health promotion condition. Although there were no significant effects of the HIV risk-reduction intervention on self-reports of unprotected coitus at the three-month follow-up, at the six-month follow-up adolescents who had received the HIV risk-reduction intervention reported fewer days on which they had coitus without using a condom in the previous three months than did those who had received the health promotion intervention, controlling for preintervention self-reports.

There was evidence for the generality of the effects of the intervention across race of the facilitator, gender of the facilitator, gender of the participants, and gender composition of the intervention groups. Despite the relatively large number of interactions tested—which would have increased the likelihood of a type I error—these factors did not moderate facilitators' reports of how the participants reacted to the intervention or participants' own reports of their reactions to the interventions: how much they liked it, how much they talked, and how much they felt they learned. In addition, these factors did not moderate effects of the intervention on AIDS knowledge, prevention beliefs, hedonistic beliefs, perceived self-efficacy, intentions, or self-reports of unprotected coitus. The effects of the HIV risk-reduction intervention were about the same irrespective of the race of the facilitator, the gender of the facilitator, the gender of the participants, and the gender composition of the intervention group. Our initial study on black male adolescents (Jemmott, Jemmott, & Fong, 1992) also found that matching the gender of participant and facilitator did not enhance intervention effects. The lack of effects of race of facilitator may reflect the fact that the facilitators received common training in the intervention that was culturally sensitive. It may well be that if an intervention is culturally sensitive and the facilitators are well trained, the characteristics of the facilitators are not important determinants of the efficacy of intervention implementation. This, of course, is an empirical question.

Contrasting Different Intervention Strategies for Changing Intentions

The vast majority of HIV risk-reduction studies have contrasted two groups, typically a group that receives the intervention and a group that receives no treatment. Relatively few studies have attempted to test the effectiveness of more than one HIV risk-reduction intervention. A study by Jemmott et al. (1992), in a preliminary way, tested the effects of two HIV risk-reduction interventions. The HIV risk-reduction intervention used in the Jemmott, Jemmott, and Fong (1992, 1993) studies attempted to have an impact on a variety of theory-derived variables that might affect behavior. These variables included hedonistic beliefs, AIDS knowledge, prevention beliefs, and perceived self-efficacy. The question that Jemmott et al. (1992) addressed was whether it would be more effective to use interventions that emphasized hedonistic beliefs and perceived self-efficacy or interventions that emphasized prevention beliefs and AIDS knowledge.

The study compared the effects of three interventions on intentions to use condoms: (1) a social cognitive intervention designed to increase perceived self-efficacy/behavioral control to use condoms and hedonistic beliefs favorable to condom use; (2) an information-alone intervention designed to increase general AIDS knowledge and specific prevention beliefs; and (3) a general health promotion intervention designed to provide information about health problems other than AIDS.

The subjects were 19 sexually active black adolescent women from an inner-city family planning clinic. All interventions lasted 105 minutes and involved the use of culturally appropriate videotapes and small-group exercises, games, and discussions. Participants' evaluations of the interventions did not differ among the conditions. Adolescents in the social cognitive condition, however, registered greater postintervention intentions to use condoms than did those in the two control conditions. In addition, participants in the social cognitive condition scored higher in perceived self-efficacy and favorable hedonistic expectancies—the two hypothesized mediators of the intervention effect. Although participants who received the information-alone intervention scored higher in AIDS knowledge and in the specific beliefs that condoms prevent pregnancy, STDs, and AIDS than did those in the health promotion condition, they did not express greater intentions to use condoms. What this study suggests is that in addition to having adequate knowledge about AIDS and the risk of certain sexual practices, it is necessary to affect adolescents' beliefs about the consequences of condom use for sexual enjoyment, their perceived skill at negotiating with their partner to use condoms, and their technical skill on how to use condoms correctly to make them pleasurable. The limitation of the study is the relatively small sample size. Although significance tests take sample size into account by making it more difficult to achieve statistical significance with small samples, additional studies are needed to demonstrate the generalizability of these findings in larger samples.

The theory of planned behavior suggests that in addition to beliefs about the consequences of engaging in behavior and perceptions of behavioral control or self-efficacy, there are normative influences on adolescents' sexual behavior. One potentially important but underutilized normative influence is the adolescent's parents. A recent study by Jemmott, Jemmott, Braverman, Lerman, Fong, Boccher-Lattimore, McCaffree, and Hacker (1993) tested the effects on intentions to influence daughters' HIV risk-associated sexual behavior of a social cognitive intervention for parents of black inner-city female adolescents. The subjects were 50 mothers of black female adolescents recruited from an adolescent medicine clinic of a children's hospital serving a low-income, inner-city, ethnic minority community. The participants were randomly assigned to: (1) an AIDS social-cognitive intervention designed to increase perceived self-efficacy to influence their daughter's sexual behavior; or (2) one of two control conditions—an AIDS information-alone intervention designed to increase AIDS knowledge or a general health promotion intervention that provided information about important health problems other than AIDS. All interventions lasted 3.5 hours and involved films and small-group exercises. All of the interventions were designed to encourage the mothers to influence their daughters' health-related behaviors but the behaviors that were targeted depended on the condition to which they were randomly assigned (AIDS conditions versus general health promotion). Participants' evaluations of the interventions did not differ among the three conditions. As hypothesized, participants in the social-cognitive condition registered greater postintervention intentions to influence their daughters' sexual behavior than did those in the two control conditions. In addition, participants in the social-cognitive condition scored higher in perceived self-efficacy—the hypothesized mediator of the intervention effect. Although participants who received the information-alone intervention subsequently had greater AIDS knowledge than did those in the health promotion condition, they did not express greater intentions to use condoms. These results highlight the potential value of a social-cognitive approach to helping parents influence their children's AIDS risk behavior. In additional research, we and our colleagues are studying whether the social cognitive intervention affects mothers' behavior toward their daughters and their daughters' HIV risk associated behavior.

Translating Findings into Community-Based Programs

Often the results of intervention research remain buried in the pages of scientific journals, where they are unlikely to come to the attention of the community people who could make the best use of them. Unfortunately, the ideal of translating research results into practical community-based programs is seldom realized. Recently, we attempted to address this issue by adapting our HIV risk-reduction interventions for use in a program implemented by a community based organization, the Urban League of Metropolitan Trenton (Jemmott & Jemmott, 1992).

The AIDS prevention program drew upon our experiences with the Jemmott, Jemmott, and Fong (1992) study and the Jemmott et al. (1992) study and used many of the same activities. It was designed to be meaningful and culturally appropriate for the specific population of inner-city African-American adolescent women who would receive it. Prior to implementing the program, individual and focus group interviews were conducted with adolescents from Trenton. These interviews suggested that many of the adolescents had a strong sense of identification with Africa. Posters used to advertise the program were colored red, black, and green (the black liberation colors) and bore a map of Africa and the motto "Respect Yourself, Protect Yourself—Because You Are Worth It." When the adolescents completed the program they were given T-shirts with the phrase "Respect Yourself, Protect Yourself" and a map of Africa colored in red, black, and green on the front and the phrase "Because I am Worth It" on the back.

The program was six hours long. Taking into account the constraints within which the community-based organization had to work, however, it was designed to be implemented in three two-hour sessions, which included 30-minute preintervention and postintervention assessments, rather than our usual one session. The first session focused on factual information about the cause, transmission, and prevention of AIDS and the risks faced by black women of childbearing age in New Jersey. The second session focused on beliefs regarding partner reactions and hedonistic beliefs. The third session focused on skill building and self-efficacy to use condoms. Videotapes, games, and exercises were used to reinforce learning and to encourage active participation. The participants received the intervention in small groups of 6 to 10 adolescents led by a specially trained African-American female health educator who was a native Trenton resident.

The participants in the program were 109 sexually experienced African-American female adolescents (mean age = 16.8 years). About 72% reported that they had had coitus in the past three months. As in previous research on inner-city African-American adolescents, the chief risky sexual behavior was the failure to use condoms. About 19% of those who had had coitus in the past three months reported that condoms were never used on those occasions and only 29% reported that condoms were always used on those occasions. Analyses revealed that the adolescents scored higher in intentions to use condoms, AIDS knowledge, hedonistic beliefs, prevention beliefs, and self-efficacy to use condoms after the intervention compared with before the intervention

(Jemmott & Jemmott, 1992). In addition, increased self-efficacy and more favorable hedonistic beliefs and beliefs regarding sexual partner's support for condom use were significantly related to increased condom-use intentions, but increases in general AIDS knowledge and specific prevention-related beliefs were not.

One weakness of the study is that the changes in intentions might not reflect intervention effects, but history. Jemmott and Jemmott (1992) reasoned that history is an unlikely explanation because the women participated in intervention groups that were run sequentially over a six-month period. In this view, it is unlikely that events besides the intervention activities could have occurred between preintervention and postintervention and increased scores for these multiple intervention groups. Although history cannot account for the differential predictive power of perceived self-efficacy and hedonistic beliefs as compared with AIDS knowledge and prevention beliefs, the fact that the study did not include a control group that did not receive HIV risk-reduction interventions limits the ability to draw causal inferences about intervention effects.

METHODOLOGICAL AND LOGISTICAL ISSUES IN HIV RISK-REDUCTION INTERVENTIONS WITH INNER-CITY AFRICAN-AMERICAN ADOLESCENTS

In this section, we will describe some of the important methodological and logistical issues that arise in HIV risk-reduction intervention research on adolescents in community settings. This will include both internal and external validity. We will discuss the limitations of self-report data, the problem of generalizing from nonrandom samples, and the relative merits of using incentives in intervention studies. Our discussion will also center on such additional challenges as subject recruitment, attrition from intervention and follow-up sessions, and enlisting community cooperation. Although these comments on methodological and logistical issues are specifically directed at HIV risk-reduction research on African-American adolescents in community settings, many of them are relevant to HIV risk-reduction research and to intervention research in general.

Internal Validity

True Experiments

Internal validity has to do with the ability to draw causal inferences about the effects of the HIV risk-reduction intervention. The most rigorous design for ensuring internal validity is the true experiment in which individuals are randomly assigned to receive or not to receive the intervention. This design has been used in several intervention studies on black adolescents in community settings (e.g., Jemmott, Jemmott, & Fong, 1992; Schinke et al., 1990). Despite its rigor, one potential problem with implementing the true experiment in community settings is that it involves the withholding of the HIV risk-reduction intervention from some adolescents. This may raise ethical issues regarding withholding a valuable treatment from people who need it. In addition, the adolescents or their advocates may be disappointed because the AIDS education they desired will not be made available to them. The adolescents may drop out of the project because of this; and they may seek AIDS education elsewhere. In any event, the integrity of the experiment would be compromised.

There are a number of approaches to handling this problem. A common solution in other areas of research is to assign adolescents in the control group to a waiting list to receive intervention at some period of time after the adolescents in the experimental group receive it. Another common solution is to give the adolescents in the control group "usual care," the standard AIDS education programming they would have received had they not been in the study. Although often reasonable solutions, a frequent drawback of these two approaches is that the no-treatment control condition and even the usual-care control condition differ from the HIV risk-reduction intervention, not only in content, but in the amount of intervention time. This is problematic from the standpoint of understanding the mechanism of intervention effects because it becomes difficult to determine conclusively whether differences between the effects of the HIV risk-reduction intervention and the control condition are due to the content of the HIV risk-reduction intervention or the amount of time and attention the two groups received. For some purposes, this confound may be relatively unimportant, but what may matter is not why an intervention works, but whether or not it works.

Another possible solution is to use a placebo control group in which adolescents receive an intervention that is structurally similar to the HIV risk-reduction intervention, but focused on important risks other than AIDS that the adolescents may have. An advantage of this approach is that it controls for content as well as amount of intervention time, which often is not possible with the other approaches to the problem. The Jemmott, Jemmott, and Fong (1992) study is an example of this approach. Based on the premise that unemployment is a major risk for inner-city African-American adolescent men, the control-condition participants in that study were given an intervention on career opportunities. In Jemmott et al. (1992) the control group received an intervention targeted at other important behavior-relevant health risks of inner-city African-American women. To reduce the likelihood that adolescents would be disappointed because they were receiving an intervention other than the HIV risk-reduction intervention, these studies did not recruit subjects for an AIDS study. Instead the adolescents were recruited for a "risk-reduction project" (Jemmott, Jemmott, & Fong, 1992) or a "healthy living program" (Jemmott et al., 1992) and the control interventions were designed to be valuable and enjoyable. In this way, the likelihood that adolescents in the control condition would feel disappointed was reduced.

Quasi-Experimental Design

Under certain circumstances, it may not be feasible to use a true experimental design and a quasi-experimental design may be more appropriate (Cook & Campbell, 1979). Although quasi-experimental designs do not provide a rigorous basis for causal inferences because they fail to rule out a number of alternative interpretations, it is sometimes possible to establish that these alternative interpretations are implausible based on accepted theory, common sense, statistical evidence, or other nondesign considerations (Cook & Campbell, 1979). An example of this type of reasoning can be found in Jemmott and Jemmott (1992) in which the authors discussed the plausibility of alternative explanations of putative intervention effects in terms of history, maturation, testing, and statistical regression for their tests of an intervention using a quasi-experimental design.

In some cases a nonequivalent control group design is used because it is impractical to randomly assign individuals to intervention and control conditions. For example, there may be concern about contamination of subjects in the control condition. In the Lanier and McCarthy (1989) study, for example, all the adolescents in a given juvenile correction institution were assigned to the same condition. Had the adolescents within a given institution been assigned to different conditions, there is the possibility that they would talk to one another about the interventions they received and hence the adolescents in the control condition might have received some of the intervention programming. This might have biased the study against finding significant intervention effects. By reducing differences between the intervention and control conditions, it could have reduced the likelihood that the intervention condition would have shown greater improvement than the control condition.

Jemmott, Jemmott, and Fong (1992) directly assessed the potential for contamination in their study and found no evidence that it had any effect. About 18% of the black male adolescents said they discussed their small group's activities with someone from another group in the study. Adolescents in the AIDS condition and career condition were equally likely to talk to someone from another group. Analyses on AIDS knowledge, attitudes, intentions, and risky sexual behavior at the three-month follow-up revealed no significant interaction between experimental condition and whether or not the adolescents reported discussing the study with someone from another group. Thus, the intervention's effects were not significantly weaker among the subsample of adolescents who talked with participants from other groups.

Clearly, the plausibility of contamination as an important alternative explanation should be considered carefully. It would seem to be a more important factor to the extent that the adolescents in different conditions are likely to be in frequent, close contact with one another over nontrivial amounts of time. Such might certainly be the case in an institution, which was the situation of Lanier and McCarthy (1989), but may be less likely outside of an institution, which was the situation of Jemmott, Jemmott, and Fong (1992). Also potentially relevant is the extent to which the essential element of the intervention is simply information as opposed to experientially acquired skills and affective changes. In the latter case, it may be more difficult for interactions between subjects in different conditions to translate into contamination. In cases where there is reason to believe that contamination may occur, efforts should be made to assess the extent of between-group interaction and to take contamination effects, if any, into account in statistical analyses.

The particular version of the nonequivalent control group design in the Lanier and McCarthy study involved the collection of only posttest data. Although the use of the nonequivalent control group design may be useful to address the possibility of contamination effects, the absence of pretests in the Lanier and McCarthy study means that posttest differences among the groups may be attributed to the interventions or to preexisting group differences.

In some situations it may be necessary to use a one-group pretest–posttest design because it is not possible to withhold the intervention, even for a period of time, from some adolescents. In such situations, it may be necessary to evaluate the intervention without using a control group. For instance, Jemmott and Jemmott (1992) evaluated the HIV risk-reduction intervention program of the Urban League in Trenton using the prepost design. The trouble with this design is that in the absence of a control group, differences between pretest and posttest scores may be attributed to the intervention or to history, statistical regression, maturation, and testing.

In general, a more readily interpretable quasi-experimental design is the pretest–posttest nonequivalent control group design, which combines features of the two designs just described. For example, one intact group might receive the intervention, whereas another intact group does not, but both groups complete pretest and posttest measures. Although it was not used in any of the studies we reviewed on adolescents in community settings, it is among the most internally valid of the quasi-experimental designs (Cook & Campbell,

1979). The ideal would be to always use random assignment of individuals to conditions, but where this is not feasible, the use of the pretest–posttest nonequivalent control group design would be highly recommended.

Regardless of whether a true experiment or one of the quasi-experimental designs is used, an important potential threat to the internal validity of HIV risk-reduction intervention studies is differential attrition. In any intervention study that follows individuals longitudinally, there is the possibility that the attrition rate at data collection points after the intervention may be significantly different between the intervention condition and the control condition. From the standpoint of internal validity, this raises the possibility that differences between the intervention and control conditions may be due, not simply to the intervention content, but to self-selection—differences between those who remained in the study and those who dropped out. Another way in which attrition can cloud causal interpretation is in cases where multiple-session interventions are used and some subjects are absent from some of the sessions. Deleting from the analyses subjects who have not received the full dose of the intervention would introduce a potential self-selection bias, making results difficult to interpret. Including such subjects in the analyses (the intention-to-treat approach) could create a bias against finding intervention effects because the subjects have not received the full intended intervention. In this latter case, however, if a significant effect were obtained, it might be considered an underestimation of the potential effects of the intervention. Cook and Campbell (1979) have described a number of ways of analyzing the potential biasing effects of differential attrition. Needless to say it is preferable to reduce the likelihood of differential attrition, which may be more likely to occur when there are differences in how appealing the subjects perceive their condition to be.

External Validity

One issue that arises with HIV risk-reduction intervention studies in community settings is external validity or the ability to generalize the results beyond the participants and implementation involved in the study. The ability to generalize to a population is maximized when subjects are randomly selected from the population, but this ideal situation is extremely rare in practice. No HIV risk-reduction intervention studies have been done on randomly selected samples; instead all HIV risk-reduction intervention studies have used convenience samples. Short of random sampling there are some steps that can be taken to clarify the population to which the results might generalize. Thus if subjects are recruited from an STD clinic and the goal is to generalize to the clinic population, it would be important to know whether the subjects who actually participated in the study are similar to the clinic population on important characteristics. If the sample is significantly different from the clinic population on important characteristics, it may be possible to estimate the type of population that the sample might be representative of. This will improve the plausibility of generalizability, though generalizing from nonrandom samples is still problematic. Attrition can also cause problems for generalizability. Statistical analysis may reveal that the intervention had significant effects, but generalizability to the population of interest may be limited by attrition. The results may not generalize to subjects who dropped out of the study, for their outcomes are unknown. A number of procedures described by Cook and Campbell (1979) can be used to assess the potential impact of attrition on generalizability.

In addition to considering the population to which results may generalize, it is important, some would say more important given the difficulty of random sampling (Cook & Campbell, 1979), to consider whether results generalize across different populations and circumstances. A focus on this type of external validity would clarify whether interventions are more or less effective with subpopulations of adolescents and might suggest tailoring interventions to subpopulations. In addition, it would clarify whether particular ways of implementing the intervention are differentially effective. Often assumptions are made about generalizability across populations, but there has been virtually no effort to establish empirically this type of external validity in HIV risk-reduction research. One exception is the Jemmott, Jemmott, and Fong (1993) study, which examined whether HIV risk-reduction intervention effects generalized across gender of participants, gender of facilitators, race of facilitators, and gender composition of intervention groups.

The Use of Incentives

A number of questions often arise regarding whether to use incentives in intervention research in community settings and what effects incentives might have on generalizability. Incentives can be used to increase the likelihood that adolescents will participate in interventions; hence, incentives may increase sample size. In addition, when incentives are used, a more diverse population may be reached: The project might include people who are participating because they have an intrinsic interest in the topics (these are people who would be involved without the incentives) as well as those who are involved because of the incentives (people who might not participate without an incentive). In this way, the use of incentives can permit a test of the intervention with a larger sample of a broader population, and can open the possibility of generalizability beyond simply those who have an intrinsic interest in the topic. Another advantage of the use of incentives is that it can reduce the likelihood of attrition at follow-up postintervention data collection sessions and the associated problems of generalizability.

Although incentives are not limited to money, community-based organizations not involved in funded research projects may not have the resources to provide strong incentives for participating in HIV risk-reduction programs. An important question, then, is whether HIV risk-reduction interventions that proved to be effective using monetary incentives would also be effective without monetary incentives. First, we would argue that community-based organizations may be able to provide participants with relatively inexpensive nonmonetary incentives, tokens that would be valuable to the population. For example, appropriately designed T-shirts, key chains, and so on might be used, as in the Urban League of Metropolitan Trenton's AIDS prevention program. The use of such incentives could broaden the reach of the AIDS prevention program. Of course, another way to broaden the reach is to present a program as not simply on AIDS and sexually transmitted disease, but on male–female relationships and other issues of interest to adolescents. Second, we would argue that if an intervention is effective with the use of monetary incentives, it is likely to be effective also when monetary incentives are not used. This is because the use of monetary incentives may provide a more stringent test of HIV risk-reduction interventions. It may be easier to change the sexual behavior of a population of adolescents that has a specific interest in a behavior-change intervention (those willing to participate without monetary incentives) than to change the behavior of a population of adolescents with a mix of motives for participating.

SELF-REPORTS OF SEXUAL BEHAVIOR

Given its private nature, it is not possible to directly measure sexual behavior. Consequently, research must rely upon self-reports of sexual behavior, but they may be intentionally or unintentionally inaccurate. A number of approaches to dealing with this problem are possible. One approach is to use other indirect measures of sexual behavior that do not share the same problems as self-report measures. For example, condom-coupon redemption (Rickert, Gottlieb, & Say, 1990; Solomon & DeJong, 1989) has been used as an unobtrusive measure of protected sexual behavior (or at least behavior that would seem to emanate from intentions to practice safer sex). Because condom coupons are redeemed outside of the intervention setting, there is less demand for socially desirable responses. In addition, more effort would be required to make a socially desirable response.

There is an important ambiguity inherent in the condom coupon redemption measure, however (Jemmott & Jones, 1993), especially when used in populations where some individuals may practice abstinence whereas others may use condoms (e.g., adolescent samples). Unclear is whether adolescents who participate in an AIDS prevention program should be predicted to redeem greater or fewer numbers of coupons than those who do not participate. Participants might be expected to redeem fewer coupons because they would have sexual intercourse less often (and therefore have less need for condoms) than the nonparticipants. Of course, redeeming fewer coupons could also mean they are having more unprotected sex. On the other hand, participants might be expected to redeem more coupons because they would be expected to use condoms more consistently when they have sexual intercourse. Of course, redeeming more coupons could also mean they are having sex more frequently even though their consistency of condom use does not differ from those who did not participate in the intervention.

The results of tests for sexually transmitted infections are another indirect measure of sexual behavior. Unfortunately, such tests may be feasible only in limited circumstances. They seem most feasible when the adolescents are clients at a clinic that provides family planning services and does such testing. In some AIDS prevention studies, particularly with young adolescents, many of the participants will not have had sexual intercourse, and STD testing on such individuals may be unacceptably intrusive. Moreover, it should be noted that STD testing is not a perfect measure of unprotected sexual intercourse because it *underestimates* the actual frequency of unprotected sexual intercourse. Although a positive STD test establishes that unprotected sexual intercourse has occurred, a negative test result does not establish that unprotected sexual intercourse has not occurred. The test could be negative, not because of the practice of safer sex or abstinence, but because of unprotected sex with a partner who was not infected.

In addition to seeking alternative indirect measures of sexual behavior, researchers have attempted to increase the accuracy of self-reports. To reduce problems in memory, adolescents might be asked to recall sexual behaviors over a relatively brief period of time, which would facilitate their ability to recall their behavior. It is more difficult to recall accurately behavior that occurred 12 months ago as opposed to two weeks ago (Kauth, St. Lawrence, & Kelly, 1991). It is important to consider, however, the frequency of the behavior and the length of the recording interval. A two-week interval may be too brief because of the frequency of the behavior among adolescents. If a behavior is relatively infrequent, some reporting intervals may be too brief to capture sufficient behavior for a statistically powerful analysis. In addition, it may be easier to remember vivid infrequent events over longer periods of time than a large number of events over the same period of time. Although many African-American adolescents are sexually experienced, that is, they have had coitus at least once, their sexual activity is sporadic and relatively infrequent. Thus, to maximize recall and likelihood of capturing a reasonable amount of behavior, a three-month reporting interval is often used. To further increase accuracy of recall, it may be useful to provide participants with a calendar with the dates clearly marked. This will make salient to respondents the dates that are included when they are asked to recall their behavior over a specific temporal interval.

To reduce the likelihood that the participants will minimize or exaggerate reports of their sexual experiences, efforts should be made to motivate them to respond honestly. Participants could be informed that their responses will be used to help improve programs for other black youths like themselves and that optimum programs will be created to the extent that they answer the questions as truthfully as possible. Needless to say, participants should be assured that their responses will be kept confidential. To reduce the likelihood of demand characteristics from giving their responses to the same individuals from whom they received an intervention, different people should serve as data collectors and as AIDS educators.

Another approach to the problem of self-report bias is to statistically evaluate it by testing hypotheses about its impact. In this connection, Jemmott, Jemmott, and Fong (1993) found that preintervention and follow-up self-reports of condom use and the change in reported condom use were unrelated to social desirability response bias as indexed by the Marlowe-Crowne Social Desirability Scale (Crowne & Marlowe, 1964). It might be argued that need for social approval should be most strongly related to self-reported condom use among participants in the HIV risk-reduction condition in which condom use was specifically encouraged. However, need for social approval did not interact with experimental condition to affect self-reported condom use. Need for social approval was also unrelated to self-reported condom use among the subsample of adolescents in the HIV risk-reduction condition.

COMMUNITY COOPERATION

Although there is a great need for additional research to develop, implement, and test HIV risk-reduction interventions for African-American adolescents in community settings, such efforts may encounter substantial obstacles. Because of the legacy of racism, many inner-city African-American adolescents and their advocates in the community may distrust researchers who seek to recruit them for studies. Some African Americans may believe that researchers are trying to exploit rather than improve the health of their community. They may be suspicious that research findings will be used to support insidious stereotypes of African-American adolescents or, more generally, that researchers will draw interpretations that disparage African Americans.

There has been great concern that psychological testing and research has been used inappropriately to label African-American adolescents as pathological or intellectually inferior (Williams, 1980). There is also distrust of medical research. Inner-city African Americans may believe that they are being used as guinea pigs in experiments. One often-cited example of medical research that has exploited blacks is the infamous Tuskegee study. In that study, begun in 1934, treatment for syphilis was withheld from 412 black male sharecroppers from Tuskegee, Alabama as part of a study on the natural course of the disease. For 40 years, researchers observed the men as they suffered and died from the disease, without telling them that they had syphilis or treating them for it. A *New York Times*/CBS telephone poll (DeParle, 1990) conducted in New York City in June 1990 revealed evidence of distrust regarding AIDS among African Americans. About 10% of black respondents said that the AIDS virus was deliberately created in a laboratory to infect black people. Another 19% felt that the theory might possibly be true.

In addition to distrusting researchers, African Americans may distrust HIV risk-reduction information and recommendations provided by government officials and health professionals. African Americans may perceive ulterior motives in behavior change messages. For example, the message that condoms should be used or that HIV-positive pregnant women should have abortions might be seen, not simply as a benign effort to reduce the spread of HIV, but as a cynical strategy to reduce the number of African Americans. Similarly, African Americans might be skeptical about other recommendations regarding the value of early testing to detect HIV and the use of drugs to treat AIDS.

These possibilities present formidable challenges to those who would seek to implement HIV risk-reduction interventions for African-American adolescents in community settings. To enlist support for behavior change interventions, researchers must be aware of the issues and must be sensitive to the values, beliefs, and concerns of the population of African Americans that will be the target of intervention efforts. This may mean seeking community input in the planning and implementation of HIV risk-reduction studies. The use of individual and focus group interviews and meetings with community opinion leaders may be useful in this connection. In addition, there is a need for more African-American scientists who are actively involved in HIV risk-reduction research in community settings.

IMPLICATIONS FOR DEVELOPMENT OF EFFECTIVE INTERVENTIONS

The present review of the literature suggests that interventions to increase African-American adolescents' use of condoms need to address hedonistic beliefs regarding the consequences of safer sex practices for sexual enjoyment. For example, Jemmott et al. (1992) found that an intervention that incorporated hedonistic beliefs was especially effective at changing intentions to use condoms. Jemmott and Jemmott (1992) reported evidence that changes in hedonistic beliefs were a mediator of changes in intentions to use condoms. Thus, interventions should attempt to weaken the common belief that sexual enjoyment is curtailed if condoms are used.

Quite apart from adolescents' beliefs about condoms, HIV risk-reduction interventions need to address the reactions of adolescents' sexual partner, particularly the sexual partner's approval or disapproval of safer sex practices, including abstinence. Unlike many health behavior interventions, HIV risk-reduction interventions have to take into account the fact that the adolescent may not have complete control over the targeted behavior. Protected sexual intercourse is interpersonal behavior and hence the sexual partner's beliefs are important. Trust is an issue that often arises during intervention-group discussions regarding convincing sexual partners to use condoms. Asking a partner to use condoms may suggest to the partner that the adolescent does not trust the partner. This is particularly likely if the partner has an established or long-term relationship with the adolescent. In contrast it may be easier to establish condom use at the beginning of new relationships. Clearly, HIV risk-reduction interventions have to take this barrier to condom use into account.

Several studies also suggested that interventions should address skills and perceived self-efficacy. Although skills and perceived self-efficacy are likely to be correlated—people who have the skills are also likely to feel efficacious—they are not identical and it is unclear which of the two is more important to behavior change. A number of types of skills and efficacy have been highlighted in the literature. Perhaps the most widely recognized type of skill or perceived efficacy is negotiation or resistance skill—the ability of the adolescent to convince a sexual partner to practice protected sexual intercourse or to resist partner pressure to practice unprotected sexual intercourse. Much less attention has been paid to technical skill in condom use, particularly skill at using condoms without ruining the mood, but, this type of skill may be just as important as negotiation skills (Jemmott, Jemmott, & Hacker, 1992). HIV risk-reduction interventions must teach adolescents how to use condoms. It is not enough to simply tell them they should use condoms. By increasing technical skill at using condoms it may be possible to allay the adolescents' sexual partner's concerns about the adverse impact of condom use on sexual enjoyment. Clearly, if an adolescent successfully negotiates condom use, but then implements it in a clumsy manner, the experience may decrease the likelihood that the adolescent will attempt to use condoms in the future or may make it more difficult to negotiate future use with that sexual partner. Role-plays are one way to enhance negotiation skills; condom exercises can be used to rehearse use of condoms. Because of the importance of negotiation and technical skills and perceived self-efficacy it is important to use well-trained facilitators who are comfortable with sexual matters. A facilitator who is uncomfortable with sexual matters may give the skills short shrift. Yet these skills are a critical feature of the intervention.

A clear implication of the literature on HIV risk-reduction interventions with African-American adolescents is that a focus on AIDS knowledge is an ineffective way of changing behavior. Although all of the AIDS prevention interventions we reviewed covered the facts about the etiology, transmission, and prevention of HIV infection, interventions that focused only on these facts were less effective than those that focused on other potential mediators of behavior change. A study that demonstrated this effect was the Jemmott et al. (1992) study in which an AIDS information-alone intervention had weaker effects on intentions to use condoms than did an intervention focusing on perceived self-efficacy and hedonistic beliefs. Similarly, the Jemmott and Jemmott (1992) study suggested that changes in intentions to use condoms were not associated with changes in knowledge.

The goal of HIV risk-reduction interventions is to decrease unprotected sexual intercourse so as to reduce risk of exposure to HIV. Empirical evidence does not clarify whether the best strategy to accomplish this goal is to stress decreases in sexual activity (e.g., abstinence) or to stress the consistent use of condoms during sexual activity. Although interventions should emphasize that the decision to practice abstinence or to have sexual intercourse is one that the adolescent has to make, they should make clear that abstinence is an acceptable choice that many adolescents make and that abstinence is the only way to eliminate completely the potential for sexually transmitted HIV infection. In addition, interventions should emphasize that adolescents who decide to have sexual intercourse should use condoms to reduce their risk of sexually transmitted infection. The issue of birth control may arise. Adolescents are often far more concerned about pregnancy than about STDs, though this may be changing. Adolescents may believe that condoms are unnecessary because of the use of contraceptive pills. It should be emphasized that both pregnancy prevention *and* STD prevention are important, that even if the female partner uses contraceptive pills, it is still necessary to use a latex condom to prevent sexually transmitted infection.

FUTURE RESEARCH

The literature on HIV risk-reduction interventions for African-American adolescents is relatively small. There are a number of significant questions that remain to be addressed in future studies. Although it is important to use culturally appropriate educational materials, one question that is unanswered is whether there are limits to the gains that can be achieved with tailoring interventions to the target population's culture. For example, many of the interventions were culturally appropriate, but none of them were Afrocentric. If a culturally appropriate intervention is effective, would an Afrocentric intervention be measurably more effective? Studies are needed to develop, implement, and contrast the effects of Afrocentric interventions with those of culturally sensitive interventions.

More broadly, we need a series of studies that contrast different types of interventions to determine which interventions are most effective. At this point we know that it is possible to change HIV risk-associated behavior among African-American adolescents. What we need is empirical evidence regarding what types of intervention strategies will bring about the greatest changes in behavior. Studies are also needed to further clarify the circumstances that lead to the greatest changes in behavior. Only two studies focused on this issue. Although these studies considered gender of facilitator, race of facilitator, gender of participant, and gender composition of small-group effects, additional studies are needed to replicate these results and to consider other features of interventions. For example, peers are thought to have an important impact on adolescents' risk behavior. In the literature on smoking and substance abuse, peer educators have been utilized; however, this approach was not used in any of the studies of interventions with African-American adolescents we reviewed. In particular, it would be interesting to compare effects of interventions implemented by peers with those implemented by adults.

CONCLUSIONS

In conclusion, there is ample evidence of the risk of sexually transmitted HIV infection among inner-city African-American adolescents, but little progress has been made toward scientific knowledge regarding how to reduce this risk. We did find that some studies on African-American adolescents have evaluated interventions to change HIV risk-associated sexual behavior, but there have been relatively few such studies.

Our review of the literature suggested a number of avenues that future studies should pursue. Particularly valuable would be experiments that test theory-based interventions. But the use of theory should not be limited to the design of intervention procedures. Theory should also drive the selection of variables to be assessed. By measuring the putative theory-based mediators of behavior change, a better conceptual understanding of risk behavior will emerge. Thus, statistical analyses might focus on whether the effects of an intervention are mediated by the conceptual variables it was designed to influence. We would conjecture that it is the conceptual variables or mediating mechanisms that are likely to generalize from study to study rather than the details of intervention protocols. Thus, for example, the best approach for changing hedonistic beliefs may vary from population to population, but the importance of changing hedonistic beliefs may be invariant. In addition, if a theory-based intervention fails to change behavior, an examination of the putative mediators might shed light on why change did not occur or might suggest that the hypothesized variables are not important mediators. In this way, the key variables that risk-reduction interventions should target might be identified.

Finally, research on HIV risk-reduction among African-American adolescents in community settings is in an early stage of development. Few intervention studies have been conducted, and, accordingly, the inferences that can be drawn are limited. There is clearly a need for additional, methodologically rigorous, studies in this area, but there are also potential obstacles to such studies. These obstacles include logistical problems and community distrust of researchers and skepticism about behavior change recommendations. We are optimistic that by being sensitive to the values, beliefs, and concerns of the community it may be possible to conduct the theory-based, methodologically sound studies that are necessary to inform HIV risk-reduction efforts aimed at African-American adolescents in community settings.

ACKNOWLEDGMENT. The authors gratefully acknowledge the helpful comments of Carla Lewis, Ph.D. on a previous version of this chapter. Preparation of this chapter was supported in part by grant R01 MH45668 from the National Institute of Mental Health, grant R01 NR03123 from the National Center for Nursing Research, and grants R01 HD24921 and U01 HD30145 from the National Institute of Child Health and Human Development.

REFERENCES

Ajzen, I. (1985). From intentions to actions: A theory of planned behavior. In J. Kuhl & J. Beckmann (Eds.), *Action-control: From cognition to behavior* (pp. 11–39). Heidelberg, Germany: Springer.

Ajzen, I. (1991). The theory of planned behavior. *Organizational Behavior & Human Decision Processes, 50,* 179–211.

Ajzen, I., & Fishbein, M. (1980). *Understanding attitudes and predicting social behavior.* Englewood Cliffs, NJ: Prentice-Hall.

Bandura, A. (1982). Self-efficacy mechanism in human agency. *American Psychologist, 37,* 122–147.

Bandura, A. (1986). *Social foundations of thought and action: A social cognitive theory.* Englewood Cliffs, NJ: Prentice-Hall.

Bandura, A. (1989). Perceived self-efficacy. In V. M. Mays, G. W. Albee, & S. F. Schneider (Eds.), *Primary prevention of AIDS: Psychological approaches* (pp. 128–141). Newbury Park, CA: Sage.

Belcastro, P. A. (1985). Sexual behavior differences between Black and White students. *Journal of Sex Research, 21,* 56–67.

Bell, T. A., & Holmes, K. K. (1984). Age-specific risks of syphilis, gonorrhea, and hospitalized pelvic inflammatory disease in sexually experienced U.S. women. *Sexually Transmitted Diseases, 7,* 291.

Brown, S. V. (1985). Premarital sexual permissiveness among Black adolescent females. *Social Psychology Quarterly, 48,* 381–387.

Catania, J. A., Dolcini, M. M., Coates, T. J., Kegeles, S. M., Greenblatt, R. M., Puckett, S., Corman, M., & Miller, J. (1989). Predictors of condom use and multiple partnered sex among sexually-active adolescent women: Implications for AIDS-related health interventions. *Journal of Sex Research, 26,* 514–524.

Cates, W., Jr. (1987). Epidemiology and control of sexually transmitted diseases: Strategic evolution. *Infectious Disease Clinics of North America, 1,* 1–23.

Centers for Disease Control and Prevention. (1988). Condoms for the prevention of sexually transmitted diseases. *Morbidity and Mortality Weekly Report, 37,* 133–137.

Centers for Disease Control and Prevention. (1991). Premarital sexual experience among adolescent women—United States, 1970–1988. *Morbidity and Mortality Weekly Report, 39,* 929–932.

Centers for Disease Control and Prevention (CDC). (1993). *HIV/AIDS Surveillance Report, February,* 1–23. Atlanta, GA: National Center for Infectious Diseases, Centers for Disease Control and Prevention.

Coates, T. J., McKusick, L., Kuno, R., & Stites, D. P. (1989). Stress reduction training changed number of sexual partners but not immune function in men with HIV. *American Journal of Public Health, 79,* 885–887.

Cook, T. & Campbell, D. (1979). *Quasi-experimentation: Design and analysis for field settings.* Chicago.

Crowne, D., & Marlowe, D. (1964). *The approval motive.* New York: Wiley.

DeParle, J. (1990, October 29). Talk of government being out to get blacks falls on more attentive ears. *New York Times,* p. B7.

Fishbein, M., & Ajzen, I. (1975). *Belief, attitude, intention and behavior.* Boston: Addison-Wesley.

Fishbein, M., & Middlestadt, S. (1989). Using the theory of reasoned action as a framework for understanding and changing AIDS-related behaviors. In V. Mays, G. Albee, & S. Schneider (Eds.), *Primary prevention of AIDS: Psychological approaches* (pp. 93–110). Newbury Park, CA: Sage.

Fox, G. L., & Inazu, J. K. (1980). Patterns and outcomes of mother-daughter communication about sexuality. *Journal of Social Issues, 36,* 7–29.

Furstenberg, F. F. (1971). Birth control experience among pregnant adolescents: The process of unplanned parenthood. *Social Problems, 19,* 192–203.

Gillum, R. F. (1982). Coronary heart disease in black populations. I. Mortality and morbidity. *American Heart Journal, 104,* 839–843.

Handelsman, C. D., Cabral, R. J., & Weisfeld, G. E. (1987). Sources of information and adolescent sexual knowledge and behavior. *Journal of Adolescent Research, 2,* 455–463.

Hatcher, R. A., Stewart, F. H., Trussell, J., Kowal, D., Guest, F., Stewart, G. K., & Cates, W. (1990). *Contraceptive technology 1990–1992.* New York: Irvington Publishers.

Hingson, R. W., Strunin, L., Berlin, B., & Heeren, T. (1990). Beliefs about AIDS, use of alcohol and drugs, and unprotected sex among Massachusetts adolescents. *American Journal of Public Health, 80,* 295–299.

Hofferth, S. L., & Hayes, C. D. (Eds.). (1987). *Risking the future: Adolescent sexuality, pregnancy, and childbearing* (Vol. 2). Washington, DC: National Academy Press.

Hofferth, S., Kahn, J., & Baldwin, W. (1987). Premarital sexual activity among U.S. teenage women over the past three decades. *Family Planning Perspectives, 19*(20) 46–53.

Hogan, D. P., & Kitagawa, E. M. (1985). The impact of social status, family structure, and neighborhood on the fertility of Black adolescents. *American Journal of Sociologym, 90,* 825–855.

Hogan, D. P., Astone, N. M., & Kitagawa, E. M. (1985). Social and environmental factors influencing contraceptive use among Black adolescents. *Family Planning Perspectives, 17,* 165–169.

Ibrahim, M., Chobanian, A. V., Horan, M., & Roccella, E. J. (1985). Hypertension prevalence and the status of awareness, treatment, and control in the United States: Final report of the Subcommittee on Definition and Prevalence of the 1984 Joint National Committee on Detection, Evaluation, and Treatment of High Blood Pressure. *Hypertension, 7,* 453–468.

Jemmott, L. S., & Jemmott, J. B. III. (1990). Sexual knowledge, attitudes, and risky sexual behavior among inner-city black male adolescents. *Journal of Adolescent Research, 5,* 346–369.

Jemmott, L. S., & Jemmott, J. B., III. (1991). Applying the theory of reasoned action to AIDS risk behavior: Condom use among black women. *Nursing Research, 40,* 228–234.

Jemmott, L. S., & Jemmott, J. B. III. (1992). Increasing condom-use intentions among sexually active inner-city black adolescent women: Effects of an AIDS prevention program. *Nursing Research, 41,* 273–279.

Jemmott, J. B. III, Jemmott, L. S., & Fong, G. T. (1992). Reductions in HIV risk-associated sexual behaviors among Black male adolescents: Effects of an AIDS prevention intervention. *American Journal of Public Health, 82,* 372–377.

Jemmott, J. B. III, & Jemmott, L. S., & Fong, G. T. (1993). *Reducing the risk of AIDS in Black adolescents: Evidence for the generality of intervention effects.* Manuscript under editorial review.

Jemmott, J. B. III, Jemmott, L. S., Braverman, P., Boccher-Lattimore, D., Fong, G. T., Lerman, C., McCaffree, K., & Hacker, C. I. (1993). *Training mothers to reduce their daughters' HIV risk behavior: A social cognitive intervention.* Paper presented at the Annual Meeting of the Society of Behavioral Medicine, San Francisco, CA, April.

Jemmott, J. B. III, Jemmott, L. S., & Hacker, C. I. (1992). Predicting intentions to use condoms among African American adolescents: The theory of planned behavior as a model of HIV risk associated behavior. *Journal of Ethnicity & Disease, 2,* 371–380.

Jemmott, J. B. III, Jemmott, L. S., Spears, H., Hewitt, N., & Cruz-Collins, M. (1992). Self-efficacy, hedonistic expectancies, and condom-use intentions among inner-city black adolescent women: A social cognitive approach to AIDS risk behavior. *Journal of Adolescent Health, 13,* 512–519.

Jemmott, J. B. III, & Jones, J. M. (1993). Social psychology and AIDS among ethnic minority individuals: Risk behaviors and strategies for changing them. In J. Pryor & G. Reeder (Eds.), *Social psychology of HIV infection* (pp. 183–224). Hillsdale, NJ: Lawrence Erlbaum.

Jones, E. F., Forrest, J. D., Goldman, N., Henshaw, S., Lincoln, R., Rosoff, J. I., Westoff, C. F., & Wulf, D. (1986). *Teenage pregnancy in industrialized countries.* New Haven, CT: Yale University Press.

Kauth, M. R., St. Lawrence, J. S., & Kelly, J. A. (1991). Reliability of retrospective assessments of sexual HIV risk behavior: A comparison of biweekly, three-month, and twelve-month self-reports. *AIDS Education and Prevention, 3,* 207–214.

Keller, S. E., Barlett, J. A., Schleifer, S. J., Johnson, R. L., Pinner, E., & Delaney, B. (1991). HIV-relevant sexual behavior among a healthy inner-city heterosexual adolescent population in an endemic area of HIV. *Journal of Adolescent Health, 12,* 44–48.

Kelly, J. A., St. Lawrence, J. S., Diaz, Y. E., Stevenson, L. Y., Hauth, A. C., Brasfield, T. L., Kalichman, S. C., Smith, J. E., & Andrew, M. E. (1991). HIV risk behavior reduction following intervention with key opinion leaders of population. *American Journal of Public Health, 81,* 168–171.

Kelly, J. A., St. Lawrence, J. S., Hood, H. V., & Brasfield, T. L. (1989). Behavioral intervention to reduce AIDS risk activities. *Journal of Consulting and Clinical Psychology, 57,* 60–67.

Lanier, M. M., & McCarthy, B. R. (1989). AIDS awareness and the impact of AIDS education in juvenile corrections. *Criminal Justice and Behavior, 16,* 395–411.

Madden, T. J., Ellen, P. S., & Ajzen, I. (1992). A comparison of the theory of planned behavior and the theory of reasoned action. *Personality and Social Psychology Bulletin, 18,* 3–9.

Milan, R. J., & Kilmann, P. R. (1987). Interpersonal factors in premarital contraception. *Journal of Sex Research, 23,* 289–321.

Morrison, D. M. (1985). Adolescent contraceptive behavior: A review. *Psychological Bulletin, 98,* 538–568.

Mosher, W. D., & Pratt, W. F. (1990). *Contraceptive use in the United States, 1973–1988. Advance data from vital and health statistics* (no. 182). Hyattsville, MD: National Center for Health Statistics.

Nathanson, C. A., & Becker, M. H. (1986). Family and peer influence on obtaining a method of contraception. *Journal of Marriage & the Family, 48,* 513–526.

O'Leary, A. (1985). Self-efficacy and health. *Behavioral Research & Therapy, 23,* 437–451.

O'Leary, A., Goodhardt, F., Jemmott, L. S., & Boccher-Lattimore, D. (1992). Predictors of safer sex on the college campus: A social cognitive theory analysis. *Journal of American College Health, 40,* 254–263.

Page, H. S., & Asire, A. J. (1985). *Cancer rates and risks* (3rd ed.) (NIH Publication No. 85-691). Bethesda, MD: National Institutes of Health.

Pleck, J. H. (1989). Correlates of black adolescent males' condom use. *Journal of Adolescent Research, 4,* 247–253.

Pratt, W., Mosher, W., Bachrach, C., & Horn, M. (1984). Understanding U. S. fertility: Findings from the National Survey of Family Growth, Cycle III. *Population Bulletin, 39,* 1–42.

Reinisch, J. M., Sanders, S. A., & Ziemba-Davis, M. (1988). The study of sexual behavior in relation to the transmission of human immunodeficiency virus. *American Psychologist, 43,* 921–927.

Rickert, V. I., Jay, M. S., & Gottlieb, A. (1991). Effects of a peer-counseled AIDS education program on knowledge, attitudes, and satisfaction of adolescents. *Journal of Adolescent Health, 12,* 38–43.

Rickert, V. I., Gottlieb, A., & Jay, M. S. (1990). A comparison of three clinic-based AIDS education programs on female adolescents' knowledge, attitudes and behavior. *Journal of Adolescent Health Care, 11,* 298–303.

Schinke, S. P., Gordon, A. N., & Weston, R. E. (1990). Self-instruction to prevent HIV infection among African-American and Hispanic-American adolescents. *Journal of Consulting & Clinical Psychology, 58,* 432–436.

Solomon, M. Z., & DeJong, W. (1989). Preventing AIDS and other STDs through condom promotion: A patient education intervention. *American Journal of Public Health, 79,* 453–458.

Sonenstein, F. L., Pleck, J. H., & Ku, L. C. (1989). Sexual activity, condom use and AIDS awareness among adolescent males. *Family Planning Perspectives, 21,* 152–158.

Stone, K. M., Grimes, D. A., & Magder, L. S. (1986). Personal protection against sexually transmitted diseases. *American Journal of Obstetrics & Gynecology, 155,* 180–188.

Taylor, H., Kagay, M., & Leichenko, S. (1986). *American teens speak: Sex, myths, TV, and birth control.* New York: Planned Parenthood Federation of America.

Thomas, S. B., Gilliam, A. G., & Iwrey, C. G. (1989). Knowledge about AIDS and reported risk behaviors among black college students. *Journal of American College Health, 38,* 61–66.

Turner, C., Miller, H., & Moses, L. (1989). *AIDS: Sexual behavior and intravenous drug use.* Washington, DC: National Academy Press.

Valdiserri, R. O., Arena, V. C., Proctor, D., & Bonati, F. A. (1989). The relationship between women's attitudes about condoms and their use: Implications for condom promotion programs. *American Journal of Public Health, 79,* 499–503.

Valdiserri, R. O., Lyter, D. W., Leviton, L. C., Callahan, C. M., Kingsley, L. A., & Rinaldo, C. R. (1989). AIDS prevention in homosexual and bisexual men: Results of a randomized trial evaluating two risk reduction interventions. *AIDS, 3,* 21–26.

Williams, R. L. (1980). The death of white research in the black community. In R. L. Jones (Ed.), *Black psychology* (pp. 403–416). New York: Harper & Row.

Wyatt, G. E., Peters, S., & Guthrie, D. (1988a). Kinsey revisited, I: Comparisons of sexual socialization and sexual behavior of white women over 33 years. *Archives of Sexual Behavior, 17,* 201–239.

Wyatt, G. E., Peters, S., & Guthrie, D. (1988b). Kinsey revisited, II: Comparisons of sexual socialization and sexual behavior of black women over 33 years. *Archives of Sexual Behavior, 17,* 289–332.

Zelnik, M., Kantner, J. F., & Ford, K. (1981). *Sex and pregnancy in adolescence.* Beverly Hills, CA: Sage.

9

Preventing HIV among Runaways:
Victims and Victimization

*MARY JANE ROTHERAM-BORUS,
JULIE FELDMAN, MARGARET ROSARIO,
and EDWARD DUNNE*

INTRODUCTION

Runaway and homeless youth are an understudied and underserved population at increased risk of human immunodeficiency virus (HIV) infection. While seroprevalence data were preliminary, high rates of HIV infection among homeless and runaway adolescents throughout several major American cities indicated cause for concern. Among this adolescent subgroup, HIV seropositivity ranged from a low of 2% in Houston (Stricof, Novick, & Kennedy, 1990) to 5% in New York City (Stricof, Kennedy, Nattell, Weisfuse, & Novick, 1991) and 8% in San Francisco (Shalwitz, Goulart, Dunnigan, & Flannery, 1990). These HIV seroprevalence rates were 2 to 10 times higher than the seropositivity rates reported for other adolescent populations in this country (DiClemente, 1992; St. Louis, Hayman, Miller, Anderson, Petersen, & Dondero, 1989). The markedly higher seropositivity rates among runaway and homeless youth relative to other adolescent populations suggested that

MARY JANE ROTHERAM-BORUS • Division of Social Psychiatry, Department of Psychiatry, UCLA Neuropsychiatric Institute, Los Angeles, California 90024-1759.   *JULIE FELDMAN* • Division of Child Psychiatry, College of Physicians and Surgeons, Columbia University, New York, New York 10032.   *MARGARET ROSARIO* • Department of Psychiatry, College of Physicians and Surgeons, and School of Public Health, Columbia University, New York, New York 10032.   *EDWARD DUNNE* • Department of Psychiatry, College of Physicians and Surgeons, Columbia University, New York, New York 10032.

Preventing AIDS: Theories and Methods of Behavioral Interventions, edited by Ralph J. DiClemente and John L. Peterson. Plenum Press, New York, 1994.

HIV prevention programs for this population are an important public health priority.

PREVALENCE OF HIV SEXUAL RISK BEHAVIORS

Considerable evidence demonstrated that a sizable proportion of runaway and homeless adolescents engaged in behaviors associated with transmission of HIV (Koopman, Rosario, & Rotheram-Borus, 1993; Robertson, 1989; Rotheram-Borus et al., 1992; Pennbridge, Freese, & MacKenzie, 1992; Sugerman, Hergenroeder, Chacko, & Parcel, 1991; Yates, MacKenzie, Pennbridge, & Cohen, 1988). Runaways tended to initiate sexual intercourse two to three years earlier than national samples of adolescents (Zelnick & Shah, 1983). Among runaways in New York City, the mean age for any genital or anal sex was 12.4 years (Rotheram-Borus et al., 1992). Having multiple sexual partners was also characteristic of this adolescent subgroup. Among runaways in New York City, 47% of males and 16% of females reported having 10 or more opposite-sex partners (Rotheram-Borus et al., 1992), and 98% of male street youth in Los Angeles had multiple partners (Pennbridge et al., 1992). These findings were dramatic when compared to 7% of a national sample of older male adolescents having 11 or more sex partners and to 5% of a national sample of older female adolescents having 10 or more sex partners (Miller, Turner, & Moses, 1990).

Runaway and homeless adolescents were also more likely to engage in survival sex. Twenty-two percent of runaways in Los Angeles (Yates et al., 1988) and 26% in New York City were involved in survival sex (Rotheram-Borus et al., 1992), as compared with 1% in a national sample (Sonenstein, Pleck, & Ku, 1989). One of the most alarming risk factors among runaway and homeless adolescents was their inconsistent use of condoms. Only 24% of male street youth in Los Angeles always used condoms with opposite-sex partners and 40% never used condoms with opposite-sex partners (Pennbridge et al., 1992). Sugerman and colleagues (1991) found that among a sample of runaway and homeless adolescents in Houston, 20% reported consistent condom use and 33% reported rarely or never using condoms. In summary, approximately one-fifth of these adolescents reported using condoms consistently, while more than one-third reported never using condoms. These data were particularly worrisome considering the high rates of survival sex and multiple partners among these adolescents.

PREVALENCE OF SUBSTANCE ABUSE

The sharing of injection drug needles is a primary route of HIV infection (Miller et al., 1990). In Los Angeles, the lifetime prevalence of injection drug use among runaway and homeless adolescents was approximately 35%, and one-third (34%) of those injecting drugs in the three months prior to the study reported sharing their injection drug needles (Pennbridge et al., 1992; Yates et al., 1988). Similarly, one-fourth of homeless youth in Hollywood had injected drugs during their lifetime (Robertson, 1989). In contrast to the high prevalence of injection drug use in California, markedly lower prevalence rates of injection drug behavior were identified in New York City; between 0.3 and 5% of the runaway and homeless youth in New York City reported injection drug use (Koopman et al., 1993; Shaffer & Caton, 1984).

Nevertheless, runaway and homeless youth in New York City (Koopman et al., 1993) were far more likely to report substance use than national samples of teenagers (National Institute on Drug Abuse, 1991). For example, the runaways were 1.5 times more likely to use alcohol (71% vs. 48%); three times more likely to use marijuana (45% vs. 15%); and seven times more likely to use cocaine/crack (19% vs. 2.6%). Although alcohol and noninjection drug use are not directly linked to HIV infection, use of drugs and alcohol can greatly influence adolescents' sexual risk behaviors. For example, adolescents may engage in sex in order to fund their drug and/or alcohol habits (Fullilove, Fullilove, Bowser, & Gross, 1990). In addition, substance use can disinhibit sexual restraints and lead to unprotected sex acts (e.g., Fullilove et al., 1990). Two-thirds of the runaway and homeless youth in Los Angeles were high on drugs more than half the time during survival sex and one-fourth were high on drugs more than half the time during recreational sex (Pennbridge et al., 1992). Drug users may also be more likely to come into contact with populations associated with injection drug use. Consequently, there is an increased chance that they will have sexual encounters with injection drug users. For example, 67% of the runaway and homeless youth in Los Angeles reported having at least one sex partner who had injected drugs (Pennbridge et al., 1992).

These rates demonstrated the substantial sexual and substance use risk acts that accounted for the high HIV seroprevalence rate among homeless and runaway youth. The data also indicated the necessity: (1) to implement early intervention, given the early age of sexual initiation; (2) to provide training and practice in skills needed to negotiate sexual intercourse in the context of survival sex, a business transaction that places the youth in a vulnerable power position because it often determines whether the youth eats or sleeps comfortably over the next week; (3) to address gender differences in the pattern of sexual risk acts by tailoring programs according to gender; and (4) to curtail substance use, teach skills needed to maintain safer sex practices while under the influence of alcohol and drugs, and maintain clean injection equipment.

HIV PREVENTION FOR RUNAWAY AND HOMELESS ADOLESCENTS

Few HIV prevention programs specifically targeting runaway and homeless adolescents have been adequately evaluated. In one study, Rotheram-Borus and her colleagues (Rotheram-Borus, Koopman, Haignere, & Davies, 1991a) used a randomized control design to assess the effect of a risk-reduction intervention. Over a two-year period (from 1988 to 1990), consecutive recruitment of adolescents at two residential shelters in New York City (one designated the nonintervention site and the other the intervention site) resulted in 79 and 188 runaways available for enrollment in the program at the intervention and nonintervention sites, respectively. After attrition, the final sample was comprised of 78 adolescents in the intervention condition and 67 adolescents in the nonintervention condition.

Runaways participating in the risk-reduction program were exposed to a multiple session intervention administered by skilled trainers. The program addressed the following: general knowledge about HIV and acquired immunodeficiency syndrome (AIDS), coping skills, access to health care and other resources, and individual barriers to use of safer sex practices. General HIV knowledge was addressed by having adolescents participate in video and art workshops and review commercial HIV/AIDS videos. Coping skills training addressed runaways' unrealistic expectations regarding emotional and behavioral responses in high-risk situations. Additional medical and mental health care and other resources were made available to address specific individual health concerns. Individual barriers to adopting and maintaining safer sex practices were reviewed in private counseling sessions.

Participants in the nonintervention condition were exposed to individual counseling from staff; but this counseling did not specifically address HIV prevention. Condoms were available and staff members, on an unsystematic basis, discussed condom use.

Runaways in the risk-reduction program demonstrated a significant and dramatic increase in consistent condom use and less frequently reported engaging in a high-risk pattern of HIV-associated behaviors over six months. A high-risk pattern of sexual behavior was defined as consistent condom use occurring in fewer than 50% of sexual encounters, 10 or more sexual encounters, and/or three or more sexual partners. A greater proportion of adolescents (22%) in the control group reported this high-risk pattern of sexual behavior compared to those adolescents (9%) who received between 10 and 14 intervention sessions and those (0%) who received 15 or more intervention sessions. Reports of consistent condom use increased from about 32% of runaways at initiation of the project to 62% six months after receiving more than 15 intervention sessions.

A two-year follow-up of the same sample continued to show significant reductions in risk acts among those who received the intervention (Rotheram-Borus, 1993). The effectiveness of the intervention was not uniform. In general, however, while program effectiveness varied greatly for each gender and ethnic group (Reid, Rotheram-Borus, Rosario, & Gwadz, 1993), those who participated in the intervention continued to report fewer unprotected risk acts. Program impact was most prominent with African-American adolescents. The mean number of unprotected sexual acts was two times higher among those African-American adolescents who did not receive the intervention compared with those who did participate in the intervention (16 vs. 6 high-risk sex acts in three months). Males had significantly fewer unprotected acts compared to females (5 vs. 14 acts during the last three months). The mean number of unprotected acts for females in the control group was twice that of females in the intervention group, but females were at much higher risk two years later compared to males. The effects were similar for white adolescents (26 vs. 8 acts). High anxiety and low levels of knowledge of HIV appeared to mediate the impact of the intervention.

These results parallel changes found by programs targeting HIV risk behaviors among other adolescent populations such as runaway and homeless youth (Fritz & Shaffer, 1992), minority youth (Jemmott, Jemmott, & Fong, 1991), and gay male youth (Rotheram-Borus, Rosario, & Reid, 1993). Similar to these successful programs, this was an intensive program which included social skills training, multiple goals (e.g., reducing drug and alcohol use, increasing condom use), small groups in an institutional setting where learning could be reinforced by peers and adults, and the development of engaging and fun activities.

Although prevention programs for adolescents have been successful in changing behavior, albeit modestly, at least three major problems remain. First, a significant proportion of persons are unresponsive to intervention efforts (about 30%: Reid et al., 1993; Rotheram-Borus et al., 1991a). Second, a significant proportion relapse in their risk behaviors, usually within a year (about 8% to 18%: Reid et al., 1993; Rotheram-Borus et al., 1991a; 1993). And, finally, the programs are expensive and, therefore, will only be applied to the subgroups at highest risk, prohibiting broad scale dissemination of HIV prevention programs.

The living circumstances of adolescents and their limited resources further complicate the potential dissemination of programs. HIV prevention efforts must now meet the challenge of designing programs to address these problems.

SOCIETY'S ATTITUDES AND POLICIES
TOWARD HOMELESS YOUTH

The above recommendation cannot be addressed by HIV intervention programs alone. The success experienced with helping homeless adolescents to reduce their HIV risk behaviors has been significant; particularly when viewed within the context of the highly stressful living environments and limited available resources of runaway and homeless adolescents. To promote long-term maintenance of HIV-preventive behaviors, however, we must examine the social context of adolescents' lives in shelters and their relation to service providers.

There is broad-scale agreement that societies have a responsibility to care for their children. The international rights of children have been affirmed by the United Nations document indicating these rights (U.N. Convention on the Rights of Children, 1991). In the case of runaway and homeless youth, these basic rights of food, shelter, and health care in a safe environment clearly have been violated.

The shelters serving runaway and homeless youth are often marginalized institutions that secure financing based on "charitable" contributions from others. Some of the largest shelters in the United States are funded by private charities which solicit for funds on an ongoing basis, often obtaining up to 80% of their funds from contributions by corporations, foundations, and individuals (Covenant House, 1992). The success of these appeals is based partly on depicting runaways as victims or waifs who can be saved by financial contributions. The following quote is illustrative.

> Tonight on the streets of Hollywood—a place where dreams are made and lost— a kid wanders. It's been a week since he made his way to what he thought was the glamour of Hollywood from his mother's home in Oregon where he thought no one cared about him. Ever since he arrived, he has been on the streets, alone, terrified and hungry. It doesn't take long for a young boy like that to learn the danger . . . to know how limited his options are. He knows the places where the kids like himself end up. The question is, just how desperate is he? How long can he hold out? (Covenant House, 1992)

This description is disturbing and those reading it often have an immediate response of wanting to help this youth. As successful as they are in raising money, there are negative consequences to these types of appeals. First, the fund-raising method victimizes rather than empowers adolescents. The literature soliciting contributions paints adolescents as atypical, helpless waifs who are on the road to moral corruption, but who can be saved. Lost in such descriptions is adolescents' basic right to a stable place to live for an extended period of time while they set achievable educational and occupational goals. Second, these appeals and the services provided by charitable institutions serving homeless youth, deflect attention from the institution ultimately responsible for these adolescents and their educational, occupational, mental, and physical well-being: society. A minor without a stable family and home is a ward of the state whether or not society accepts the responsibilities associated with this charge.

Although appeals, such as the one described earlier, have been very effective in raising money essential for the maintenance of shelters for homeless and runaway adolescents, little attention has been paid to meeting these adolescents' needs for stable, long-term living conditions. Runaway and homeless adolescents are challenged to provide for themselves in a manner inconsistent with their developmental stage. They are burdened by adult responsibilities and expected by society to provide for their own food, shelter, and security. Physically these children are capable of having sex, but emotionally they are ill-prepared to cope with the consequences of sexual activity.

Runaway and homeless youth clearly have become victims, receiving neither support nor caretaking from society, and are forced to place their lives at risk in order to survive. As a consequence, some runaway and homeless youth also begin to victimize others in order to survive. Thus these youth, who are themselves victims, continue the cycle by victimizing others. Petty theft, drug dealing, or survival sex may be the only means for unskilled, isolated adolescents to secure food and shelter. In many countries, there is negative sentiment against homeless youth who are seen as hustlers taking advantage of the public because some of these youth engage in commercial sex and petty theft to survive (Luna & Rotheram-Borus, 1992). Public attitudes toward street youth have become even more negative with the advent of HIV because these young people are perceived as a potential vector for infecting the middle-class, heterosexual community.

In the face of such strong negative public sentiment, efforts to increase the awareness of public responsibility for homeless youth have again tended to portray them as hapless victims. Paradoxically, these portrayals further contribute to the deterioration of their lives by deflecting responsibility for these youth away from society and by perpetuating the victim/victimizer cycle. Consequently, their basic human rights to decent housing, sustenance, and occupational and educational opportunities are not recognized.

When the Runaway and Homeless Youth Act of 1974 was originally passed by Congress, agencies were to be full-service programs. A full-service program provides for adolescents' comprehensive needs (housing, food, medical care, safety) and it begins to address longer-term problems associated with educational needs, family crises intervention, and stable living. Today, however, very few full-service agencies for homeless youth exist. Only the shelters that are administered most effectively can piece together funding that assists youth in securing long-term stable placements.

Focus has now become centered on receiving immediate needs, rather than providing long-term care. After receiving temporary shelter, where are youth to go? For example, there are an estimated 9,000 to 12,000 homeless youth in New York City per year (Shaffer & Caton, 1984), 85% of whom will not return to their families (Rotheram-Borus et al., 1992). These youth need to find stable placements or living situations. There are about 285 short-term residential shelter beds (30-day crisis care; Empire State Coalition of Youth and Family Services, Personal communication, 1993), approximately 80 transitional residential beds (up to one year placements; Empire State Coalition, Personal communication, 1993), and slightly over 5,600 foster care group home placements which are filled predominantly by youth who are removed from their homes due to neglect and/or abuse or by emotionally disturbed youth (Child Welfare Administration [CWA], 1992; Personal communication, 1993). Clearly, there are at least 3,000 runaway and homeless children for whom no stable placement is available (conservatively assuming that all foster care group home beds are filled by runaway and homeless youth). Thus, adolescents' long-term stable placement is not a realistic alternative in the current structure of the social service delivery system for runaways in New York City. Of the few services that are available, the majority are funded through the private sector. As we have seen, these agencies resort to charitable appeals to fund these services, typically portraying homeless youth as hapless victims.

How do these structural features of the system of soliciting and receiving funding for runaway and homeless youth impact HIV prevention for youth? Reduction and maintenance of safer sex and substance use behaviors are contingent on homeless youth having long-term stable placements. If street-based and shelter programs are the primary means of providing for youth, then HIV prevention programs must be tailored to deal with this unfortunate reality. We need to develop intervention strategies anticipating that youth will leave shelters and live on the streets instead of moving into stable, long-term residences.

YOUTH'S REACTIONS TO SOCIETY

Being a victim is only one aspect of a paradox of victimization-victimizer. Homeless youth also have been found to have conduct problems and engage in delinquent acts that place them in the role of victimizing others. For example, about one-fourth of the youth have had contact with the criminal justice system in the last three months (Rotheram-Borus, Rosario, & Koopman, 1991b). In the last three months, youth report a mean of 3.2 conduct problems (i.e., lying, stealing). A diagnosis of conduct disorder requires three symptoms to meet the criterion outlined in *The Diagnostic and Statistical Manual* (DSM-III-R) (American Psychiatric Association, 1987); more than half of the youths would meet this criterion (Shaffer & Caton, 1984). Substance use among runaway and homeless youth is also high: the rate of crack cocaine use (28%) is about eight times the national average and marijuana use (42%) is about three times the national average (National Institute of Drug Abuse, 1991). Some of these youth victimize neighborhoods by dealing drugs.

This paradox of the victim being victimizer is one of the central challenges facing service providers, educators, policy-makers, and researchers. Some homeless youth do engage in illegal activities; there are no other ways to survive. Rage is the dominant emotion felt by the majority of youth in such circumstances and sometimes this rage is directed toward those more fortunate, and results in robbery. Often it is directed toward the service providers attempting to help them. It may be expressed subtly in the form of manipulation, by youth "working" the service delivery system: a few streetwise youth can involve 20 to 30 providers at one time in trying to care for them, each spending weeks trying to provide for the youth because no one agency knows the full story of the youth's condition. But whether expressed openly or more subtly, homeless youth often feel angry at being violated by the world.

SHELTER STAFF'S ROLE IN THE VICTIM/VICTIMIZER PARADOX

In New York City, shelter care workers receive salaries that are 17% lower than those of any other social service agency staff and are perceived as having little status. Since so few of these agencies are full-service agencies, the efforts of even the best-intentioned service providers are undermined. The most talented or best qualified staff members move quickly to less stressful work circumstances. The high rate of turnover results in service being provided by the least talented or qualified, in an inconsistent manner, to a population that already often receives service on an inconsistent basis. These staff members, more deeply mired in the trap, find themselves directing their frustration at the very people they are supposed to be serving. The victimization of homeless youth by providers begins with the marginalization of the service providers, paralleling that of the youth they serve.

A recent incident in a large community-based agency demonstrates how the providers of services to homeless youth can become trapped in the paradoxical position of being both victim and victimizer. A nurse at a medical clinic linked to a homeless shelter was ready to go on vacation with her family. The car was loaded with the family's suitcases, including school clothes the nurse was bringing to her grandchildren. It was a very special trip—the first family vacation in several years. The nurse herself had been raised in the neighborhood and had worked hard for many years to finish school, get a job, and raise her children. Now she wanted to contribute to society by helping those less fortunate. While she stopped by the shelter on the way out of town to pick up her paycheck, her car was broken into and burglarized. The nurse was hurt and angry and the vacation was ruined.

Nearly three weeks later, a homeless mother came into the shelter with her 3-year-old child. The child was dressed in the school clothes intended for the nurse's grandchildren. A tremendous furor ensued. The clothes were taken off the child; the child was left standing in her underwear, sobbing and not understanding why her new clothes had been stripped from her. The nurse who had been victimized became the victimizer of an innocent 3-year-old.

The paradoxical situation of homeless youth being both victims and victimizers is replicated in the way in which the delivery of service within shelters and agencies is structured, as well as in the ways the needs of this population are brought to public attention. As an example of homeless youth's dilemma, consider the following scenario: two social service agencies in a large inner-city area receive public funding from the city to provide shelter to homeless youth. One shelter is a full-service agency, employing a public health nurse who visits once each week; two social workers who attempt to resolve the youth's social service needs; and a number of experienced child care workers with diverse educational backgrounds. Although this agency has written personnel policies, codified acceptable methods for intervening with youth, and standard record-keeping procedures, untrained staff members sometimes yell at youth because they cannot implement techniques for setting limits consistently without becoming angry, and some staff inappropriately hug clients. At the other agency, the house rules are so stringent that the majority of youth, unaccustomed to structure, are expelled and denied read-mittance for an extended period of time. These youth often appear at the doorstep of the other agency, swelling the caseload at that site. Many of the staff members of both agencies have themselves endured difficult life experiences that may cause them to be indifferent to the problems of these youth or unable to place enough distance between the youth's problems and their own to act in a consistently professional manner in the best interests of those who come to them for help. For several months, the staff members of this second agency have not been paid on time. Payroll funds have been redirected to supplement other social service problems, such as programs to serve substance abusers—a group with a much higher profile in the media and the community than homeless youth. In addition, funds appropriated for building repairs and custodial service somehow never materialized. At the shelter, there are holes in the walls, holes in the bedspreads, unreliable televisions, broken light fixtures, overflowing toilets, and a stench in the hallways. Experiencing themselves as victims of a system in which they are underpaid and subject to intolerable work conditions, staff become enraged and burned out.

The victim–victimizer paradox is reflected in two contrasting belief systems common among shelter staff. In some shelters, staff behavior is guided by a belief that "all youth need is love" in order to alleviate the problems of the past. Youth are perceived as victims and social service counselors assume the role of providing a reconstructive experience where the victims recognize their own worth and feel loved unconditionally. Service providers adopting this philosophy often have difficulty setting limits with youth. Staff will sometimes take youth home with them, hug youth to express affection, and work extra hours to demonstrate their personal concern for youth. Youth may become confused and hurt when staff cross boundaries. For example, what if some youth feel excluded when they are not taken to a staff member's home or if a staff member crosses boundaries inconsistently. This philosophy can also be harmful for workers; burnout among staff espousing this philosophy is high.

In contrast, shelters which recognize that runaway and homeless youth sometimes victimize others, often operate on a belief system that "all they need is discipline." This opposite position is sometimes adopted in shelters which feel that homeless and runaway youth have difficulty following rules. These shelters enforce rigid and consistent regulations. Youth who break a rule in these shelters will typically be suspended and prevented from receiving services at the shelter for a specified period of time. This type of philosophy is often too rigid and does not accommodate to these youth's often unpredictable lives. Youth are more likely to respond more favorably to a disciplined yet flexible atmosphere.

CONCLUSIONS

HIV prevention programs can only be successful when runaway and homeless youth secure long-term stable living situations. In order to secure society's support for such placements and basic human rights, the victim-victimizer cycle must be stopped. We need to stop painting runaway and homeless youth as victims in order to secure funding based on appeals for charity. When victimizing strategies are abandoned and the rights of homeless youth are recognized, the funding priorities will shift. Although the task is formidable, researchers and service providers must still address HIV prevention among youth, prior to economic change being implemented. Despite researchers' acknowledgements that the context of youth's daily lives should play a critical role in shaping prevention efforts, research in this domain has been limited. We must recognize that satisfying sexual safety needs is not likely to be high on youth's personal agenda until more basic needs such as food and shelter are met. Why would adolescents care about dying in 10 years from AIDS, if they do not know when they will eat next or where they will sleep? Risk for HIV cannot be examined in isolation from risk for multiple negative outcomes or from the necessity of comprehensive health care for youth. Even when food and shelter are provided during the intervention program, many of these youth's needs are still unmet. We must acknowledge that the success of our intervention programs, no matter how elegant, is likely to be undermined by the circumstances in which these youth live.

No person, government, or society wants youth to go homeless. Homelessness is an outcome of fundamental national and international socioeconomic problems. It is critical that service providers and researchers acknowledge those aspects of their work they can and cannot change. Service providers must end their own victimization of the youth they are trying to serve. We must ask the hard questions: do our shelters and street outreach programs replicate the problems experienced by youth? Are those who work with homeless youth treated humanely and with sensitivity, or do they become victims of a system that underpays and ignores their contributions? How can the anger and frustration of youth and service providers be channeled in a manner that is constructive? How can we increase the visibility of the issues and concerns of homeless youth without further marginalizing and victimizing these children? Although future research evaluating HIV interventions must address these issues, economic and social policies are the foundation for addressing these paradoxes on a long-term basis.

ACKNOWLEDGMENT. This chapter was completed with support by grants to the HIV Center for Clinical and Behavioral Studies, Anke Ehrhardt, Principal Investigator, and Mental Health Research Grant ME30903-07 from the National Institutes of Mental Health and a career development award from the William T. Grant Foundation.

REFERENCES

American Psychiatric Association (1987). *Diagnostic and Statistical Manual of Mental Disorders* (3rd ed., rev.). Washington, DC: American Psychiatric Press.

Child Welfare Administration (1992). *Congregate Care Programs at a Glance and Program Profile.* New York: Author.

Covenant House (1992). *A place for second chances.* Covenant House 1992 Annual Report. New York: Author.

DiClemente, R. J. (1992). Epidemiology of AIDS, HIV seroprevalence and HIV incidence among adolescents. *Journal of School Health, 62,* 325–330.

Fritz, R., & Shaffer, T. (1992, July). *How effective are AIDS education programs for high-risk populations? An evaluation of 4 AIDS prevention programs in Chicago, U.S.A.* Paper presented at the 13th International Conference on AIDS, Amsterdam, the Netherlands.

Fullilove, R. E., Fullilove, M. T., Bowser, B. P., & Gross, S. A. (1990). Risk of sexually transmitted disease among black adolescent crack users in Oakland and San Francisco, California. *Journal of the American Medical Association, 263,* 851–855.

Jemmott, J. B., Jemmott, L. S., & Fong, G. T. (1991). Reductions in HIV risk-associated sexual behaviors among black adolescents: Effects of an AIDS prevention intervention. *American Journal of Public Health, 82,* 372–377.

Koopman, C., Rosario, M., & Rotherman-Borus, M. J. (1993). *Alcohol and drug use and sexual behaviors placing runaways at risk for HIV infection.* Manuscript submitted for publication.

Luna, G. C., & Rotheram-Borus, M. J. (1992). Street youth and the AIDS pandemic. *AIDS Education and Prevention, Suppl.,* 1–13.

Miller, H. G., Turner, C. F., & Moses, L. E. (1990). *AIDS: The second decade.* Washington, DC: National Academy Press.

National Institute on Drug Abuse (1991). *National household survey on drug abuse: Population estimates 1990.* Washington, DC: Government Printing Office (DHHS Pub. No. (ADM)91-1732).

Pennbridge, J., Freese, T., & MacKenzie, R. (1992). High-risk behaviors among male street youth in Hollywood, California. *AIDS Education & Prevention* (Fall supplement), 24–33.

Reid, H. M., Rotheram-Borus, M. J., Rosario, M., & Gwadz, M. (1993, June). *Effectiveness of HIV prevention with homeless youth over two years.* Paper presented at the 9th International Conference on AIDS, Berlin.

Robertson, M. (1989). *Homeless youth in Hollywood: Patterns of alcohol use.* A report to the National Institute on Alcohol Abuse and Alcoholism, Alcohol Research Group, School of Public Health, University of California, Berkeley.

Rotheram-Borus, M. J. (1993, March). HIV prevention with adolescents. Paper presented at the HIV Center for Clinical and Behavioral Studies, Columbia University, New York City.

Rotheram-Borus, M. J., Koopman, C., Haignere, C., & Davies, M. (1991). Reducing HIV sexual risk behaviors among runaway adolescents. *Journal of the American Medical Association, 266,* 1237–1241.

Rotheram-Borus, M. J., Meyer-Bahlburg, H. F. L., Koopman, C., Rosario, M., Exner, T. M., Henderson, R., Matthieu, M., & Gruen, R. S. (1992). Lifetime sexual behaviors among runaway males and females. *Journal of Sex Research, 29,* 15–29.

Rotheram-Borus, M. J., Rosario, M., & Koopman, C. (1991). Minority youths at high risk: Gay males and runaways. In S. Gore & M. E. Colton (Eds.), *Adolescent stress: Causes and consequences* (pp. 181–200). Hawthorne, NY: Aldine de Gruyter.

Rotheram-Borus, M. J., Rosario, M., & Reid, H. (1993). *Reducing HIV sexual risk behaviors among gay/bisexual male adolescents.* Manuscript submitted for publication.

Shaffer, D., & Caton, D. (1984). *Runaway and homeless youth in New York City: A report to the Ittleson Foundation.* New York: Ittleson Foundation.

Shalwitz, J., Goulart, M., Dunnigan, K., & Flannery, D. (1990, June). *Prevalence of sexually transmitted diseases (STD) and HIV in a homeless youth medical clinic in San Francisco* (Abstract no. SC571). Abstracts from the 6th International Conference on AIDS, San Francisco, California.

Sonenstein, F. L., Pleck, J. K., & Ku, L. C. (1989). Sexual activity, condom use and AIDS awareness among adolescent males. *Family Planning Perspectives, 21,* 152–158.

St. Louis, M., Hayman, C., Miller, C., Anderson, J., Petersen, L., & Dondero, T. (1989, June). *HIV infection in disadvantaged adolescents in the U.S.: Findings from the Jobs Corps Screening*

Program (Abstract no. MDPI). Abstracts from the 5th International Conference on AIDS, Montreal, Quebec, Canada.

Stricof, R., Kennedy, J., Nattell, T., Weisfuse, I., & Novick, L. (1991). HIV seroprevalence in a facility for runaway and homeless adolescents. *American Journal of Public Health, 81* (supple.): 50–53.

Stricof, R., Novick, L., & Kennedy, J. (1990, June). *HIV seroprevalence in facilities for runaway and homeless adolescents in four states: Florida, Texas, Louisiana, and New York.* Paper presented at the 7th International Conference on AIDS, San Francisco, CA.

Sugerman, S. T., Hergenroeder, A., Chacko, M., & Parcel, G. (1991). Acquired immunodeficiency syndrome and adolescents: Knowledge, attitudes, and behaviors of runaway and homeless youths. *American Journal of the Diseases of Children, 145,* 431–436.

United Nations. (1991). United Nations Convention of the Rights of the Child: Unofficial summary of articles. *American Psychologist, 46,* 50–52.

Yates, G., MacKenzie, R., Pennbridge, J., & Cohen, E. (1988). A risk profile comparison of runaway and non-runaway youth. *American Journal of Public Health, 78,* 820–821.

Zelnick, M., & Shah, F. K. (1983). First intercourse among young Americans. *Family Planning Perspectives, 15,* 64–70.

10

Behavioral Interventions for In-Treatment Injection Drug Users

LAURIE ROEHRICH, TAMARA L. WALL, and JAMES L. SORENSEN

INTRODUCTION

An estimated one million individuals in the United States inject drugs (Institute for Health Policy Studies, 1990). Injecting drug users (IDUs) represent the second largest group at risk for human immunodeficiency virus (HIV) infection, and are the primary source for heterosexual and perinatal HIV transmission (Centers for Disease Control, 1991). Drug injection is more highly concentrated among poor and socially marginal groups. Rates of HIV infection among IDUs vary according to geographical location and generally range from 0% to about 20% (Centers for Disease Control, 1991). In areas such as New York City and Newark, New Jersey, however, over 50% of all IDUs may have been infected (Caussy et al., 1990; Lee et al., 1990). Therefore, the reduction of high-risk behavior is a critical issue in the drug treatment field.

Drug abuse treatment can not only restrict the spread of HIV directly by reducing needle use, but can also have secondary beneficial effects by serving as a platform for other services. Many reports, consequently, have called for increasing the availability of drug abuse treatment in the United States to slow the spread of HIV (Public Health Service, 1988; Sisk, Hatziandreu, & Hughes, 1990; Turner, Miller, & Moses, 1989).

LAURIE ROEHRICH, TAMARA L. WALL, and JAMES L. SORENSEN • Department of Psychiatry, University of California, San Francisco, and Substance Abuse Services, San Francisco General Hospital, San Francisco, California 94110.

Preventing AIDS: Theories and Methods of Behavioral Interventions, edited by Ralph J. DiClemente and John L. Peterson. Plenum Press, New York, 1994.

By decreasing the level of needle use, patients can lower their risk of HIV infection. Numerous studies of HIV seroprevalence in treatment programs using opiate substitution (usually methadone) have found that being in treatment is associated with lower seropositivity rates (Abdul-Quader et al., 1987; Bliz & Grondbladh, 1988; Grimm, Wolf, Bornemann, & Bschor, 1989; Hartel, Selwyn, Schoenbaum, Klein, & Friedland, 1988; Tidone, Sileo, Goglio, & Borra, 1987; Williams et al., 1990). Other studies have found much lower HIV seroprevalence among patients in methadone maintenance treatment (MMT) for longer times (Barthwell, Senay, Marks, & White, 1989; Novick et al., 1989).

Drug treatment can have secondary beneficial effects by providing a base for mounting other services such as medical treatment, psychiatric care, job training, and social services. Across the country, for example, a small number of drug treatment programs have begun to provide medical care for HIV-infected patients within methadone treatment programs (see Selwyn et al., 1989). Other treatment programs have initiated AIDS education programs for their clientele and their sexual partners (for reviews see Sorensen, 1991; Wermuth, Ham, & Robbins, 1991).

This chapter provides an overview of treatment-based interventions that can help to slow the spread of HIV and to provide care to drug users with HIV infection. The chapter begins with a discussion of the many dilemmas faced by researchers in the field of HIV and substance abuse. The next sections focus on interventions that can be employed during drug treatment: HIV risk assessments and testing, psychoeducational interventions, medical care, and psychological treatments. We conclude with a list of suggestions for further research.

CULTURAL AND PHILOSOPHICAL DILEMMAS IN THE STUDY OF HIV AND SUBSTANCE ABUSE

The AIDS epidemic links two behaviors—sexual activity and drug use. In the United States, public attitudes about sex and drugs have been ambivalent. History shows periods of relative acceptance, as well as dramatic swings toward intolerance (analyses can be found in Musto, 1987, 1991; Tannahill, 1989). According to Musto (1991), periods of intolerance are marked by severe legal or social penalties and attempts to prevent the dissemination of information about the "taboo" substance or behavior. Indeed, during the past 10 years, obstacles prevented the presentation of certain AIDS awareness messages, and opposition prevailed toward federal funding for bleach distribution, the establishment and evaluation of needle exchange programs, and studies of sexual behavior. The specter of AIDS has also forced us to confront another taboo subject: death. For example, in early January 1993, the AIDS death toll in San Francisco had reached 10,000 people (Russell, 1993).

IDUs as a Subculture

The illegal nature of injection drug use and other illicit activities, such as prostitution and exchanging sex for drugs, serve to define the subculture of IDUs. These are the behaviors that researchers need to understand in order to help IDUs institute effective risk reduction techniques; mainstream society, however, has punished and denigrated IDUs for exhibiting these same behaviors. Thus many IDUs lead secretive and transient life-styles, and only a minority of these users actually enter treatment (Watters & Cheng, 1991). This set of circumstances has resulted in the following research limitations: (1) a reliance on in-treatment samples of IDUs because this group is easiest to access; (2) a reliance on cross-sectional designs because finding and following IDUs over time is extremely difficult and; (3) a reliance on self-report data about drug use and sexual behavior.

It is essential for researchers and treatment providers to recognize that working with and gaining the trust of drug users can be an arduous, but rewarding, task. These individuals have often endured many years of multiple stigmatization: drug use, low socioeconomic status, and discrimination as members of minority groups. Therefore, for many IDUs, issues such as the assessment and reduction of HIV risk behaviors or HIV testing may elicit fear, anxiety, and anger. Clients may feel that acceptance of their HIV risk status means confronting yet another stigma.

Injecting drug users can display rather cynical views regarding the benefits of both drug treatment and participation in research. Many IDUs believe HIV/acquired immunodeficiency syndrome (AIDS) is a plot designed to rid the country of drug users, gays, and minorities; this belief is common and widespread. Attempts to dissuade IDUs from this idea can be met with both hostility and distrust. Instead, researchers and treatment staff are encouraged to exhibit sensitivity toward this issue and in many cases, empathic listening and reflection are the most effective tools.

DRUG TREATMENT PROGRAMS

Most drug treatment programs in the United States have traditionally emphasized abstinence from all drugs as a primary treatment goal and expect clients to adhere to this orientation. However, some of the most promising methods for HIV risk reduction (e.g., needle exchange programs, cleaning injection equipment with bleach, and condom distribution) are rooted in harm reduction models and may potentially arouse conflict and discomfort in drug treatment staff (Sorensen, Costantini, & London, 1989).

"Harm reduction" refers to the education and support of IDUs in their efforts to become more responsible as drug users and as sexual partners (Stimson & Lart, 1991). The focus is on personal safety and public health; a person with an alcohol problem may be encouraged to take thiamine supplements, or an IDU may be provided with sterile injection equipment. These techniques ensure that active drug users have some contact with the treatment system. While this approach has been adopted in Holland and England, it has met with some resistance in the United States (Oppenheimer, 1991; Stimson & Lart, 1991). Harm reduction models may offer several benefits for drug abuse treatment programs. For example, total abstinence regarding drug use and sexual behavior is an ideal treatment outcome, but probably is not a realistic goal for many IDUs. In addition, this can be a frustrating goal for treatment staff. In contrast, the harm reduction model emphasizes that even small changes in drug use practices and sexual behavior may save lives. Cognitive–behavioral techniques can be used by clients and staff to identify problem behaviors, to monitor these behaviors, and to see concrete evidence for behavioral change. These methods can increase the self-efficacy of IDUs and may instill feelings of hopefulness in IDUs who have been unsuccessful in traditional 12-step or medical model treatments. Harm reduction may be the initial goal for some clients who eventually move toward abstinence.

The link between HIV and substance abuse has forced the treatment field to reexamine traditional treatment philosophies and to consider adjustments in the perception of what constitutes an acceptable treatment outcome. Dissonance in treatment aims can be distressing and frustrating for both staff and clients; treatment staff may experience burnout, high turnover, and demoralization. Clients may react with anger, alienation from the health care system, refusal to engage in treatment, and high drop-out rates.

Although many researchers advocate harm reduction approaches, clinical staff may not always agree. For example, a survey of treatment goals endorsed by staff ($N = 549$; Price et al., 1991) showed high agreement among treatment professionals that not only were improvements in physical and psychological health important treatment goals, but also that complete abstinence should be a primary goal. Staff members disagreed with the goal of "socially responsible use of alcohol or drugs." Thus the introduction of harm reduction techniques must be handled in a sensitive way. Involvement of treatment staff in these decisions is critical. Researchers who refuse to deal with these areas of potential friction may find they either cannot mount new interventions successfully, or their interventions are adopted in name only (Rappaport, Seidman, & Davidson, 1979).

HIV TESTING AND RISK ASSESSMENT

For many drug users, the outpatient drug treatment program represents their sole contact with the health care system. Drug treatment facilities, however, have traditionally not been involved in the delivery of medical care. The HIV/AIDS epidemic and the reemergence of tuberculosis have forced the drug treatment field to reconsider the rationale suggesting that medical care and drug treatment should be independent. Injecting drug users are often without the necessary social and financial resources to receive adequate health care. In this sense, a community drug treatment program may be able to provide services clients are unlikely to receive elsewhere. In addition, these services may encourage clients to remain in drug treatment and may result in more positive treatment outcomes (Childress, McLellan, Woody, & O'Brien, 1991). We will explore the impact of HIV testing in this section, as an example of one service that can be provided during drug treatment. For seropositive individuals, interventions may include routine CD4 counts, the administration of AZT, pneumocystis carinii pneumonia (PCP) prophylaxis, or PAP smears (see section entitled "Medical Interventions and HIV Secondary Prevention").

The Centers for Disease Control (1986, 1987) recommend voluntary HIV testing, routinely offered to all clients. We feel, in addition, that risk assessments should become a routine aspect of drug treatment. In this context, HIV testing is offered as one aspect of a complete HIV/AIDS risk assessment. Unfortunately, standardized risk assessment instruments, including measures of injection drug use practices, other drug use such as alcohol and cocaine, and sexual behavior are not widely available at present. One potential measure, however, appears to be in development (see Metzger, 1992). Also, some research suggests that injection drug users may evaluate their personal risk for HIV primarily in terms of their drug use, and they may underestimate their risk of sexual transmission (Feucht, Stephens, & Gibbs, 1991; Sibthorpe, Fleming, Tesselaar, & Gould, 1991). Clearly a need exists for psychometrically sound instruments that combine all types of HIV risk behavior.

IMPACT OF TESTING ON DRUG ABUSE TREATMENT

Drug treatment providers may be concerned that HIV risk assessments and/or HIV testing could act as a stressor and possibly undermine drug treatment efforts. Is this fear justified? Studies of gay men (see review by Jacobsen, Perry, & Hirsch, 1990) suggest we must look at all steps of the process: (1) What influences a client's decision to seek testing? Unfortunately, no research is available in this area. If we knew more about what motivates people to be tested, this might ultimately lead to new interventions. (2) What influences the client's decision to receive or not receive test results? Studies reviewed by Jacobsen, Perry, and Hirsch (1990) indicated that clients who elected to receive their test results believed that knowledge of their HIV status would be useful for themselves or for their partners. Clients who avoided notification tended to fear a positive test result would be too overwhelming. Thus, it may be critical for pretest counseling to include situations where clients role-play or imagine what it might be like to receive HIV test results. Counselors would then have an opportunity to help clients problem solve and prepare for the notification process. (3) What is the psychological impact of notification? Several prospective studies have examined this issue. Ostrow and colleagues (Ostrow et al., 1989) found positive test results were related to increased distress, and negative test results were associated with decreased distress levels. Another study, however, which included a number of injection drug users, found no significant increases in distress for clients who received intensive prepost counseling (Perry et al., 1990). Casadonte, Des Jarlais, Friedman, and Rostrosen (1990) studied a sample of injection drug users. Their prepost design indicated that seropositive clients experienced increased anxiety several weeks after notification, followed by anxiety reduction, and behavioral change. Seronegative individuals responded with feelings of relief and also exhibited positive behavior changes. Anxiety about HIV increased for subjects who were not tested. So far, results suggest testing does not appear to have an adverse impact upon clients. In fact, the assessment and testing process may lead to positive outcomes for a majority of clients.

Another recent study examined the impact of standard versus enhanced prepost counseling, and HIV notification among injection drug users in a methadone detoxification program (Gibson, Young, & Lovelle-Drache, 1992). Follow-ups conducted at 6-month and 12-month intervals noted significant reductions in risky injection practices and risky sexual behavior across the treatment conditions. No differences were found between standard and enhanced types of prepost counseling. The authors suggested that simply interviewing subjects about risk behavior may lead to behavioral changes (see also Calsyn, Saxon, Freeman, & Whittaker, 1992). Farley, Cartter, Wassell, and Hadler (1992) examined the records of 594 clients attending methadone maintenance in Connecticut to determine the impact of HIV counseling and testing on: (1) risk for discontinuation of drug treatment, and (2) illicit drug use. Human immunodeficiency virus testing and counseling did not increase the probability of treatment drop-out, and clients who received HIV counseling showed lower overall levels of drug use compared to clients who did not receive HIV counseling.

In summary, HIV risk assessments and voluntary testing have become a necessary component of drug treatment. These interventions do not appear to have overwhelmingly negative effects on drug treatment. They may instead create a forum where clients and counselors can engage in important discussions surrounding drug use and sexual behavior, they may potentially lead to behavioral changes for clients, and they provide treatment staff with opportunities to initiate early medical interventions with seropositive drug users. Clearly the period of time surrounding the risk assessment, the decision to seek testing, and awaiting test results can elicit anxiety for many clients; it may also elicit urges to use drugs. Counseling sessions should address these issues directly. For example, clients can practice relaxation techniques, engage in pleasant activities that help to distract them and reduce negative affect, as well as attend additional 12-step or recovery oriented meetings.

TREATMENT-BASED PSYCHOEDUCATIONAL INTERVENTIONS

Providing education about AIDS is important in managing HIV issues in addiction treatment programs. The authors use a "levels of defense" approach to preventing the spread of HIV, which emphasizes both drug use and sexual behaviors (see Fig. 1). In drug use, the less risky behaviors are: abstinence, not using needles, not sharing needles (or other equipment such as cookers and cotton), and always cleaning needles between users (Sorensen, Heitzmann, & Guydish, 1990). These behaviors appear in the figure as increasingly permeable lines between HIV-infected drug users and their drug-sharing partners. The increasingly risky defenses in sexual activities include abstinence, mutual monogamy, and always using condoms/spermicides. We caution that a mutually monogamous relationship does not provide protection for the sexual partner of the drug user, because the drug user could become infected through unsafe needle use. Education can aim at promoting the most impermeable defenses, while it also recognizes that less effective defenses are still better than none at all.

Educational interventions to encourage safe sex involve more than just distributing condoms. Human immunodeficiency virus-infected drug users can benefit from discussions of the risks of having sex, as well as counseling about how to introduce condoms into intimate relationships, and how to use condoms and spermicides. Our impression is that education may have greater potential if it includes hands-on instruction demonstrating proper condom use (Sorensen et al., in press).

Research teams around the country have had some success with small-group psychoeducational AIDS prevention interventions, totaling between 6 and 20 hours, in New York (Dengelegi, Weber, & Torquato, 1990; Magura, Shapiro, Grossman, & Lipton, 1989; El-Bassel & Schilling, 1992); New Orleans (Corrigan, Thompson, Malow, & Sorensen, 1992); and Westboro, Massachusetts (McCusker, Stoddard, Zapka, Morrison, Zorn, & Lewis, 1992). Most of

DRUG USE

Abstinence

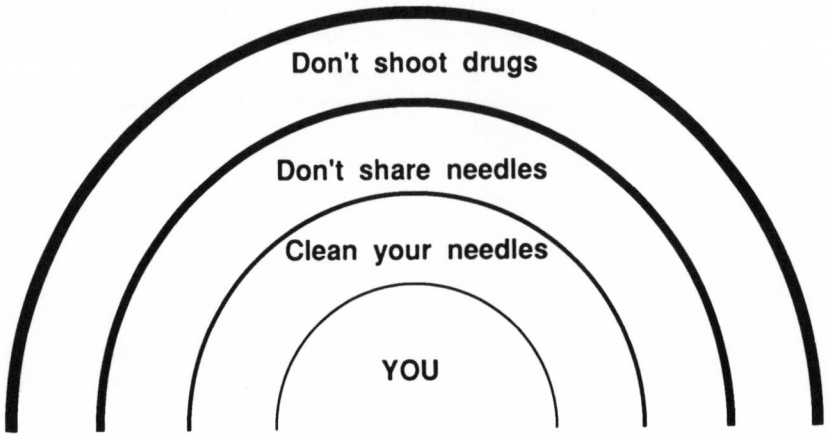

SEXUAL ACTIVITY

Abstinence

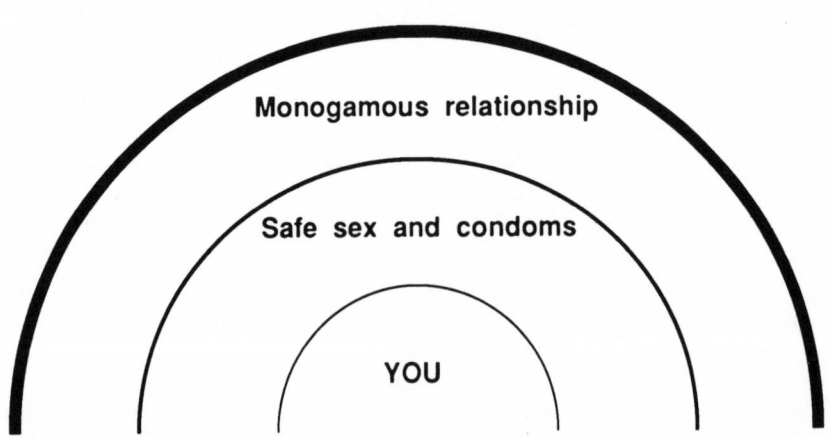

Figure 1.   Defenses against AIDS: Drug use and sexual activity (Sorensen, Heitzman, & Guydish, 1990). Copyright 1990 by the Clinical Psychology Publishing Company. Adapted by permission.

these studies involved the random assignment of subjects to either a small-group intervention or an intervention thought to be less powerful (e.g., brochures, information only, or no intervention). Follow-up times tend to be short, usually less than six months. The majority of these studies have found improvements in knowledge, attitudes, intentions, or skills; the impact on actual behavior appears to be less powerful. Viewed together, however, this research indicates that the group approach is significantly more effective than giving brochures or other information to clients on an individual basis. The group approach fits well into the traditions and mores of addiction programs; this approach is an efficient way for a small number of staff to reach a large number of patients. Additionally, the intimate atmosphere gives a chance for participants to build mutually committed relationships to change their drug use and sexual activities.

Psychoeducational interventions for the prevention of AIDS in IDUs, however, should not be regarded as a panacea. As noted with other types of interventions, increases in knowledge and skills may not necessarily lead to significant behavioral change. Knowledge levels may decay over time, and new research findings about HIV and AIDS appear daily. Booster sessions may be needed in order to achieve longer lasting effects and to keep IDUs up to date regarding new developments (El-Bassel & Schilling, 1992). Interventions may have high attrition rates and low attendance rates, leading some researchers to conclude that AIDS prevention education should: (1) be required for all clients in drug treatment or (2) use incentives to increase attendance rates (Magura et al., 1989). Other strategies that may help to increase the efficacy of psychoeducational interventions with IDUs include peer led groups, and interventions specifically targeted and designed for female and minority IDUs.

MEDICAL INTERVENTIONS AND HIV SECONDARY PREVENTION

Drug abuse treatment programs faced with the AIDS epidemic can also expand to include HIV-related medical services. Methadone treatment programs, in particular, offer an excellent opportunity for providing medical care for several reasons. Addicts who may distrust traditional medical systems, and who may not want to attend AIDS clinics for fear of stigmatization, can be medically treated at the same sites where they receive methadone treatment. Minority groups (especially African Americans and Hispanics), who are disproportionately represented among all AIDS cases and especially among IDUs, can be offered easier access to medical care that is often impeded because of problems associated with cultural differences and low socioeconomic status. Finally, methadone programs have daily contact with patients who have chaotic life-styles and are often erratic in their compliance with medical regimens. On-site medical care can provide flexibility by allowing patients to be seen on a "drop-in" basis rather than by appointment. This may be particularly helpful for female IDUs who find it difficult to arrange child care. In addition, potential exists for the staff who dispense methadone also to dispense other medications, as well as monitor compliance and follow-up.

Even among the general population, noncompliance with medical care is a common problem. Scheduled appointments with health care providers are kept only about 50% of the time; compliance with medications prescribed over many weeks or months also averages about 50% (Eraker, Kirscht, & Becker, 1984). A recent study randomly assigned patients at admission to a methadone clinic to on-site medical care versus referral to a nearby clinic (Umbricht-Schneiter, Ginn, Pabst, & Bigelow, 1992). Further medical care was received by significantly more patients in the on-site group (92%) compared to the referred group (35%). This demonstrates that providing medical care at the drug treatment site increases compliance of appointment keeping over the usual referral procedure.

At least two other methadone programs have implemented on-site medical services in geographic areas of the United States particularly hard hit by the AIDS epidemic: New York and San Francisco. These programs now provide primary medical care for patients with, or at high risk for, HIV infection (Batki et al., 1990; Selwyn et al., 1989). The medical care includes routine admission and annual physical examinations required in all methadone programs, PAP tests for women, treatment for acute HIV-related illness and prophylactic regimens, as well as referrals and consultation with specialized AIDS clinics.

Increasing compliance with antiretroviral treatments, such as zidovudine (AZT), may be especially urgent since AZT can delay progression of HIV disease and improve the quality of life (Fischl et al., 1991; Volberding et al., 1990); but, because of its short half-life that necessitates multiple daily dosages, and its severe side effects, it may be a regimen to which it is particularly difficult for patients to adhere. In addition, AZT is offered as often, but is accepted *less* often by IDUs compared to HIV-infected patients in other risk groups (Broers, Hirschel, Gabriel, & Morabia, 1992). IDUs, then, begin AZT treatment later in the course of disease progression. Significantly lower rates of AZT compliance have been noted, moreover, for patients with a history of IDU (Fischl, 1991; Samet et al., 1992). To address this problem at San Francisco General Hospital, we recently conducted a small intervention study ($N = 25$) to determine whether compliance with AZT increases by having one of the daily doses administered at the methadone clinic (Wall & Sorensen, unpublished data). Preliminary results suggest medication compliance, as measured by self-report and indirect biological measures, significantly improves through dispensing AZT at the clinic. When the intervention was withdrawn, however, AZT adherence was reduced. Further research is needed to establish the efficacy of this approach over other potential interventions, and to examine strategies that could lead to long-term increases in medication adherence.

On-site medical care in methadone programs can also monitor for other HIV-related diseases such as pneumocystis carinii pneumonia (PCP) and tuberculosis (TB), as well as provide prophylactic medications for these diseases. Tuberculosis, for example, is increasingly prevalent in the United States. New infections are especially common among certain high-risk groups including people with HIV disease, IDUs, and racial or ethnic minority groups. Medical treatment of tuberculin skin test positive (PPD+) patients currently consists of a standard chemoprophylaxis regimen such as six months of isoniazid (INH) or rifampin. Compliance with TB chemoprophylaxis is typically poor among IDUs. Poor compliance can lead to no treatment or incomplete treatment, both of which result in the failure to prevent TB. Active TB can rapidly spread among IDUs, particularly in persons who are HIV infected. Drug treatment programs have successfully provided PPD tests and monitored compliance with chemoprophylaxis to maximize prevention of TB (Hayden, Jereb, Dooley, Stern, & Seawright, 1991).

Methadone programs with on-site medical care can also more readily monitor the complex regimens of multiple medications and the interactions of pharmacologic treatments. A classic example is a drug such as rifampin that induces liver enzymes and may reduce the activity of several drugs, including methadone and dapsone (Amodio-Groton & Currier, 1992). In order to enhance compliance, treatment providers must appreciate the patients' difficulty in adhering to complex pharmaceutical regimens that may potentially include unpleasant side effects; patients' concerns must be addressed in a prompt and direct manner.

In review, AIDS has become a tremendous medical problem among drug abusers. Providing on-site medical care is an effective way of providing secondary prevention of common life-threatening and contagious disorders and may reduce the morbidity and cost associated with HIV disease.

PSYCHOLOGICAL INTERVENTIONS AND HIV RISK REDUCTION

Prior research indicates that between 50 and 60% of methadone maintenance (MMT) clients have a history of depressive disorders (Woody, McLellan, O'Brien, & Luborsky, 1991), and high levels of depressive symptoms may contribute to poor treatment outcomes and increased HIV risk (Batki, Sorensen, Gibson, & Maude-Griffin, 1990). Marlatt and Gordon (1985) have noted drug and alcohol relapses are often preceded by a wish to reduce negative affect or to increase positive affect. A recent report by Gibson, Lovelle-Drache, Young, and Chesney (1992) found that drug users with higher depression levels engaged in more frequent HIV risk behaviors, as compared to subjects with low symptom levels of depression. In addition, many IDUs are dealing with severe psychosocial stressors including poverty, homelessness or inadequate housing, medical problems, and legal difficulties. A large body of existing research suggests that low socioeconomic status is associated with hopelessness, demoralization, and other depressive symptoms (Lorion & Felner, 1986).

It also appears that the depressive symptoms experienced by IDUs may represent a chronic difficulty that is not always alleviated by addiction treatment alone. In contrast, clients who are in treatment for alcohol or cocaine dependence may initially present with high levels of depressive symptoms, but these symptoms tend to decrease significantly over the first four to eight weeks of drug treatment. Because depression is so common among IDUs, and because it appears to be related to other problem behaviors (i.e., relapse to drug use, HIV risk), we strongly advocate that IDUs receive a depression screening upon entry into treatment (for a thorough review of psychological assessment methods with substance abusers, see Sorensen & Wall, 1992). Additional screens at the one- and three-month points in treatment can be helpful in determining if the client's depressive symptoms are situational or chronic. Chronic symptoms may respond to antidepressants, psychotherapy, or a combination of these methods (Woody, O'Brien, McLellan, Marcovici, & Evans, 1982). Woody et al. (1983) found that clients who attended cognitive–behavioral therapy or supportive–expressive therapy, combined with MMT and drug counseling, had more positive outcomes compared with clients who received only MMT and drug counseling.

Many clients have lost friends, lovers, and family members to AIDS. A study conducted at our MMT clinic indicated that the typical client had experienced six AIDS-related losses over the past year (London, Sorensen, Roehrich, Stall, & Delucchi, 1992). More than 25% of the clients reported moderate distress in reaction to these deaths; over 50% stated they experienced considerable or extreme distress related to multiple AIDS losses. As the AIDS epidemic devastated the gay and bisexual men's communities in the United States, hopelessness emerged, and the ability of these men to take effective action against infection was reduced (McKusick & Hilliard, 1991). The degree to which this phenomenon may generalize to injection drug users is unknown and is only recently being evaluated (J. London, personal communication). Drug abuse treatment programs may consider offering individual and group support to help these patients cope with the emotional consequences of multiple and severe loss.

Mental health treatment is also frequently needed to help HIV-infected injection drug users manage their illness. During the course of HIV disease, many people suffer severe mental health difficulties, including cognitive impairment as well as mood, anxiety, and psychotic disorders. Psychiatric and psychological symptoms not only occur in the presence of HIV infection, but also depend on individual psychological characteristics such as coping and resilience, premorbid psychiatric history, and the availability of social support resources. Injecting drug users, who are more likely to have preexisting psychiatric disorders, including personality disorders, and who are often socially isolated because of their drug abuse and other antisocial behavior, are at especially high risk for psychiatric and psychological complications following HIV infection (Batki, 1986, 1990). An additional hardship is that this population frequently has less access to care. Ideally, psychological and psychiatric assessments and treatment should be available for the in-treatment injection drug user at all phases of their disease.

Anxiety and depression are almost always associated with having HIV disease, particularly with a substance abusing patient. Symptom reduction frequently can be gained through the use of medication (Ostrow, Grant, & Atkinson, 1988), but there are also effective behavioral interventions. Supportive individual and group interventions can provide these patients with the opportunity to establish greater social support (Markowitz, Klerman, & Perry, 1992). Teaching active coping skills can also be helpful in giving patients alternative ways for controlling and managing their anxiety and depression. For clients with HIV infection, these interventions could potentially lead to an improved quality and quantity of life. Cancer researchers, for example, have found that patients who received structured psychosocial interventions such as relaxation training, cognitive coping strategies, or education about their disease, experience less emotional distress and may actually live longer than their counterparts who received only standard medical treatment (for review, see Andersen, 1992).

Injection drug users infected with HIV are also at high risk for neuropsychological impairment. If a reason exists to suspect cognitive impairment, a comprehensive assessment, including neurological and neuropsychological evaluations, should be performed. After ruling out treatable conditions, a neuropsychological evaluation can be used to clarify the nature and severity of cognitive impairment and can help determine how the patient's cognitive difficulties are likely to impact on his or her everyday functioning. Appropriate recommendations can then be made. Strategies to help individuals compensate for their cognitive difficulties include slowing down, using written reminders and verbal monitoring, and avoiding fatigue and stressful situations (Boccellari, 1991). Patients with significant cognitive impairment may also need assistance with money management and applications for social services such as welfare,

Social Security income, or housing. Furthermore, patients may feel self-conscious about directly asking a treatment provider for help in these situations. Thus it may be necessary for treatment staff to inquire routinely about these issues and offer assistance in a sensitive and nonjudgmental manner.

Psychological and psychiatric treatment of the at-risk or HIV-infected patient represents an increasing challenge for the substance abuse treatment field. Drug treatment programs must be aware of the complex interaction between the substance abuse, medical, psychiatric, and psychosocial problems manifested in this population. Historically, little attention or research effort has been devoted to the development and evaluation of cognitive–behavioral interventions for IDUs. Group interventions focusing on difficulties such as depression, bereavement, and living with HIV would appear particularly cost effective. These strategies may be associated with improved drug treatment outcome and increased psychological well-being, and could ultimately lead to increases in immune function and improved survival rates for HIV-infected IDUs. At present, most existing interventions have been aimed at gay male populations; it is currently unclear if these methods will generalize to IDUs. This area appears wide open for research opportunities, and psychology has the potential to provide significant contributions to our understanding of the links between substance abuse, psychopathology, and HIV risk.

CONCLUSIONS

In this chapter, we have attempted to elucidate some of the cultural and philosophical dilemmas inherent in the study of HIV and substance abuse. We then explored some of the more recent innovations in HIV risk assessments and testing, psychoeducational, medical, and psychological interventions. This list of topics is by no means exhaustive, and other interventions may also hold promise for the future. Some additional research recommendations follow:

1. Development of psychometrically sound assessment and outcome measures should receive high priority, especially regarding sexual behaviors and injection drug use practices.
2. New interventions should be carefully evaluated; we need evidence that they will work. This includes attending to issues such as generalizability, the use of manualized treatments, and efforts to disseminate successful interventions.
3. Increased provision of on-site services and increased availability of "low threshold treatments" should be priority concerns. Low threshold programs can provide drug and HIV information to users who are

not currently in treatment via outreach programs staffed by community members, mobile units deployed in high-risk neighborhoods, or programs offered in welfare hotels and shelters (see American Psychological Association, 1991).

4. Further development of services and interventions focused on women and minority groups should be encouraged.

5. Peer led interventions and services provided by peer nominated community leaders are worthy of further exploration. Information provided by a respected peer may be perceived as more credible, and peers may serve as effective role models.

6. Increased exploration of case management strategies for low functioning IDUs and seropositive drug users in order to prevent frequent and costly hospitalizations.

7. Contingency management techniques (Stitzer, Iguchi, & Felch, 1992) may be useful for improving drug treatment outcomes and can serve as a concrete reward for IDUs who implement successful behavior changes.

ACKNOWLEDGMENT. This work was supported in part by National Institute on Drug Abuse grant # 1R18DA06097.

REFERENCES

Abdul-Quader, A. S., Friedman, S. R., Des Jarlais, D., Marmor, M. M., Maslansky, R., & Bartelme, S. (1987). Methadone maintenance and behavior by intravenous drug users that can transmit HIV. *Contemporary Drug Problems, 14,* 425–434.

American Psychological Association. (1991). Special Issue: Homelessness. *American Psychologist, 46,* 1108–1245.

Andersen, B. L. (1992). Psychological interventions for cancer patients to enhance the quality of life. *Journal of Consulting & Clinical Psychology, 60,* 552–568.

Amodio-Groton, M., & Currier, J. (1992). HIV drug interactions. *AIDS Clinical Care, 4,* 25–29.

Barthwell, A., Senay, E., Marks, R., & White, R. (1989). Patients successfully maintained with methadone escaped human immunodeficiency virus infection (letter). *Archives of General Psychiatry, 46,* 957.

Batki, S. L. (1986). Drug abuse, psychiatric disorders, and AIDS: Dual and triple diagnosis. *The Western Journal of Medicine, 152,* 547–552.

Batki, S. L. (1990). Substance abuse and AIDS: The need for mental health services. In S. M. Goldfinger (Ed.), *Psychiatric aspects of AIDS and HIV infection* (pp. 55–82). San Francisco: Jossey-Bass Inc.

Batki, S. L., London, J., Goosby, E., Clement, M., Wolfe, R., Ryan, C., French, D., Young, M., Miller, D., Christmas, R., & Sorensen, J. L. (1990, June). *Medical care for intravenous drug users with AIDS and ARC: Delivering services at a methadone treatment program.* Paper presented at the 6th International Conference on AIDS, San Francisco, CA.

Batki, S. L., Sorensen, J. L., Gibson, D. R., & Maude-Griffin, P. (1990). HIV-infected IV drug users in methadone treatment: Outcome and psychological correlates—a preliminary report. In L. S. Harris (Ed.), *Problems of drug dependence, 1989* (DHHS Publication No. ADM 90-1663, pp. 405–406). Rockville, MD: NIDA.

Bliz, O., & Grondbladh, L. (1988, June). *AIDS and IV heroin addicts: The preventive effect of methadone maintenance in Sweden.* Paper presented at the 4th International Conference on AIDS, Stockholm, Sweden.

Boccellari, A. (1991, May). Care at home for people with dementing illness: Practical suggestions that can make a difference. *Bulletin of Experimental Treatments for AIDS,* 13–21.

Broers, B., Hirschel, B., Gabriel, V., & Morabia A. (1992, July). *Compliance of drug users with Zidovudine treatment.* Poster presented at the 7th International Conference on AIDS, Amsterdam, The Netherlands.

Calsyn, D. A., Saxon, A. J., Freeman, G., Jr., & Whittaker, S. (1992). Ineffectiveness of AIDS education and HIV antibody testing in reducing high-risk behaviors among injection drug users. *American Journal of Public Health, 82,* 573–574.

Casadonte, P. P., Des Jarlais, D. C., Friedman, S. R., & Rostrosen, J. P. (1990). Psychological and behavioral impact among intravenous drug users of learning HIV test results. *International Journal of the Addictions, 25,* 409–426.

Caussy, D., Weiss, S., Blattner, W., French, J., Cantor, E., Ginzberg, H., Altman, R., & Goedert, J. (1990). Exposure factors for HIV-1 infection among heterosexual drug abusers in New Jersey treatment programs. *AIDS Research & Human Retroviruses, 6,* 1459–1467.

Centers for Disease Control and Prevention. (1986). Additional recommendations to reduce sexual and drug abuse-related transmission of human T-Lymphatropic Virus Type III/lymphoadenopathy-associated virus. *Morbidity & Mortality Weekly Report, 35,* 152–155.

Centers for Disease Control and Prevention. (1987). Public Health Service guidelines for counseling and antibody testing to prevent HIV infection and AIDS. *Morbidity and Mortality Weekly Report, 36,* 509–515.

Centers for Disease Control and Prevention. (1991, July). *HIV/AIDS surveillance report.* Atlanta, GA: Author.

Childress, A. R., McLellan, A. T., Woody, G. E., & O'Brien, C. P. (1991). Are there minimum conditions necessary to reduce intravenous drug use and AIDS risk behaviors? In R. W. Pickens, C. G. Leukefeld, & C. R. Schuster (Eds.), *Improving drug abuse treatment* (pp. 167–177). Rockville, MD: U.S. Department of Health & Human Services, NIDA.

Corrigan, S. A., Thompson, K. E., Malow, R. M., & Sorensen, J. L. (1992). A psychoeducational approach to prevent HIV transmission among injection drug users. *Psychology of Addictive Behavior, 6,* 114–119.

Dengelegi, L., Weber, J., & Torquato, S. (1990). Drug users' AIDS-related knowledge, attitudes, and behaviors before and after AIDS education sessions. *Public Health Reports, 105,* 504–510.

El-Bassel, N., & Schilling, R. F. (1992). 15 month follow-up of women methadone patients taught skills to reduce heterosexual HIV transmission. *Public Health Reports, 107,* 500–504.

Eraker, S. A., Kirscht, J., & Becker, M. H. (1984). Understanding and improving patient compliance. *Annals of Internal Medicine, 100,* 258–268.

Farley, T. A., Cartter, M. L., Wassell, J. T., & Hadler, J. L. (1992). Predictors of outcome in methadone programs: Effect of HIV counseling and testing. *AIDS, 6,* 115–121.

Feucht, T. E., Stephens, R. C., & Gibbs, B. H. (1991). Knowledge about AIDS among intravenous drug users: An evaluation of an education program. *AIDS Education & Prevention, 3,* 10–20.

Fischl, M. A. (1991, April). *Adherence in the safety and efficacy study of Zidovudine in the treatment of subjects with mildly symptomatic HIV.* Paper presented at the Conference of Adherence in AIDS Clinical Trials, San Francisco, California.

Fischl, M. A., Parker, C. B., Pettinelli, C., Wulfsohn, M., Hirsch, M. S., Collier, A. C., Antoniskis, D., Ho, M., Richman, D. D., Fuchs, E., Merigan, T. C., Reichman, R. C., Gold, J., Steigbigel, N., Leoung, G. S., Rasheed, S., Anastasios, T., & the AIDS Clinical Trials Group. (1991). A randomized controlled trial of a reduced daily dose of Zidovudine in patients with the acquired immunodeficiency syndrome. *New England Journal of Medicine, 323,* 1009–1014.

Gibson, D. R., Lovelle-Drache, J., Young, M., & Chesney, M. (1992, July). *HIV risk linked to psychopathology in IV drug users.* Paper presented at the 8th International Conference on AIDS, Amsterdam, the Netherlands.

Gibson, D. R., Young, M., & Lovelle-Drache, J. (1992). *Effects of standard versus enhanced antibody test notification on the HIV risk behavior of injection drug users.* Unpublished data, University of California, San Francisco, Department of Psychiatry and the Center for AIDS Prevention, San Francisco, CA.

Grimm, M. G., Wolf, B., Bornemann, R., & Bschor, F. (1989). *Prevention of HIV infection in parenteral drug abusers: About evaluation and efficacy of opiate-substitution treatment.* Paper presented at the 5th International Conference on AIDS, Montreal, Canada.

Hartel, D., Selwyn, P. A., Schoenbaum, E. E., Klein, R. S., & Friedland, G. H. (1988, June). *Methadone maintenance treatment and reduced risk of AIDS and AIDS-specific mortality in intravenous drug users.* Presented at the 4th International Conference on AIDS, Stockholm, Sweden.

Hayden, C. H., Jereb, J., Dooley, S., Stern, H., & Seawright, M. (1991, June). *HIV-related tuberculosis prevention in drug treatment centers and correctional facilities.* Paper presented at the 7th International Conference on AIDS, Florence, Italy.

Institute for Health Policy Studies (1990, February). *The HIV epidemic: New and continuing challenges for the public and private sectors.* Paper prepared for Funders Concerned about AIDS and the Council on Foundations, University of California, San Francisco.

Jacobsen, P. B., Perry, S. W., & Hirsch, D. (1990). Behavioral and psychological responses to HIV antibody testing. *Journal of Consulting and Clinical Psychology, 58,* 31–37.

Lee, H., Weiss, S., Brown, L., Mildvan, D., Shorty, T., Saravolatz, L., Chu, A., Ginzberg, H., Markowitz, N., & Des Jarlais, D. C. (1990). Patterns of HIV-1 and HTLV-I/II in intravenous drug users from the middle atlantic and central region of the USA. *Journal of Infectious Diseases, 162,* 347–352.

London, J., Sorensen, J. L., Roehrich, L., Stall, R., & Delucchi, K. (1992). *AIDS-related bereavement among IDUs in methadone maintenance.* Unpublished data, University of California, San Francisco.

Lorion, R., & Felner, R. D. (1986). Research on psychotherapy with the disadvantaged. In S. L. Garfield & A. E. Bergin (Eds.), *Handbook of psychotherapy and behavior change* (3rd ed., pp. 739–776). New York: John Wiley & Sons.

Magura, S., Grossman, J., Lipton, D. S., Amann, K. R., Koger, J., & Gehan, K. (1989). Correlates of participation in AIDS education and HIV antibody testing by methadone patients. *Public Health Reports, 104,* 231–240.

Magura, S., Shapiro, J. L., Grossman, J., Lipton, D. S. (1989). Education/support groups for AIDS prevention with at-risk clients. *Social Casework,* 10–20.

Markowitz, J. C., Klerman, G. L., & Perry, S. W. (1992). Interpersonal psychotherapy of depressed HIV-positive outpatients. *Hospital & Community Psychiatry, 43,* 885–890.

Marlatt, G. A., & Gordon, J. R. (1985). *Relapse prevention.* New York: Guilford.

McCusker, J., Stoddard, A., Zapka, J., Morrison, C., Zorn, M., & Lewis, B. (1992). AIDS education for drug abusers: Evaluation of short-term effectiveness. *American Journal of Public Health, 82,* 533–540.

McKusick, L., & Hilliard, R. (1991, June). *Multiple loss accounts for worsening distress in a community heavily hit by AIDS.* Paper presented at the 7th International Conference on AIDS, Florence, Italy.

Metzger, D. (1992). *Risk for AIDS behaviors.* Unpublished manuscript, University of Pennsylvania and Philadelphia VAMC, Center for Studies on Addiction, Philadelphia, PA.

Musto, D. (1987). *The American disease: Origins of narcotic control.* New York: Oxford University Press.

Musto, D. (July, 1991). Opium, cocaine, and marijuana in American history. *Scientific American,* 40–47.

Novick, D. M., Joseph, H., Croxson, T. S., Salsitz, E. E., Wang, G., & Richman, B. L. (1989, June). *Absence of antibody to HIV in long-term, socially rehabilitated methadone maintenance patients.* Poster presented at the 5th International Conference on AIDS, Montreal, Canada.

Oppenheimer, G. M. (1991). To build a bridge: The use of foreign models by domestic critics of U. S. drug policy. *Milbank Quarterly, 69,* 495–526.

Ostrow, D. G., Grant, I., & Atkinson, H. (1988). Assessment and management of the AIDS patient with neuropsychiatric disturbances. *Journal of Clinical Psychiatry, 49,* 14–22.

Ostrow, D. G., Joseph, J. G., Kessler, R., Soucy, J., Tal, M., Eler, M., Chmiel, J., & Phair, J. P. (1989). Disclosure of HIV antibody status: Behavioral and mental health characteristics. *AIDS Education and Prevention, 1,* 1–11.

Perry, S. W., Jacobsberg, L. B., Fishman, B., Weiler, P. H., Gold, J. W., & Frances, A. J. (1990). Psychological responses to serological testing for HIV. *AIDS, 4,* 145–152.

Price, R. H., Burke, A. C., D'Aunno, T. A., Klingel, D. M., McCaughrin, W. C., Rafferty, J. A., & Vaughn, T. E. (1991). Outpatient drug abuse treatment services, 1988: Results of a national survey. In R. Pickens, C. Leukefeld, & C. Schuster (Eds.) *Improving drug abuse treatment* (pp. 63–92) (DHHS Publication No. ADM 91-1754). Rockville, MD: NIDA.

Public Health Service. (1988). Report of the Second Public Health Service AIDS Prevention and Control Conference. *Public Health Representative, 193,* 66–77.

Rappaport, J., Seidman, E., & Davidson, W. S. (1979). Demonstration research and manifest versus true adoption: The natural history of a research project designed to divert adolescents from the legal system. In R. F. Munoz, L. R. Snowden, & J. G. Kelly (Eds.), *Social and psychological research in community settings: Designing and conducting programs for social and personal well-being* (pp. 101–144). San Francisco: Jossey-Bass, Inc.

Russell, S. (1993, January 7). S. F. reaching bitter AIDS milestone. *San Francisco Chronicle,* pp. A1, A8.

Samet, J. H., Libman, H., Steger, K. A., Dhawan, R. K., Chen, J., Shevitz, A. H., Dewees-Dunk, R., Levenson, S., Kufe, D., Craven, D. E. (1992). Compliance with Zidovudine therapy in patients infected with human immunodeficiency virus, type I: A cross-sectional study in a municipal hospital clinic. *The American Journal of Medicine, 92,* 495–502.

Selwyn, P. A., Feingold, A. R., Iezza, A., Satyadeo, M., Colley, J., Torres, R., & Shaw, J. F. M. (1989). Primary care for patients with human immunodeficiency virus (HIV) infection in a methadone maintenance treatment program. *Annals of Internal Medicine, 110,* 761–763.

Selwyn, P. A., Hartel, D., Lewis, V. A., Schoenbaum, E. E., Vermund, S. H., Klein, R. S., Walker, A. T., & Friedland, G. H. (1989). A prospective study of the risk of tuberculosis among intravenous drug users with human immunodeficiency virus infection. *New England Journal of Medicine, 320,* 545–550.

Sibthorpe, B., Fleming, D., Tesselaar, H., & Gould, J. (1991). Needle use and sexual practices—Differences in perception of personal risk of HIV among intravenous drug users. *Journal of Drug Issues, 21,* 699–712.

Sisk, J. E., Hatziandreu, E. J., & Hughes, R. (September, 1990). *The effectiveness of drug abuse treatment: Implications for controlling AIDS/HIV infection* (OTA background paper #6), p. 9.

Sorensen, J. L. (1991). Preventing HIV transmission in drug treatment programs: What works? *Journal of Addictive Diseases, 10,* 67–79.

Sorensen, J. L., Costantini, M. F., & London, J. A. (1989). Coping with AIDS: Strategies for patients and staff in drug abuse treatment programs. *Journal of Psychoactive Drugs, 21,* 435–440.

Sorensen, J. L., Heitzmann, C., & Guydish, J. (1990). Community psychology, drug use, and AIDS. *Journal of Community Psychology, 18,* 347–353.

Sorensen, J. L., London, J., Heitzmann, C., Gibson, D. R., Morales, E. S., Dumontet, R., & Acree, M. (In press). Psychoeducational group approach: HIV risk reduction in drug users. *AIDS Education & Prevention.*

Sorensen, J. L., & Wall, T. L. (1992). Substance abuse and AIDS: Assessment and treatment issues. In L. Vandercreek, S. Knapp, & T. L. Jackson (Eds.), *Innovations in clinical practice: A source book* (Vol. 11, pp. 541–552). Sarasota, FL: Professional Resource Press.

Stimson, G. V., & Lart, R. (1991). HIV, drugs, and public health in England: New worlds, old tunes. *International Journal of the Addictions, 26,* 1263–1267.

Stitzer, M. L., Iguchi, M. Y., & Felch, L. (1992). Contingent take-home incentive: Effects on drug use of methadone maintenance patients. *Journal of Consulting & Clinical Psychology, 60,* 927–934.

Tannahill, R. (1989). *Sex and history.* London: Cardinal Press.

Tidone, L., Sileo, F., Goglio, A., & Borra, G. C. (1987). AIDS in Italy. *American Journal of Drug and Alcohol Abuse, 13,* 485–486.

Turner, C. F., Miller, H. G., & Moses, L. E. (Eds.). (1989). *AIDS sexual behavior and intravenous drug use.* Washington, DC: National Academy Press.

Umbricht-Schneiter, A., Ginn, D. H., Pabst, K. M., & Bigelow, G. E. (1992, June). *Providing medical care to patients on methadone: A controlled study of referral versus on-site care.* Poster presented at the College on Problems of Drug Dependence, Keystone, Colorado.

Volberding, P. A., Lagakos, S. W., Koch, M. A., Pettinelli, C., Myers, M. W., Booth, D. K., Balfour, H. H., Jr., Reichman, R. C., Bartlett, J. A., Hirsch, M. S., Murphy, R. L., Hardy, W. D., Soeiro, R., Fischl, M. A., Bartlett, J. G., Merigan, T. C., Hysop, N. E., Richman, D. D., Valentine, F. T., Corey, L., & the AIDS Clinical Trials Group of the National Institute of Allergy and Infectious Diseases. (1990). Zidovudine in asymptomatic human immunodeficiency virus infection: A controlled trial in persons with fewer than 500 CDC4-positive cells per cubic millimeter. *New England Journal of Medicine, 322,* 941–949.

Watters, J. K., & Cheng, Y. (1991). Toward comprehensive studies of HIV in intravenous drug users: Issues in treatment-based and street-based samples. In P. Hartsock & S. G. Genser, (Eds.), *Longitudinal studies of HIV infection in intravenous drug users: Methodological issues in natural history research* (DHHS Publication No. ADM 91-1786, pp. 63–74). Rockville, MD: NIDA.

Wermuth, L., Ham, J., & Robbins, L. (1991). Women don't wear condoms: AIDS risk among sexual partners of IV drug users. In J. Huber & B. E. Schneider, (Eds.), *Social relations and the AIDS crisis.* Newbury Park, CA: Sage.

Williams, A., Vranizan, D., Gorter, R., Brodie, B., Meakin, R., & Moss, A. (1990, June). *Methadone maintenance, HIV serostatus and race in injection drug users (IDU) in San Francisco, CA.* Poster presented at the 6th International Conference on AIDS, San Francisco, CA.

Woody, G. E., Luborsky, L., McLellan, A. T., O'Brien, C. P., Beck, A. T., Blaine, J., Herman, I., & Hole, A. (1983). Psychotherapy for opiate addicts. *Archives of General Psychiatry, 40,* 639–645.

Woody, G. E., McLellan, A. T., O'Brien, C. P., & Luborsky, L. (1991). Addressing psychiatric comorbidity. In R. Pickens, C. Leukefeld, & C. Schuster (Eds.) *Improving drug abuse treatment* (pp. 152–166) (DHHS Publication No. ADM 91-1754). Rockville, MD: NIDA.

Woody, G. E., O'Brien, C. P., McLellan, A. T., Marcovici, M., & Evans, B. D. (1982). The use of antidepressants with methadone in depressed maintenance patients. *Annals of the New York Academy of Science, 398,* 120–127.

11

HIV/AIDS Prevention for Drug Users in Natural Settings

JOHN K. WATTERS and JOSEPH GUYDISH

INTRODUCTION

The problem of human immunodeficiency virus (HIV) infections in drug users is of global importance. The sharing of contaminated injection equipment is a major route for transmission of HIV in the United States (Allen, Onorato, & Green, 1992; National Commission on AIDS, 1991; Wodak & Moss, 1990), and is the principal means by which HIV infection has spread in Italy, Spain, Thailand, and Eastern India (Chin, 1991; Choopanya et al., 1991). In the United States, one quarter of the 44,823 acquired immunodeficiency syndrome (AIDS) cases diagnosed among adults during 1991 occurred among heterosexual injection drug users. An additional 4% (1,798) were adults whose sole risk factor was having a sexual partner who injected drugs. Of the 683 pediatric AIDS cases diagnosed in 1991, over half (54%) were attributed to HIV transmission from mothers who used injected drugs themselves or engaged in sexual activity with injection drug users (Centers for Disease Control, 1992).

Due to the illegal nature and nearly universal social condemnation of the practice, illicit drug injection is very much an underground activity. Consequently, there exists no reliable enumeration of the prevalence of injection drug use in the United States or elsewhere. Official estimates for the United States are that there are 1.2 million injection drug users (IDUs), approximately

JOHN K. WATTERS • Department of Family and Community Medicine and Institute for Health Policy Studies, School of Medicine, University of California, San Francisco, San Francisco, California 94143-1304.   JOSEPH GUYDISH • Institute for Health Policy Studies, School of Medicine, University of California, San Francisco, San Francisco, California 94143-0936.

Preventing AIDS: Theories and Methods of Behavioral Interventions, edited by Ralph J. DiClemente and John L. Peterson. Plenum Press, New York, 1994.

15% of whom are enrolled in drug treatment on any day (Wiley & Samuel, 1989). Consequently, there has been growing recognition by public health planners that if HIV prevention efforts are to effectively reach the vast majority of IDUs, these efforts must reach out to IDUs who are not enrolled in drug treatment programs. This recognition has, in the United States, led to federal funding for "outreach" programs which seek to contact IDUs in noninstitutional settings. At their peak, in 1988, over $70 million were spent on such efforts in the United States. In this chapter we discuss the emergence of HIV Prevention Programs targeting IDUs in natural settings. We first consider contextual issues by describing the major approaches to drug abuse treatment, and the limitations of drug treatment as an HIV prevention strategy. We then describe HIV prevention efforts in the natural setting and challenges involved in evaluating these programs.

MAJOR APPROACHES TO DRUG ABUSE TREATMENT AND PREVENTION

To understand the development of HIV/AIDS prevention, it is important to have some background in the philosophical traditions that define the field of drug abuse. In the United States there are three ideological poles around which intervention policy is structured. These are: (1) criminal justice; (2) recovery and medicalization; and (3) harm reduction. While these perspectives are not necessarily exclusive, proponents of these distinguishable philosophies are often at odds in terms of their definitions of the problem, program objectives, and methods of intervention selected. Drug use has long been considered an anathema in Western society. The history of attempts to reduce the negative aspects of the use of psychoactive compounds has, for the last 100 years, been one of legislating government proscription and use of the criminal justice system to enforce compliance with legal sanctions (Epstein, 1977; Musto, 1973). Concurrent with the criminal justice approach, which defines drug (or alcohol use) as criminal behavior requiring the intervention of police, courts, and prisons, has been the medical model. The medical model defines drug use as a medical problem requiring treatment. Under this rubric, we place the recovery oriented programs such as Alcoholics Anonymous (AA) and Narcotics Anonymous (NA). While there are important differences in the medical/treatment approach and the AA and NA recovery approach, both define drug and alcohol abuse as "diseases" and employ various methods containing steps or treatments to combat the "illness" of addiction. A third major approach has been termed "harm reduction." This view defines drug and alcohol use as potentially problematic and attempts to reduce, to a minimum, the amount of harm that can result from the use of psychoactive compounds in the absence of drug treatment or without reliance on the criminal justice system. Such efforts as bleach distribution and syringe exchange represent examples of applied harm reduction.

All three principal ideological perspectives offer some form of intervention in natural settings. The criminal justice approach includes police intervention directed at disrupting illegal actions of drug users (drug sales, drug use, public intoxication, possession of drugs, possession of drug paraphernalia) and the congregation of drug users in certain locations. The goal of these efforts is to remove offenders and install sufficient disincentives to drug use and sales to effectively discourage these practices. The medical/recovery model also includes prevention-oriented efforts in natural settings. In this case, activities include (in some venues) treatment/recovery services located in communities with significant drug use activities, and/or "outreach" activities that seek to recruit drug users into treatment. The goal of these approaches is to achieve abstinence from drug use among individuals who participate in treatment and/or recovery programs. The third model, and the one which we are principally concerned with in this chapter, is that of harm reduction, an approach which seeks to reduce the negative impact associated with various potentially harmful activities. Harm reduction does not have as its objective abstinence from drug use. Consequently, programs that provide harm reduction services focus on the specific behaviors associated with risk.

LIMITATIONS OF DRUG TREATMENT AS AN HIV PREVENTION STRATEGY

From the earliest days of the HIV/AIDS epidemic, drug abuse treatment has been considered a principal means by which disease prevention objectives might be attained, while simultaneously achieving the desired albeit broader societal objective of reducing or eliminating drug use (or at least injecting behavior) among drug treatment program clients. As such, drug abuse treatment addresses HIV risk behavior indirectly through changes in drug abuse behavior. In providing a point of access to the IDU population, however, treatment programs also become a platform to support HIV-specific clinic-based strategies. These include HIV counseling and testing (Higgins et al., 1991), individual counseling concerning HIV risk (Gibson, Wermuth, Lovelle-Drache, Ham, & Sorensen, 1989), and HIV education/counseling using group therapy models (Malow, Corrigan, Pena, Calkins, & Bannister, 1992; Sorensen, London, & Morales, 1991). The impact of clinic-based HIV prevention may extend beyond drug treatment, since the IDU may provide prevention information to family, friends, or IDUs not enrolled in treatment (Bixler, Palacios-Jimenez, & Springer, 1987). In one program, for example, IDUs entering drug treatment were used to enroll female sexual partners in HIV prevention counseling (Wermuth, Robbins, Choi, & Eversley, 1991). Women who are sexual partners of IDUs do not form natural social groupings or congregate in areas where they can be easily identified and offered HIV prevention messages, so clinic-based outreach may represent an important avenue in reaching this target population.

As desirable as drug abuse treatment is for those willing and able to utilize such resources, there are three fundamental problems with reliance on drug treatment as a sole means of HIV primary prevention. These are: (1) many IDUs do not wish to enter drug treatment (Watters, Feldman, Biernack, & Newmeyer, 1986; Watters & Cheng, 1991); (2) addiction has been shown in many studies to be a chronic and relapsing condition that can be refractory to conventional drug treatment in many individuals (Ball & Ross, 1991; Brown, Watters, Igelart, & Akins, 1982–1983; Cooper, Altman, Brown, & Czechowicz, 1983; D'Aunno & Vaughn, 1993); and (3) the cost of expanding drug treatment to an adequate level to permit treatment of *half* of the estimated 1.2 million IDUs in the United States would require at least a tripling of the current number of drug abuse treatment slots. Although a laudable goal, other means of behavior change in drug users are necessary while work is launched to increase the nation's drug treatment capacity. In addition to the time and resources it would take to triple the number of drug treatment slots in this country is the issue of cost. While there have been some efforts on the part of local, state, and federal authorities to expand drug treatment capacity between 1986 and 1992, these efforts have made no appreciable influence on the sizable number of drug injectors who remain outside drug treatment. Moreover, the drug abuse treatment field is struggling with treatment technologies that often cannot prevent relapse and that tend to be most effective with heroin addicts—a shrinking minority in the larger spectrum of injection drug users (Kozel & Adams, 1986; Watters, Cheng & Lorvick, 1991). Consequently, while the improvement of drug treatment technologies and the expansion of the treatment capacity are vital objectives, their short-term or intermediate impact on HIV transmission among drug users is unlikely to be substantial.

PREVENTION EFFORTS IN NATURAL SETTINGS

The AIDS pandemic has, to a significant degree, altered the way in which intervention and research efforts for IDUs are conceived and delivered. Prior to 1986, nearly all studies of IDUs were studies of individuals who were enrolled in drug treatment programs. Studies of IDUs outside of drug clinics, courts, and prisons were very rare. Interventions designed to address issues of drug use and health promotion and delivered in natural social settings of IDUs were nearly nonexistent. The need to reach beyond the traditional settings where IDUs could be easily found changed rapidly in the mid-1980s as the AIDS caseload among heterosexual IDUs grew to unforseen proportions. Independent of the early Dutch experiments with syringe exchange in 1984, several early programs in New Jersey, New York, Baltimore, and San Francisco began to reach IDUs with AIDS prevention messages on the streets of inner city neighborhoods. These early efforts were followed by programs in Chicago and other major U.S. cities supported largely with funding from the National Institute on Drug Abuse (NIDA) and the Centers for Disease Control and Prevention (CDC). Many of these intervention efforts contained research components that permitted data collection among out-of-treatment drug users. These studies represent the first generation of research efforts that have sought to systematically understand the characteristics, behaviors, drug and sexual practices of, and HIV infection rates among, IDUs outside of institutional settings.

Community Health Outreach

In part, because of a perceived need to directly address HIV prevention for IDUs out of treatment, community health outreach began in the United States in the mid-1980s (Watters et al., 1986). These efforts have focused on AIDS prevention and education and have been supplemented by the use of distribution tactics such as dissemination of bleach (used to decontaminate syringes) and condoms. These programs have sought to apply principles of harm reduction as rapidly as possible, and provide a stopgap method of interrupting the spread of HIV while other treatments and behavioral interventions could be developed.

These programs are distinguished from other "field efforts" in that their central objective is to provide information and prevention materials in a nonjudgmental context that will result in the lowering of behavioral risk among the targeted population. In order to attain this objective, individuals, often known as "community health outreach workers" (CHOWs) are trained to enter high-risk communities, develop relationships with members of social groupings of IDUs, and begin the process of education. In some ways, what the CHOWs *don't* do is as important as what they *do.* For example, in San Francisco, CHOWs participating in our early HIV/AIDS prevention projects were instructed to adhere to these cardinal rules: (1) never ask about illegal activities and change the subject if they came up; (2) never proselytize abstinence from drugs or push drug treatment, make referrals only if requested by the client; (3) always avoid situations that are unstable, where violence or illegal activities (e.g., drug deals) might be occurring. These rules were included

to help CHOWs develop a safe and clear relationship with the target population. This could not happen if the CHOW was perceived as (1) a police
informant (too interested in illegal activities); (2) a "do gooder" intent on
lecturing on the evils of drug use and the roads to "salvation"; or (3) a "running
partner" who is a participant in illegal dealings. The role of the CHOW was
one of knowledgeable helper. The issues to be dealt with were health concerns:
CHOWs could, did, and still do make referrals to various services upon request.
This has even involved direct assistance in negotiating the professional bu-
reaucracies with which IDUs must interact in order to obtain needed services.
This is distinct, however, from the role of outreach workers whose objective
is to recruit individuals into drug treatment. For CHOWs in these outreach
programs, the IDU is viewed as a client who has made a set of choices about
his or her own life. The role of helper and educator involves providing additional options together with an even-handed explanation of consequences.
This nonjudgmental orientation has made it possible for CHOWs from vastly
different walks of life and experiential backgrounds to safely and effectively
enter social groupings of IDUs in some of San Francisco's most dangerous
neighborhoods and effectively carry out their life-saving mandate (Broadhead, 1991).

Outreach programs originally conducted in San Francisco, Chicago, New
York City, and Baltimore were expanded and the technology disseminated
across the United States with the financial support of the Centers for Disease
Control and the National Institute of Drug Abuse. Since 1990 federal support
for these programs has been flagging. With the absence of a constituency, no
clear leadership for these programs at the federal level, lack of coordination
among federal agencies, and competing priorities, the funding level for these
programs has dropped substantially. For example, the National Institute on
Drug Abuse invested approximately $50 million per year in HIV prevention
outreach demonstration projects in 1988. In the 1992 budget, this amount
was approximately $11 million. While it is true that a significant portion of
NIDA's former demonstration resources have been transferred to the new
Center for Substance Abuse Treatment, the portfolio of programming from
this agency that supports outreach activities is pitched at a vastly reduced
level (approximately $15 million) and is no longer dedicated to primary HIV
prevention for out-of-treatment IDUs, but also funds efforts directed at at-
tracting IDUs into treatment programs that often have waiting periods of
over 30 days. Despite these problems of funding and leadership, outreach
programs have been shown to be highly effective in increasing knowledge and
lowering risk.

For example, in a survey of 1584 IDUs in five U.S. cities (Miami, Chicago,
Philadelphia, Houston, and San Francisco), substantial differences were found
between IDUs interviewed at baseline and six months later (Centers for Disease

Control, 1990). At initial interview, 65% reported sharing injection equipment. At follow-up, 37% reported sharing. At baseline, 11% of those who admitted sharing needles and syringes reported consistent use of bleach. This had increased to 43% six months later. Increases were also seen in reported use of condoms from 10 to 27%. In a related study among IDUs in San Francisco (Watters, Downing et al., 1990), drug treatment programs were the leading source of AIDS information among 438 IDUs surveyed prior to implementation of outreach programs. One year later (six months after San Francisco CHOWs first began to distribute bleach), the leading source of AIDS information was outreach workers. This same study also found evidence of significant dissemination of the "don't share," "use bleach" message from other sources, most notably friends and associates. This dissemination of knowledge occurred in a context where significant changes in behavior were likewise reported. Among those who reported syringe sharing (90% in 1986, 79% in 1987), 3% said they used bleach in 1986, compared to 55% in 1987. Subsequent follow-up surveys in semiannual cross sections have shown increases in the use of bleach and condoms, and reductions in the proportion of IDUs who report sharing over time (Watters, Cheng et al., 1990). By 1988, 86% of those who reported needle sharing used bleach.

Syringe and Needle Exchange

A more controversial approach to HIV prevention has been the use of needle exchange programs which seek to discourage sharing of syringes by making injection equipment available to drug users. Opponents of syringe exchange programs believe they encourage drug use, increase the supply of syringes in the community, and will not impact the sharing behavior they seek to reduce. Despite these concerns, programs have been established which provide sterile injection equipment to drug users in exchange for their used and potentially contaminated equipment. This approach to harm reduction is based on the assumption that the primary factor associated with HIV infection among IDUs is the shared syringe, and focuses on the direct removal of contaminated syringes, their safe disposal, and their replacement with sterile ones. While the primary focus of most exchange programs is this simple replacement, syringe exchange programs can also provide an initial point of contact between IDUs and health service providers, including, for those who are so motivated, access to drug treatment (Hagan, Des Jarlais, Purchase, Reid, & Friedman, 1991a).

Previous studies have reported some benefits associated with syringe exchange. In prior research, investigators have reported that syringe exchange programs have played a significant role in lower rates of needle-sharing in Amsterdam (Hartgers, Buning, van Santen, Verster, & Coutinho, 1989; van den Hoek, van Haastrecht, & Coutinho, 1989); Sweden (Ljungberg et al., 1991); Australia (Buzolic, 1988); and the United Kingdom (Pye, Kapila, Buckley, & Cunningham, 1989; Hart et al., 1989; Stimson, 1989). Other studies have reported that syringe exchange programs have served as sources of referrals into social services, medical services, and drug treatment (Carvell & Hart, 1990; Kaplan & Heimer, 1992). The U.S. General Accounting Office (GAO) recently reviewed evaluation studies of needle exchange programs in the United States (Tacoma, WA, and New Haven, CT) and in five foreign countries (U.S. General Accounting Office, 1993). Studies were reviewed by the GAO only if they had received scientific peer review and only if they reported statistical significance at the .05 level. The GAO review team reported that, based on the studies reviewed, needle exchange may reduce needle-sharing behavior, does provide a means for IDUs to access health care services, and does not increase drug use or frequency of injection among IDUs (U.S. General Accounting Office, 1993). The GAO study is a landmark not only for the findings reported, but because it is the first needle exchange research in the United States supported by federal funds.

The first U.S. needle exchange program was implemented in Tacoma in November 1988 (Purchase, Hagan, Des Jarlais, & Reid, 1989). In one study of Tacoma exchangers, participants (n = 154) reported HIV-related risk behavior for the month before they began using the exchange, and for the most recent month in which they attended the exchange program (Hagan et al., 1991a). Participants reported a decrease in the frequency of borrowing used needles from others, from 57 times per month to 36 times per month, over the two time periods. Frequency of loaning used needles to others also decreased, from 100 times per month to 65 times per month, and use of bleach to clean needles increased from 71 to 106 times per month. In a subsequent study (Hagan, Des Jarlais, Purchase, Reid, & Friedman, 1991b), HIV seroprevalence and risk behavior was compared for exchange users (n = 265) and nonexchange users (n = 93). In the exchange group HIV seroprevalence was 2% and in the nonexchange group 7%, and nonexchangers were more likely to report unsafe injection practices (45% vs. 21%). In an ecological study (Hagan, Reid et al., 1991), researchers reported a dramatic decrease in the incidence of hepatitis B among Tacoma IDUs in the years after needle exchange was instituted.

In New Haven, Connecticut, researchers employed a "syringe tracking and testing system" to evaluate the exchange program. All needles distributed by the exchange program are affixed with an identification number, and each exchange client has his or her own client code. Each time a client visits the exchange, the client code is recorded along with the needle identification numbers for those needles that are returned by the client, and those that are given to the client (O'Keefe, Kaplan, & Koshnood, 1991). Needles returned to the exchange are tested for the presence of HIV using laboratory procedures. Using these strategies, Kaplan (1991) reported that needles distributed by the exchange, and returned, were less likely to be HIV positive than those that came from other sources (50.3% vs. 67.5%). Similarly, needles that were apparently not shared (taken and returned by the same person) were less likely to be positive than those needles that were apparently shared (taken and returned by different people; 45% vs. 57%). Based on this system, and using mathematical modeling techniques and several assumptions about unknown variables, New Haven researchers estimated that needle exchange lowered the rate of new HIV infections among their clients by one-third (Kaplan & Heimer, 1992; O'Keefe et al., 1991).

In San Francisco, the Urban Health Study, an ongoing cross-sectional study of out-of-treatment IDUs begun in 1985 has shown interesting and positive results (Watters, Clark, Estilo, & Lorvick, unpublished manuscript). The "Prevention Point" syringe exchange program was begun in November 1988. By Spring 1992, the largest proportion (45%) of Urban Health Study participants reported "typically" acquiring syringes from syringe exchange. Sixty-one percent reported having used the needle exchange program within the past year. The number of injections per day, at the 50th percentile, declined from 1.4 to .7 between 1987 and 1992. The mean age of cross-section samples increased over time from 36 to 42, suggesting that IDUs in San Francisco represent an aging cohort. The proportion of new initiates into injection drugs decreased from 3 to 1%, suggesting that the needle exchange did not increase the number of new initiates to injection drug use. In multivariate analysis of IDUs recruited into the study from Fall 1991 to Spring 1992 (n = 752), excluding duplicate observations, self-reported exchange users were less likely to share syringes than were nonexchange users. The effectiveness of needle-exchange use varied with age, with the largest effect seen in younger users. African-American ethnicity, and regular condom use were associated with not sharing needles; reported daily injection drug use, crack cocaine use, and injected cocaine use within the past 30 days were positively associated with syringe sharing. Use of syringe exchange was rapidly adopted by the target population. Frequent use of syringe exchange was strongly associated with abstinence from sharing injection equipment.

In a study specifically designed to evaluate the potential negative effects of needle exchange (Guydish et al., 1993), researchers reviewed data for all drug treatment admissions in San Francisco County over a four-year period (N = 35,460). Admissions for the two years preceding implementation of the exchange program (1987–1988) were compared to those for the two years following implementation (1989–1990). In this analysis of drug treatment data, the existence of the exchange program was *not* associated with increased injection drug use or needle sharing behavior, or with shifting from drug use by noninjection routes to drug use by the injection route. Consequently, at the same time that positive effects of needle exchange were documented by Watters et al. (unpublished manuscript), potential negative effects were not observed.

Despite these findings, syringe and needle exchange continues to be a bitterly contested issue among community groups with differing philosophies and objectives. The specter of Tuskegee haunts policy-makers and researchers (treatment was withheld from a group of black men suffering from syphilis). They point to the outcomes of the studies previously discussed, and suggest the need for more definitive research than that provided by the studies currently available. Intervention researchers and activists have had measurable success in a limited number of communities. The success of future efforts will be contingent on the ability of researchers to develop broad-based coalitions in the communities where they seek to create and deploy such programs. In addition, without adequate resources, these efforts stand little likelihood of fulfilling their promise. The cold crushing facts of public sector budgets and the volatility of the syringe exchange debate have thus far intersected at a point where symbolic progress has been made in the United States, but nothing yet on a scale required to have measurable epidemiological impact on a regional or national scale.

CHALLENGES IN EVALUATING PROGRAMS
IN NATURAL SETTINGS

The methodologies available for the evaluation of prevention programs in natural settings present researchers with significant challenges. While a critical review of formal evaluations of HIV/AIDS interventions for drug users in natural settings is beyond the scope of this chapter, there are several methods of conducting evaluation research that may be discussed. Under most conditions, the outcome variables used to evaluate interventions in natural settings will be based on self-report. Self-report data is subject to numerous biases including drug and alcohol detoxification, problems of recall, and socially desirable responses given to interviewers by respondents who wish to portray themselves in the best possible light. These problems are exacerbated when interview staff overlap with direct service delivery staff. Since, as we have seen above, funding for outreach demonstration projects has been seriously curtailed in recent years, programs charged with both delivering services and conducting research must, in order to survive, have staff wear both the CHOW hat and the evaluator hat. This inevitably compounds the problems of observational bias, since outreach workers may perceive a significant stake in making their own efforts (or those of their program) appear in the most positive light. Respondents in such settings may have difficulty in distinguishing between these roles and in offering information that they believe their CHOW most wants to hear. One way to reduce this problem is to involve research staff who do not carry an inherent role-conflict with them into the field (Lampinen, Wiebel, & Watters, 1989; Watters & Cheng, 1991; Anthony et al., 1991). However, the costs of maintaining separate research and service delivery staffs are often prohibitive.

Many intervention efforts were initially implemented with public health objectives as primary, and evaluation objectives as secondary. This has resulted in a situation where the more powerful (and expensive) research designs have not been implemented. This is due in part to the availability of resources, and the need to establish priorities that emphasize disease prevention objectives. Rigorous demands for data collection have not been easily absorbed into the day-to-day administration of programs which have goals that are primarily prevention oriented. Typically, intervention studies and service programs share neither the same objectives or methods. Consequently, efforts to evaluate outreach programs rarely utilize rigorous experimental or quasi-experimental designs which result in intervention studies in natural settings being methodologically compromised (Watters & Biernacki, 1989).

As a consequence, the available literature evaluating HIV prevention in natural settings is long on program description but short on definitive research regarding impact on behavior change that can be attributed to the intervention. Most of the studies of outreach programs and syringe exchange programs tend to rely on self-report data which are subject to numerous sources of bias (Huang, Watters, & Case, 1988). Recall errors, for example, are more likely to create problems in *internal reliability*. If investigators are willing to conduct systematic test–retest reliability trials on their data collection instruments, the magnitude of this problem can be reduced by making appropriate adjustments. If adjustment is not possible, knowledge of reliability of key items is highly useful in selecting and constructing variables for quantitative analysis, and interpretation of results.

A greater problem is that of the *external validity* of the data collected and the impact that invalid data may have on research findings. In the context of HIV/AIDS prevention programs, IDUs may seek to present themselves in the best possible light. This may mean that there is systematic exaggeration in the direction of falsely inflating compliance with the desired outcome. In other words, after the outreach workers tell IDUs not to share needles, the IDUs may be more likely to tell evaluators that they don't share needles to avoid negative judgment in the eyes of an outside observer. Should this source of bias be operating, it is far more difficult to detect than problems in recall and is more likely to be systematic in the direction of the desired effect.

Another evaluation method that does not rely on self-report data is the use of biological markers of infection, either as seroprevalence/seroconversion studies or as indicators of HIV in shared injection equipment. Interest in seroprevalence as an outcome variable has been expressed in policy contexts. Seroprevalence tends, however, to be more useful at the beginning stages of HIV epidemics. Once HIV is well established in a population, it may become increasingly difficult to correlate the effects of interventions with rates of seroprevalence. This is true due to the relatively long latency of HIV, and the fact that in the case of evaluating HIV prevention programs, the majority of IDUs participating in such programs were likely to have been infected prior to the implementation of prevention programs. Moreover, mature or long-running seroprevalence studies have the risk of *underestimating* seroprevalence rates. This occurs when there is differential attrition among seropositive members of cross-sectional studies. In later stages of HIV epidemics, this may result from morbidity and mortality of seropositive respondents. But this may also result from seropositive respondents electing not to return for testing at a rate that is different from seronegative participants who may wish to see if their serostatus has changed.

Seroincidence studies require substantial cohorts of IDUs. Cohort studies of IDUs not enrolled in drug treatment programs are expensive and difficult to conduct. Differential attrition of high-risk persons from such studies may tend to bias results. While overall rates of seroincidence can be correlated with the implementation of interventions, it is extremely difficult to control for historical artifacts in such studies (e.g., Magic Johnson or Arthur Ashe announcing they have HIV infections). Nevertheless, both prevalence and incidence studies can provide extremely useful information regarding interventions on a community scale, but analysis of these data must be tempered with a thorough understanding of the historical and contextual factors that may also play a role in changes (or lack of changes). Finally, incidence and prevalence studies can help provide clues as to the specific epidemiology of HIV infection in various subpopulations of IDUs. Such studies are, however, typically based on multivariate analyses in an attempt to identify factors that are independently associated with the attribute of interest (in this case HIV or other infectious diseases). Such studies, while interesting and of potential value in directing prevention efforts, are usually too vague to give rise to specific technologies needed for prevention efforts and are always subject to problems associated with the use of self-report data as discussed above.

A third method for research in natural settings is the use of qualitative approaches such as ethnography. Such approaches to research in natural settings have provided the foundation for survey oriented activities that have followed. While survey efforts can provide profiles of drug abuse trends among subgroups, risk behavior typologies, and estimates of the prevalence of various characteristics in a population, surveys are weak in developing knowledge as to how events are viewed and what meaning they have to group members of interest. Qualitative efforts, on the other hand, are extremely powerful tools for understanding how behavior reported in surveys occurs. For example, while surveys of IDU risk behavior in the United States tend to show increased compliance with health preservation methods, little is known about how these methods are actually applied. Through direct observation in field settings, a fuller understanding of the specific behavioral dynamics and risk practices can be developed. For example, while frequent use of bleach is routinely reported among IDUs in surveys, the specific details of how cleaning is actually accomplished is not known. This is an especially important evaluative concern. Bleach is not a magic bullet that kills HIV on contact. Emerging studies suggest that bleach use may not always be effective under all conditions. For example Vlahov et al. (1991) found bleach to have a nonsignificant protective effect on HIV[†] seroincidence among a cohort of IDUs in Baltimore. This finding may have resulted from reporting errors, or from inadequate application of the bleach rinsing protocol. Alternatively, it may be that under certain circumstances, use of bleach as recommended (two rinses with full-strength bleach followed by two rinses with water) does not inactivate HIV. Field studies using qualitative interviews and direct observation could help shed much needed light on how well the protocol is actually followed. While such techniques are, themselves, not immune from interactive effects of observation and observed behavior, these methods can contribute substantially to our knowledge about how well programs work.

SUMMARY

In this chapter we have discussed some of the philosophy, history, programmatic content, research, and challenges in evaluating HIV/AIDS prevention programs for IDUs in natural settings. Drug use, and in particular drug use by injection, is a major risk factor for HIV infection. Drug users can be a difficult group to identify due to the illegal and clandestine nature of their activity. The majority of IDUs remain outside of drug treatment programs, compounding difficulties in access. Historically, there have been three major approaches to dealing with substance abuse: (1) through the criminal

---

[†] There is some evidence that suggests that at least 30 seconds of exposure time to full-strength bleach is required to inactivate HIV in pelleted virus in laboratory settings (Shapshak et al., 1993). Minimum exposure time in a standard U-100 insulin syringe is about 15–20 seconds when the process is carried out at maximum speed.

justice system; (2) through the medicalization of addiction and recovery oriented programs; and (3) through harm reduction programs which seek to minimize the damage of drug use without condemning it. Programs for HIV/AIDS prevention amongst IDUs in natural settings have depended heavily on community outreach to IDUs in inner-city neighborhoods. Key to these efforts has been the education of IDUs to lower their risk through the avoidance of needle sharing and the use of bleach and condoms. Support for outreach programs has diminished substantially from its 1988–1989 peak. Research has demonstrated that outreach programs can be a highly cost-effective means to modify risk behavior among IDUs. Syringe and needle exchange has become an emerging technology that seeks to reduce the transmission of HIV by removing contaminated equipment from the environment and by reducing the need for IDUs to share equipment. Research in numerous venues has demonstrated that syringe exchange programs provide a useful prevention strategy to reach many IDUs. Fears that bleach distribution and syringe exchange would increase problems associated with drug use have not been supported by research.

Efforts to evaluate prevention programs in natural settings have been hampered by the complexity and expense of conducting controlled trials of intervention under natural conditions. Consequently, most studies of interventions in natural settings represent a compromise between what should be done and what can be done given the constraints of funding, human resources, and differing goals of interventionists and researchers. Most evaluative studies depend on self-reported data that are sensitive to recall errors and other sources of bias. Additional attention to development of instrumentation, and to addressing problems of internal reliability and external validity are needed. Studies that depend on biological markers are also subject to problems. Mature seroprevalence studies may underestimate rates due to differential attrition of living seropositives. Qualitative approaches can help provide a foundation for survey approaches and help provide meaning to quantitative results.

ACKNOWLEDGMENT. This work was supported in part by grants from the National Institute on Drug Abuse (U01-DA 6908 and R18-DA06979) and support from the U.S. Centers for Disease Control and Prevention, and the San Francisco Department of Public Health AIDS Office.

REFERENCES

Allen, D. M., Onorato, I. M., Green, T. A. (1992). HIV infection in intravenous drug users entering drug treatment, United States, 1986–1989. The Field Services Branch of the Centers for Disease Control. *American Journal of Public Health, 82,* 541–546.

Anthony, J. C., Vlahov, D., Celentano, D. D., Menon, A. S., Margolick, J. B., Cohn, S., Nelson, K. E., & Polk, B. F. (1991). Self-report interview data for a study of HIV-1 infection among intravenous drug users: Descriptions of methods and preliminary evidence on validity. *Journal of Drug Issues, 231,* 739–757.

Ball, J. C., & Ross, A., (1991). *The effectiveness of methadone treatment.* New York: Springer-Verlag.

Bixler, R. E., Palacios-Jiminez, L., & Springer, E. (1987). *AIDS prevention for substance abuse treatment programs.* Albany, NY: Narcotics and Drug Research, Inc. (251 New Karner Road).

Broadhead, R. S. (1991). Social construction of bleach in combating AIDS among injection drug users. *Journal of Drug Issues, 21,* 713–737.

Brown, B. S., Watters, J. K., Igelhart, I., Akins, C. (1982–1983). Methadone maintenance dosage levels and program retention. *American Journal of Alcohol & Drug Abuse, 9,* 129–139.

Buzolic, A. (1988, June). *Needle and syringe availability and AIDS prevention: Modifications of existing legislation.* Report to the Queensland, Australia, Ministerial Task Force on Drug Strategy.

Carvell, A. M., & Hart, G. J. (1990). Help-seeking and referrals in a needle exchange: A comprehensive service to injecting drug users. *British Journal of Addiction, 85,* 235–240.

Centers for Disease Control and Prevention (1990). Update: Reducing HIV transmission in intravenous drug users not in treatment—United States. *Mortality & Morbidity Weekly Report, 39,* 529–538.

Centers for Disease Control and Prevention. (1992, January). *HIV/AIDS Surveillance Report,* 1–22.

Chin, J. (1991, June). Epidemiology keynote speech. Seventh International Conference on AIDS, Florence, Italy.

Choopanya, K., Vanichsensi, S., Plangsringarm, Sonchai, W., Carballo, M., Friedmann, P., Friedman, S. R., & Des Jarlais, D. C. (1991). Risk factors and HIV seropositivity among injecting drug users in Bangkok. *AIDS, 5,* 1509–1514.

Cooper, J. R., Altman, F., Brown, B. S., & Czechowicz, D. (Eds.). (1983). *Research on the treatment of narcotic addiction: State of the art.* Rockville, MD: National Institute on Drug Abuse.

D'Aunno, T., & Vaughn, T. E. (1983). Variations in methadone treatment practices. *Journal of the American Medical Association, 267,* 253–258.

Epstein, E. J. (1977). *Agency of fear: Opiates and political power in America.* New York: Putnam Press.

Gibson, D. R., Wermuth, L., Lovelle-Drache, J., Ham, J., & Sorensen, J. L. (1989). Brief counseling to reduce AIDS risk in intravenous drug users and their sexual partners: Preliminary results. *Counselling Psychology Quarterly, 2,* 15–19.

Guydish, J., Bucardo, J., Young, M., Woods, W., Grinstead, O., & Clark, W. (1993). Evaluating needle exchange: Are there negative effects? *AIDS, 7,* 871–876.

Hagan, H., Des Jarlais, D. C., Purchase, D., Reid, T., & Friedman, S. R. (1991a). The Tacoma syringe exchange. *Journal of Addictive Diseases, 10,* 81–88.

Hagan, H., Des Jarlais, D. C., Purchase, D., Reid, T., & Friedman, S. R. (1991b, June). *Lower HIV seroprevalence, declining HBV and safer injection in relation to the Tacoma syringe exchange.* Poster presented at the 7th International Conference on AIDS, Florence (Abstract W.C. 3291).

Hagan, H., Reid, T., Des Jarlais, D. C., Purchase, D., Friedman, S. R., & Bell, T. (1991). The incidence of HBV infection and syringe exchange programs. *Journal of the American Medical Association* (Letter), 266, 1646–1647.

Hart, G. J., Carvell, A. L., Woodward, N., Johnson, A. M., Williams, P., & Parry, J. V. (1989). Evaluation of needles exchange in central London: Behaviour change and anti-HIV status over one year. *AIDS, 3,* 261–265.

Hartgers, C., Buning, E. C., van Santen, G. W., Verster, A. D., & Coutinho, R. A. (1989). The impact of the needle and syringe-exchange programme in Amsterdam in injecting risk behavior. *AIDS, 3,* 571–576.

Higgins, D. L., Galavotti, C., O'Reilly, K. R., Schnell, D. J., Moore, M., Rugg, D. L., & Johnson, R. (1991). Evidence for the effects of HIV antibody counseling and testing on risk behaviors. *Journal of the American Medical Association, 266,* 2419–2429.

Huang, K. H. C., Watters, J. K., & Case, P. (1988). Psychological assessment and AIDS research with intravenous drug users: Challenges in measurement. *Journal of Psychoactive Drugs, 20,* 191–195.

Kaplan, E. (1991). Evaluating needle-exchange programs via syringe tracking and testing (STT). *AIDS & Public Policy Journal, 6,* 109–115.

Kaplan, E. H., & Heimer, R. (1992). HIV prevalence among intravenous drug users: Model-based estimates from New Haven's legal needle exchange. *Journal of Acquired Immune Deficiency Syndromes, 5,* 163–169.

Kozel, N. J., & Adams, E. H. (1986). Epidemiology of drug abuse: an overview. *Science, 21,* 970–974.

Lampinen, T., Wiebel, W. W., & Watters, J. K. (1989). Intravenous drug users, HIV testing and counseling. *Journal of the American Medical Association* (Letter), *262,* 1331.

Ljungberg, B., Christensson, B., Tunving, K., Andersson, B., Landvall, B., Lundberg, M., & Zall-Friberg, A. (1991). HIV prevention among injecting drug users: Three years experience from a syringe exchange program in Sweden. *Journal of the Acquired Immune Deficiency Syndromes, 4,* 890–895.

Malow, R., Corrigan, S., Pena, J., Calkins, A. M., & Bannister, T. (1992). Effectiveness of a psychoeducational approach to HIV risk behavior reduction. *Psychology of Addictive Behaviors, 6,* 120–125.

Musto, D. F. (1973). *The American disease: Origins of narcotics control,* New Haven, CT: Yale University Press.

National Commission on AIDS (1991, July). *The twin epidemics of substance abuse and HIV.* Washington, DC: National Commission on AIDS.

O'Keefe, E., Kaplan, E., & Koshnood, K. (1991, July). *Preliminary Report: City of New Haven needle exchange program.* New Haven CT: New Haven Health Department.

Purchase, D., Hagan, H., Des Jarlais, D. C., & Reid, T. (1989, June). *Historical account of the Tacoma syringe exchange.* Paper presented at 5th International Conference on AIDS, Montreal (Abstract Th. D.P.74).

Pye, M., Kapila, M., Buckley, G., & Cunningham, D. (1989, June). *A comparative study of local AIDS programs in the United Kingdom.* Paper presented at 5th International Conference on AIDS, Montreal (Abstract M. E. P. 46).

Shapshak, P., McCoy, C. B., Rivers, J. E., Chitwood, D. D., Mash, D. C., Weatherby, N. L., Inciardi, J. A., Shah, S. M., & Brown, B. S. (1993). Inactivation of human immunodeficiency virus-1 at short time intervals using undiluted bleach. *Journal of Acquired Immune Deficiency Syndromes, 6,* 218–129.

Sorensen, J. L., London, J., & Morales, E. (1991). Group counseling to prevent AIDS. In J. L. Sorensen, L. Wermuth, D. R. Gibson, K. Choi, J. Guydish, & S. Batki (Eds.), *Preventing AIDS in drug users and their sexual partners* (pp. 99–115). New York: Guilford.

Stimson, G. V. (1989). Editorial Review: Syringe-exchange programmes for injecting drug users. *AIDS, 3,* 253–260.

U.S. General Accounting Office (1993, March). *Needle exchange programs: Research suggests promise as an AIDS prevention strategy.* Washington, DC: United States General Accounting Office.

van den Hoek, J. A., van Haastrecht, H. J., & Coutinho, R. A. (1989). Risk reduction among intravenous drug users in Amsterdam under the influence of AIDS. *American Journal of Public Health, 10,* 1355–1357.

Vlahov, D., Munoz, A., Celentano, D. D., Cohn, S., Anthony, J. C., Chilcoat, H., & Nelson, K. E. (1991). HIV seroconversion and disinfection of injection equipment among intravenous drug users, Baltimore, Maryland. *Epidemiology, 2,* 444–446.

Watters, J. K., & Biernacki, P. (1989). Targeted sampling: Options for the study of hidden populations. *Social Problems, 36,* 416–430.

Watters, J. K., & Cheng, Y.-T. (1991). Toward comprehensive studies of HIV in intravenous drug users: Issues in treatment-based and community-based samples. In P. Hartsock, & S. Genser (Eds.), *Longitudinal studies of HIV infection in intravenous drug users: Methodologic issues associated in natural history research* (pp. 63–73). Rockville, MD: National Institute on Drug Abuse. NIDA Research Monograph 109.

Watters, J. K., Cheng, Y-T., & Lorvick, J. J. (1991). Drug use profiles, race, age, and risk of HIV infection among intravenous drug users in San Francisco. *International Journal of the Addictions, 26,* 1247–1262.

Watters, J. K., Cheng, Y-T., Segal, M., Lorvick, J., Case, P., & Carlson, J. (1990, June). *Epidemiology and prevention of HIV in heterosexual IV drug users in San Francisco, 1986–1989.* Paper presented at the 6th International Conference on AIDS, San Francisco, CA (Abstract F. C. 106).

Watters, J. K., Clark, G., Estilo, M., & Lorvick, J. J. (unpublished manuscript). *Syringe and needle exchange as HIV/AIDS prevention for injecting drug users: Results of the San Francisco experience.* Available from first author.

Watters, J. K., Downing, M., Case, P., Lorvick, J., Cheng, Y-T., & Fergusson, B. (1990). AIDS prevention for intravenous drug users in the community: Street-based education and risk behavior. *American Journal of Community Psychology, 18,* 587–596.

Watters, J. K., Feldman, H. W., Biernacki, P., & Newmeyer, J. A. (1986). Street-based AIDS prevention for intravenous drug users in San Francisco: Prospects, obstacles and options. In: *Community Epidemiology Work Group Proceedings* (pp. 37–43), Department of Health and Human Services, National Institute on Drug Abuse, Rockville, MD.

Wermuth, L. A., Robbins, R., Choi, K., & Eversley, R. (1991). Reaching and counseling women sexual partners. In J. L. Sorensen, L. Wermuth, D. R. Gibson, K. Choi, J. Guydish, & S. Batki (Eds.), *Preventing AIDS in drug users and their sexual partners* (pp. 130–149). New York: Guilford Press.

Wiley, J. A., & Samuel, M. C. (1989). Prevalence of HIV infection in the USA. *AIDS, 3*(Suppl. 1), 71–78.

Wodak, A., & Moss, A. (1990). HIV and injecting drug users: from epidemiology to public health. *AIDS, 4*(suppl), S105–S109.

12

Interventions for Sexual Partners of HIV-Infected or High-Risk Individuals

NANCY S. PADIAN, JANNEKE H. H. M. VAN DE WIJGERT, and THOMAS R. O'BRIEN

INTRODUCTION

Worldwide, sexual intercourse between men and women is the most common mode of transmission of human immunodeficiency virus (HIV) (World Health Organization, 1990). In the United States, heterosexuals represent the fastest growing group at risk for HIV infection, and women who are partners of HIV-infected or high risk individuals (especially injection drug users) represent the fastest growing group (Ellerbock et al., 1992). Twenty-nine percent of all cases of HIV in women were attributed to heterosexual transmission in 1986 compared to 34% in 1991. As the HIV epidemic continues to expand, a growing population is at risk because of an ongoing sexual relationship with an HIV-infected person.

In the absence of an effective vaccine, behavior change remains the most effective means to prevent the spread of HIV (Hinman, 1991). Although in the United States there are programs to counsel and test HIV-infected or at-risk individuals (Cleary et al., 1991; Higgins, Galavotti, & O'Reilly, 1991; Wenger, Linn, Epstein, & Shapiro, 1991), and some partner notification pro-

NANCY S. PADIAN and JANNEKE H. H. M. VAN DE WIJGERT • School of Medicine, University of California, San Francisco, and San Francisco General Hospital, San Francisco, California 94110.   *THOMAS R. O'BRIEN* • Viral Epidemiology Section, National Cancer Institute, Rockville, Maryland 20892.

Preventing AIDS: Theories and Methods of Behavioral Interventions, edited by Ralph J. DiClemente and John L. Peterson. Plenum Press, New York, 1994.

grams that locate, counsel, and test the partners of HIV-infected individuals (Giesecke et al., 1991), few, if any, programs provide couple counseling in which infected individuals and their sexual partners are counseled and educated at the same time about effective behavior change. The effectiveness of couple counseling has been suggested by Higgins and associates (1991) who reported that after counseling, reductions in unprotected sex were greater among discordant couples than among cohorts of high-risk individuals.

Few interventions actually involve both partners in the intervention protocol. Nevertheless, the results of partner notification programs and HIV antibody testing and counseling programs are relevant because they are often geared at partners of HIV-infected or at-risk heterosexual individuals. In this manuscript we review both of these programs and discuss in detail the design and results from a couple counseling protocol from one study. We conclude with a discussion of the limitations and strengths of all of these approaches.

REVIEW OF RELEVANT INTERVENTIONS

In an effort to minimize heterosexual HIV transmission, several interventions have been proposed and introduced in a variety of study populations. These study populations include several African communities, intravenous drug users, prostitutes, and the sex partners of transfusion recipients, hemophiliacs and bisexual men. In an effort to understand sexual behavior and to evaluate the efficacy of these interventions, knowledge, attitude, and behavior (KAB) surveys about the risky aspects of sexual intercourse have been conducted in these study populations. A consistent finding of these KAB surveys is that education and information campaigns generally result in high levels of knowledge about HIV transmission and its prevention but that this knowledge is not necessarily translated into safer sex behavior. Only a handful of studies have actually attempted to evaluate the effect of interventions on identifying HIV infected persons and on behavior change. These intervention studies will be reviewed here and the methodological limitations of these studies will be discussed.

Partner Notification

In early 1985, the Centers for Disease Control mandated creation of HIV counseling and testing sites to serve as anonymous screening places for persons wishing to be tested for HIV antibodies. Public health officials advocated HIV antibody testing on the assumption that HIV seropositive individuals could change their behaviors to prevent reexposure to the virus and transmission to other people, and that seronegative individuals will change their behaviors to protect themselves from HIV infection (Francis & Chin, 1987). Partner notification programs identify HIV-infected persons who might otherwise be missed by screening programs. (The term *partner* refers to homosexual and heterosexual sexual partners as well as needle-sharing partners.) Voluntary and confidential HIV antibody testing programs and partner notification programs have allowed health care workers to identify and target intensive interventions to HIV-infected persons and their partners. Infected persons are the source of new infections of others and represent links and opportunities for breaking transmission chains.

The partner notification approach always depends on the voluntary cooperation of the index patient in providing names of partners. The notification of partners is accomplished in two possible ways: by patient referral (also called self-referral) and provider referral. With the patient referral method, HIV positive persons are asked to notify their partners themselves and refer them to the health department for testing and counseling. With the provider referral method, trained public health counselors locate and notify the partners, based on the information given to them by the index patient. The name of the index patient will not be disclosed to the partners, although there have been circumstances where the identity of the index patient could be deduced even if he or she was not named.

Success in Identifying Partners

Several partner notification programs in the United States have been evaluated to determine the efficacy and cost effectiveness of patient and provider referral approaches. Both because of the long incubation period of HIV and because of the often large numbers of anonymous partners, it is impossible to find all partners. Furthermore, the success of partner notification programs depends to a large extent on the cooperation of the index patients. While it is extremely difficult to identify, counsel, educate, and test partners, several studies have shown that partner notification programs are very efficient in identifying previously untested and uneducated individuals.

In 1988, the Centers for Disease Control summarized the results of partner notification activities in four states (Centers for Disease Control, 1988). In Colorado, where provider referral is emphasized as the preferred method of notifying partners, 282 index cases named 508 partners in a two-year period. Of the 414 partners who were located, all were counseled and 80% were tested. The program identified 45 new cases of HIV infection. In Idaho, where provider referral is also emphasized, 120 index cases named 118 partners in a three-year time period. Of the 59 partners who were located, all accepted counseling and testing and 23 were found to be infected with HIV. Virginia provided provider referral in 1988 but did not emphasize it: 44 new cases of

HIV infection were identified in 15 months. In South Carolina (Wykoff et al., 1991), partner notification through provider referral is offered to all individuals with a confirmed HIV antibody positive test result. The results of the first 30 months of partner notification were reviewed in 1991. Of the 485 partners of 42 index cases and of their HIV positive contacts, 280 (58%) were tested for HIV antibody and 49 were seropositive. Only 3 of the 49 seropositive contacts had previously been tested, which indicates that partner notification can be an efficient way of identifying HIV positive individuals. The percentage of individuals tested and tested positive was similar for homo- and bisexual men, intravenous drug users, and heterosexuals.

In North Carolina (Landis et al., 1992), both patient and provider referral programs are available within the three public health departments and partner notification is mandatory by law. Seventy-four index cases were recruited into a study. They named 310 contacts of whom 130 were notified. Of these 130 contacts, 61 accepted HIV antibody testing and 13 tested positive. The overall effectiveness of this partner notification program in identifying HIV positive partners was therefore much lower than the programs that were mentioned above. When provider referral was compared to patient referral, profound differences were found in efficacy. In the provider referral group, 78 of the 157 partners were notified; 36 accepted HIV antibody testing of whom 9 were seropositive. In the patient referral group, only 10 of 153 partners were notified by the index patient; 5 accepted HIV antibody testing, and one was seropositive. An additional 42 partners were notified by public health counselors after one month; 20 accepted HIV antibody testing and 3 were seropositive. The authors conclude that, despite the fact that partner notification was mandatory by law and violation of this law was a misdemeanor, patient referral was quite ineffective in this study. In contrast, provider referral was quite effective in that it reached 50% of the partners in that group.

The type of partner notification services provided by different health departments depends on local resources and the number of seropositive persons identified. In San Francisco (Rutherford et al., 1991), high rates of infection among homosexual men made partner notification in this group infeasible. However, the health department did notify heterosexual partners of AIDS patients to identify infected women of childbearing age. Thirty-four opposite-sex sexual partners of 51 index cases were tested for HIV and 7 new cases of HIV infection were identified. The authors conclude that, although partner notification was more expensive than more general AIDS prevention and education efforts, its ability to target case finding, education, and counseling to women at highest risk for infection makes it cost-effective for prevention of vertically transmitted HIV infection.

In general, individuals who agree to be tested for HIV are less likely to be HIV positive than individuals who decline testing (Lee, Branan, Hoff,

Datwyler, & Bayer, 1990). Therefore, many cases of HIV infection will be missed in a voluntary HIV antibody testing program. However, the previous studies suggest that partner notification programs, in particular through provider referral, can be very efficient in identifying, testing, counseling, and educating at-risk individuals, who otherwise might have been missed by screening programs of high risk populations.

Confidentiality

Partner notification has been used for four decades for other infectious diseases, including sexually transmitted diseases, and has often proved to be highly effective in limiting the spread of disease and treating contacts (Bayer & Toomey, 1992; Francis et al., 1989). Partner notification in HIV/AIDS is different, however, because no cure can be offered for those partners who test HIV positive and because of the severe stigma attached to being HIV infected. Therefore, the need for protection of confidentiality was immediately recognized by those at risk for HIV infection and by many public health officials who believed that loss of confidentiality would reduce the likelihood that patients would cooperate, thus driving the disease underground (Bayer et al., 1992; "Partner Notification," 1991). Others believed that HIV antibody testing should be mandatory (Lee, Branan, Hoff, Datwyler, & Bayer, 1990) and that the physician, in certain circumstances, should be obligated to warn partners at risk, even if that would violate the patient's right to confidentiality. Disagreements arose over the limits of the principle of confidentiality, distrust over the motives of public health officials and the government, and doubts about the efficacy of partner notification.

Thus, fear of losing confidentiality makes partner notification programs unacceptable for some at-risk individuals. A study in South Carolina (Jones et al., 1990) showed, however, that almost all contacts identified through the health department's partner notification program were highly supportive of the program. When 132 partners were asked whether they thought the health department did the right thing in telling them about their exposure, 87% responded "yes." When asked if the health department should keep notifying persons exposed to HIV, 92% responded "yes." Similar percentages were found for HIV positive and HIV negative partners, and for homosexuals, bisexuals, heterosexuals, and intravenous drug users. The authors concluded that the health department could create a highly supportive environment and a sense of trust between at-risk individuals and the counselors. They believed that the high participation rates were mainly due to (1) the willingness of health department staff to meet partners at the time and location of their choice; (2) an honest, unbiased approach and sincere concern for the client demonstrated by the counselors; and (3) a complete respect for the clients' privacy and confidentiality. In Kansas City (Lee et al., 1990), a high level of voluntary acceptance of confidential HIV antibody testing was reached in a STD (sexually transmitted disease) clinic (92%) and in the partner notification program (80%), even though clients were informed that should they test positive they would be reported by name, demographics, and risk factors to the Missouri Department of Health in accordance with state law.

THE EFFECT OF HIV ANTIBODY TESTING, COUNSELING, AND AIDS EDUCATION ON BEHAVIOR CHANGE

Regardless of the success with which HIV-infected individuals or their partners are identified, the most important question is whether HIV antibody testing, counseling, and AIDS education actually result in a reduction of high-risk behaviors and, ultimately, in the spread of HIV. Once HIV infected persons have been identified, interventions to change the risk behaviors can take place. The only options currently available are AIDS education and counseling: AIDS education generally focuses on knowledge about ways in which HIV is transmitted; counseling can be accomplished in many different ways. Thus far no clear definition and characterization of HIV/AIDS counseling has been developed (Carballo & Miller, 1989), although the importance of counseling in HIV infection and AIDS is well-accepted throughout the world (Green, 1989).

The most important objective of AIDS education and counseling is to change risk behaviors and thereby prevent HIV transmission. In addition, many public health officials feel that counseling should be provided for all HIV-positive individuals, their partners, and families to help them cope with this life-threatening infection and to help them make important life decisions.

Several studies in the United States have examined the effect of AIDS education and counseling on behavior change. In South Carolina (Wykoff et al., 1991), partners received a 45- to 60-minute educational session about personal risk and protection at the time of notification. All tested partners also received a one-hour posttest counseling session to review the test results and reinforce the educational message. Everyone was encouraged to return at six-month intervals for educational reinforcement, reinterviewing, and re-testing if necessary. For the 36 seropositive individuals who were reinterviewed at least once, the number of named sexual and needle-sharing contacts decreased from a mean of 5.6 at the initial interview to 1.1 at the most recent interview (at 6, 12, 18, or 24 months after the initial interview). For the 101 seronegative individuals who were reinterviewed, this decrease was from a mean of 4.0 to 2.0. This suggests that the combination of counseling and testing resulted in a reduction of high-risk behavior immediately after the intervention.

Cleary and associates (1991) studied short-term behavior changes in blood donors who were notified that they were HIV antibody positive. At the time of notification, the blood donors were counseled and educated about HIV, and 243 of them completed a baseline questionnaire. One hundred ninety-six (72%) participants returned for the two-week follow-up visit. The study population was very heterogeneous and the majority of the donors was unaware that their blood would be tested for HIV. A surprisingly high number of participants did not report a major HIV risk factor and many men who described themselves as exclusively heterosexual reported having had sex with another man. At the initial interview, 88.5% of the men and 86.5% of the women reported having sexually active in the previous week whereas at the two-week follow-up, these percentages were reduced to 63.6% and 68.9% respectively. At the initial interview, 68.1% of the men and 57.7% of the women reported engaging in unsafe sex in the previous week whereas at the two-week follow-up, these percentages were reduced to 40.4% and 37.8% respectively. The authors concluded that even if the reported reduction was true, it is disconcerting that about 40% of the participants still engaged in unsafe activities at follow-up.

To assess sexual behavior changes after voluntary HIV antibody testing and routine counseling, Landis and associates (Landis, Earp, & Koch, 1992) interviewed 235 persons at two anonymous test sites in North Carolina. Volunteers were of mixed race, gender, educational level, and risk-factor groups. They were interviewed and counseled after having their blood drawn but before receiving the test results; approximately two weeks later they received posttest counseling. They were reinterviewed after one year. No significant changes were found between pre-HIV antibody testing behaviors and one-year follow-up behaviors in the number of sexual partners in the previous month, the prevalence of receptive anal intercourse without a condom, condom use during anal intercourse, vaginal intercourse or oral intercourse, mutual masturbation, and withdrawal prior to ejaculation. The proportion of persons with anonymous sex partners increased from 9% to 19%.

One randomized trial of HIV antibody testing on sexually active heterosexual adults was conducted by Wenger and associates in a Los Angeles STD clinic (Wenger, Linn, Epstein, & Shapiro, 1991). Participants randomized to the intervention received HIV antibody testing and counseling. Participants randomized to the control group were offered a list of locations for free, anonymous HIV antibody testing. Participants were interviewed at entry and after eight weeks. At follow-up, there were no differences between intervention and control groups in measures of AIDS knowledge, mental health, or health/ worry. Compared with individuals in the control group, however, more intervention subjects worried more about getting AIDS even though they received a negative test result (45% vs. 26%). Intervention subjects were also more likely to have asked partners about AIDS risk factors (41% vs. 24% for HIV antibody testing, 50% vs. 34% for injecting drugs, and 57% vs. 53% for number of sexual partners). HIV antibody testing was also associated with a decrease in unprotected vaginal and anal intercourse (27% vs. 13%). Even though the results suggest positive behavior change, the majority of the participants continued to engage in high-risk behavior.

El-Bassel and Schilling (1992) randomly assigned 91 methadone maintained women to information-only or skills-building conditions. Study participants were followed for 15 months. In comparison with the information-only group, the skills-building group felt more comfortable talking about safe sex and perceived themselves as more able to reduce their exposure to HIV, but were more likely to attribute AIDS risk to luck. No associations were found between group conditions and number of sexual partners or frequency of buying and carrying condoms.

McCusker, Stoddard, Zapka, and Zorn (1993) studied 301 heterosexually active intravenous drug users. Participants were randomly assigned to two different interventions: a two-session informational intervention by a health educator in small groups, or an "enhanced intervention" that contained the same elements as the informational intervention but emphasized skills training. Participants were also offered HIV antibody testing. Both interventions were ineffective in increasing condom use, even though they included condom use demonstrations. The study indicated that condom use was greatly influenced by the male partner.

COUPLE COUNSELING IN THE CALIFORNIA PARTNER STUDY

In 1985 Padian and associates began a cross-sectional study in which they enrolled HIV-infected individuals (index cases) and their heterosexual partners to examine risk factors for heterosexual HIV transmission (Padian et al., 1987; Padian, Shiboski, & Jewell, 1991). After enrollment, if the couple was discordant for HIV serostatus and was still having sexual relations, they were enrolled in a prospective study with (on average) biannual visits to examine HIV seroconversions and associated risk factors as well as behavior change over time. Detailed results of this prospective phase of the study are available elsewhere (Padian, O'Brian, Chang, Glass, & Francis, 1993).

One hundred seventy-five couples were eligible for follow-up (i.e., they were discordant, had a current partner, and had been in the study for at least an intake visit). Of these, 20 couples (11%) were lost to follow-up before their first follow-up visit due to poor locating information; seven couples (4%)

moved away from the study area; and four couples (2%) did not wish to continue in the study. The rest of this discussion will be limited to those 144 with at least one follow-up visit. No differences existed between couples lost to follow-up and couples who remained in the study according to sexual practices reported at intake, duration of the relationship, age of the female partner, risk group, gender of the index case, or year of entry into the study. A smaller proportion of Latino couples participated in follow-up, however, than couples of other racial/ethnic backgrounds.

Over two-thirds of the participants were white. The mean age of the women was 34 years, ranging from 19 to 61 years of age. No single risk group was predominant among the index cases. In 36% of the couples the index cases had AIDS or another symptomatic manifestation of HIV infection at enrollment. Most of the couples were recruited during or after 1988. The mean duration of a relationship was 5.6 years, ranging from 1 month to almost 40 years.

Nature of the Intervention

At each visit, each member of the couple was interviewed separately to obtain epidemiologic information (including sexual practices), and this same interviewer offered couple-counseling about safer sex practices. Both partners were present together for one counseling session per visit, although counseling was reinforced after the interview during separate follow-up visits for each partner. Counseling focused on how to purchase, store, and use condoms, refraining from the practice of anal sex, choosing abstinence, and not entering into sexual relations with new partners. Couples were also provided with condoms. Study staff used male and female genital models to educate couples about HIV transmission, contraception, and conception. The models provided a reference point for couples to talk about sex without referring to their own bodies. Sessions also included role-play to build self-esteem and confidence, and discussions of social, financial, and legal issues associated with infection with HIV (e.g., what the index case would do if the other partner or a child became infected; child care if a parent becomes ill). Although practicing protected intercourse was the goal of the counseling, nonjudgmental support rather than persuasion was offered so as not to interfere with truthful answers about behavior. On average, a counseling session lasted about one hour. Although many index cases had received HIV counseling before enrollment, more than 90% of the HIV-negative partners had not. Time between learning of infection in the index case and entry into the study ranged from a few weeks to two years.

Counseling was conducted on average every six months at each follow-up visit (although not necessarily by the same staff member), and couples were encouraged to ask questions and describe any problems in practicing safer sex. Follow-up visits were scheduled one to two months before the follow-up visit, and couples were reminded again one or two days before the visit. Study staff were also available to participants at other times by telephone. Other sources of social support included a "buddy" system in which individual participants were matched with other participants and phone numbers and addresses were exchanged, quarterly social gatherings, and information nights. Because of issues of anonymity and confidentiality, about half of the couples participated in the buddy system and information nights, and approximately one-third came to the social gatherings. We also published a quarterly newsletter for participants that included scientific information and articles by participants.

Effects of the Intervention

Among the 144 couples, follow-up ranged from three months to 5.5 years per couple (mean = 1.34 years, median = 1.5 years). The mean frequency of penile–vaginal intercourse among couples who were not abstinent at their most recent follow-up (n = 109) was two to three contacts per month. We observed no seroconversions during 193 couple-years of follow-up.

Most couples who reduced their risk did so by consistent condom use, but 17% were abstinent by their first follow-up visit (24% were abstinent at their most recent follow-up visit). Results of condom use at intake are compared to condom use at the most recent follow-up visit for each couple. Couples who abstained at their most recent follow-up (n = 35) were excluded. Substantially more couples (85%) who did not use condoms at intake did so by their most recent follow-up, whereas only 13% of couples who used condoms at entry were not using them at follow-up.

Most behavior change occurred between intake and the first follow-up. Forty-nine percent of all couples reported they consistently used condoms at intake, whereas 88% reported they consistently used condoms by their first follow-up with no other significant changes in use over time noted throughout the remainder of follow-up. Couples who used condoms at follow-up did not differ from couples who did not use condoms according to race/ethnicity, age, risk group, gender, or diagnostic status of the index case at entry into the study, year at entry into the study, or duration of the relationship.

Seventy-eight percent of the 144 couples were monogamous at intake and at each follow-up visit; 86% of all couples were monogamous at entry into the study (4 partners and 16 index cases had other partners); and 92% of all couples were monogamous at their last follow-up visit. Overall, 13 couples who were not monogamous at entry became so during the follow-up period, but 11 couples who were initially monogamous did not remain so during follow-up. In 9 couples, only the women had other partners (one of these women was abstinent with her HIV-infected partner in the study); in one of these 11 couples both partners had multiple partners; and in another couple only the man had multiple partners. Four of the 12 participants who had sex with additional partners during follow-up were HIV-positive (3% of all HIV-infected individuals in the study). The visit(s) in which multiple partners were reported were not associated with disease status of the index case, or whether the couple had abstained from sexual relations with each other during the time covered by that visit. Similarly, these 11 couples did not differ from couples remaining monogamous according to any other predictors.

Twenty-six percent of all couples had engaged in anal sex at least once before enrollment. During the follow-up period two of these couples (5%) reported practicing anal intercourse; no couples initiated this practice at follow-up.

Couples who consistently engaged in safer sex practices were compared with couples who engaged in more risky practices. There were 105 couples (73%) who said they always practiced safer sex (consistent condom use, no anal intercourse, no new partners) at each follow-up visit, and 39 couples who either did not consistently use condoms, practiced anal intercourse, or had multiple partners for at least one follow-up visit. The couples who engaged in risky practices did not differ from couples practicing safer sex with respect to any of the independent variables considered except year of entry into the study. A substantial proportion of couples (43%) who entered the study during its first three years practiced risky behavior during follow-up compared to 22% for the later three years.

Fifteen of these 39 couples who practiced risky sex had only one follow-up visit. Twenty-four had multiple follow-up visits (median = 3 visits). Five of these 24 couples who never practiced safer sex reported engaging in at least one of these high risk behaviors during every follow-up visit: They practiced anal intercourse, did not use condoms, or had multiple partners (for the infected index case only) during the follow-up period. As part of the follow-up interview, couples were asked why they did not practice safe sex (if applicable). Reasons the five couples gave for engaging in risky behavior included a sense of shared fate, feelings of invulnerability (i.e. if they were not yet infected, they were probably not susceptible), and the fear that safer sex interferes with intimacy.

LIMITATIONS OF INTERVENTIONS

There are several limitations to the interventions reviewed. Although prospective studies are necessary to evaluate the efficacy of behavioral interventions, by design, examination of those individuals for whom the intervention was unsuccessful is difficult. In the California Partner Study, because the vast majority of participating couples or individuals continued or began safer sex practices after enrollment, it is hard to characterize the small number of couples that persisted in high-risk behavior. Thus, although we may know when interventions work, we may not be able to understand why they fail.

External Validity

An experimental design with a control group that received no counseling would be a more powerful test of an intervention than the paired comparison in the California Partner Study. Few studies maintained this design, in large part because ethical considerations when the intervention was known to be at least somewhat efficacious precluded implementation. Furthermore, there are no studies in which subjects constitute a random sample of heterosexual participants; thus, results from studies of partners of infected individuals cannot be generalized to the greater heterosexual population. Individuals who live with the constant knowledge that they are at risk for infection constitute a unique sample. Results are difficult to generalize even to other couples similarly at risk. Individuals who agree to participate are likely to be more motivated to change their behavior to protect themselves and others than individuals who do not agree to participate. Study couples might be more willing to change their behaviors than couples who were not recruited or who were lost to follow-up.

Even the protocols for implementation of these studies are not necessarily generalizable to other populations. Wykoff and associates (1991) pointed out that differences in available resources, the preexisting level of trust between at-risk individuals and health-care providers, the level of HIV-related education in the community, and the dedication and motivation of the professional staff may all affect the success of HIV antibody testing and counseling in different communities.

Subject Recruitment and Attrition

In the California Partner Study, 18% of all eligible couples did not participate in follow-up mainly due to insufficient locating information, although four couples who were contacted chose not to participate. Over the five-and-a-half years of follow-up, three additional couples voluntarily dropped out, and another 68 couples became ineligible for continued follow-up over time. Locating information became invalid (the couple moved or could no longer be located) for 28 of these couples; 20 of the couples broke up or were divorced; in 20 of the couples the infected partner died. Such attrition highlights the problems associated with conducting prospective research, and limits generalizations about those couples who remained in the study. Participation rates are low in all studies and self-selection bias is very likely.

Internal Validity

The specific behaviors studied, as well as the interventions used, varied enormously between the studies reviewed in this chapter, which makes comparisons between the studies difficult and reliability hard to assess. One obstacle for all of these studies is selection of an appropriate outcome variable. In general, predicted rates of HIV seroconversion, even in the absence of an intervention, are quite low among heterosexuals in the United States, making this an unsuitable dependent variable. Furthermore, HIV seroconversion may be of limited value as a biological marker to corroborate behavior change because transmission may never occur in many couples. Thus, most studies rely on behavioral data which are based on self-report, and subjects may have had problems in remembering certain behaviors. Another problem with self-report data is that after intensive counseling and education, social desirability in response is also very likely where respondents are likely to provide responses they thought researchers were seeking. Even reported behavior change may not be due to the study intervention; it may simply result from individuals or couples who are adjusting to HIV infection or AIDS in one partner. Finally, it remains to be determined whether behavior change can be sustained over longer periods of time and whether such changes can be sustained in the absence of continued counseling should funding constraints result in termination of the study.

CONCLUSIONS

Based on the above studies and scientific developments in the last decade, several public health officials argue that partner notification is important ("Partner Notification," 1991). Partner notification programs are effective in identifying new cases of HIV infection. Although there is no curative treatment yet and positive behavior change is very difficult to achieve, early treatment with zidovudine might be beneficial (Graham, Zeger, & Park, 1991; Volberding, Lagakos, & Koch, 1990) and prophylaxis against *Pneumocystis carinii* has shown to decrease the severity and frequency of infection (Girard, Landman, & Gaudebout, 1989; Leoung, Feigal, & Montgomery, 1990). Additional antiretroviral therapies might become available in the identification of symptomless infection which could give women access to early therapy for disease manifestations that would otherwise be misdiagnosed. It would also give women access to clinical trials, in which they have been underrepresented. Reproductive issues can be discussed with HIV positive women early in infection to prevent perinatal transmission. Attitudes of society toward infection cannot be overlooked and HIV-infected persons still face severe discrimination. Appropriate health care and support cannot be guaranteed to every new case of HIV infection. Partner notification must therefore be done in a voluntary, confidential, and supportive manner.

Identifying infected or at-risk individuals is only the first step. The efficacy of counseling and education is paramount. Three of the studies discussed above suggest that HIV antibody testing, AIDS education, and counseling did result in positive behavior changes, but these changes were assessed shortly after the intervention, and were only of marginal significance (Cleary et al., 1991; Wenger et al., 1991; Wykoff et al., 1991). In contrast, the study by Landis and associates (Landis, Earp, & Koch, 1992) and the two studies on intravenous drug users (El-Bassel, & Schilling, 1992; McCusker et al., 1993) found no positive behavior changes after the intervention.

The results of the California Partner Study are more promising. Significant behavior change and no HIV seroconversion were recorded over the follow-up period. In spite of the above limitations in behavioral interventions for partners of infected or at-risk individuals, to our knowledge, the lack of seroconversion in the California Partner Study has not been demonstrated in other studies. Therefore, we suggest that intensive couple counseling and social support offered through the study may represent an effective way to promote and maintain safer sex practices among individuals who are at risk for HIV transmission from an infected partner. Results were better in all studies that included both partners in the intervention. If these findings are confirmed in additional studies, couple counseling should be considered for incorporation into HIV prevention programs including partner notification programs.

REFERENCES

Bayer, R., & Toomey, K. E. (1992). HIV prevention and the two faces of partner notification. *American Journal of Public Health, 82,* 1158–1164.

Carballo, M., & Miller, D. (1989). HIV counseling: Problems and opportunities in defining the new agenda for the 1990s. *AIDS Care, 1,* 117–123.

Centers for Disease Control (1988). Partner notification for preventing human immunodeficiency virus (HIV) infection—Colorado, Idaho, South Carolina, Virginia. *Morbidity and Mortality Weekly Report, 37,* 393–403.

Cleary, P. D., Van Devanter, N., Rogers, T. F., Singer, E., Shipton-Levy, R., Steilen, M., Stuart, A., Avorn, J., & Pindyck, J. (1991). Behavior changes after notification of HIV infection. *American Journal of Public Health, 81,* 1586–1590.

El-Bassel, N., & Schilling, R. F. (1992). 15-month follow-up of women methadone patients taught skills to reduce heterosexual HIV transmission. *Public Health Reports, 107,* 500–504.

Ellerbock, T. V., Lieb, S., Harrington, P. E., Bush, T. J., Schoenfisch, S. A., Oxtoby, M. J., Howell, J. T., Rogers, M. F., & Witte, J. J. (1992). Heterosexually transmitted human immunodeficiency virus infection among pregnant women in a rural Florida community. *New England Journal of Medicine, 327,* 1704–1709.

Francis, D. P., Anderson, R. E., Gorman, M. E., Fenstersheib, M., Padian, N. S., Kizer, K. W., & Conant, M. A. (1989). Targeting AIDS prevention and treatment toward HIV-1 infected persons. *Journal of the American Medical Association, 262,* 2572–2576.

Francis, D. P., & Chin, J. (1987). The prevention of acquired immunodeficiency syndrome in the United States: An objective strategy for medicine, public health, business and the community. *Journal of the American Medical Association, 257,* 1357–1366.

Giesecke, J., Ramstedt, K., Granath, F., Ripa, T., Rado, G., & Westrell, M. (1991). Efficacy of partner notification for HIV infection. *The Lancet, 338,* 1096–1100.

Girard, P. M., Landman, R., & Gaudebout, C. (1989). Prevention of pneumocystis carinii pneumonia relapse by pentamidine aerosol in zidovudine-treated AIDS patients. *The Lancet, 334,* 1348–1353.

Graham, N. M. H., Zeger, S. L., & Park, L. P. (1991). Effect of zidovudine and pneumocystis carinii pneumonia prophylaxis on progression of HIV-1 infection to AIDS. *The Lancet, 338,* 265–269.

Green, J. (1989). Counseling for HIV infection and AIDS: The past and the future. *AIDS Care, 1,* 5–10.

Higgins, D., Galavotti, C., & O'Reilly, K. (1991). Evidence for the effects of HIV counseling and testing on risk behaviors. *Journal of the American Medical Association, 266,* 2419–2429.

Hinman, A. (1991). Strategies to prevent HIV infection in the United States. *American Journal of Public Health, 81,* 1557.

Jones, J. L., Wykoff, R. F., Hollis, S. L., Longshore, S. T., Gamble, W. B., & Gunn, R. A. (1990). Partner acceptance of health department notification of HIV exposure, South Carolina. *Journal of the American Medical Association, 264,* 1284–1286.

Landis, S. E., Earp, J. L., & Koch, G. G. (1992). Impact of HIV testing and counseling on subsequent sexual behavior. *AIDS Education and Prevention, 4,* 61–70.

Landis, S. E., Schoenbach, V. J., Weber, D. J., Mittal, M., Krishan, B., Lewis, K., & Koch, G. G. (1992). Results of a randomized trial of partner notification in cases of HIV infection in North Carolina. *New England Journal of Medicine, 326,* 101–106.

Lee, J. H., Branan, L., Hoff, G. L., Datwyler, M. L., & Bayer, W. L. (1990). Voluntary human immunodeficiency virus testing, recidivism, partner notification, and sero-prevalence in a sexually transmitted disease clinic: A need for mandatory testing. *Sexually Transmitted Diseases, 17,* 169–174.

Leoung, G. S., Feigal, D. W., & Montgomery, A. B. (1990). Aerolized pentamidine for prophylaxis against *pneumocystis carinii* pneumonia: The San Francisco community prophylaxis trial. *New England Journal of Medicine, 323,* 769–757.

McCusker, J., Stoddard, A. M., Zapka, J. G., & Zorn, M. (1993). Use of condoms by heterosexually active drug abusers before and after AIDS education. *Sexually Transmitted Diseases, 20,* 81–88.

Padian, N., Marquis, L., Francis, D., Anderson, R. E., Rutherford, G. W., O'Malley, P. M., & Winkelstein, W. (1987). Male-to-female transmission of human immunodeficiency virus. *Journal of the American Medical Association, 258,* 788–790.

Padian, N. S., O'Brian, T. R., Chang, Y., Glass, S., & Francis, D. P. (1993). Prevention of heterosexual transmission of human immunodeficiency virus through couple counseling. *Journal of AIDS, 6,* 1043–1048.

Padian, N., Shiboski, S., & Jewell, N. (1991). Female-to-male transmission of human immunodeficiency virus. *Journal of the American Medical Association, 266,* 1664–1668.

Partner notification for prevention of HIV infection (1991) *The Lancet* [Editorial], *338,* 1112–1113.

Rutherford, G. W., Woo, J. M., Neal, D. P., Rauch, K. J., Geoghegan, C., McKinney, K. C., McGee, J., & Lemp, G. F. (1991). Partner notification and the control of human immunodeficiency virus infection. *Sexually Transmitted Diseases, 18,* 107–110.

Volberding, P. A., Lagakos, S. W., & Koch, M. A. (1990). Zidovudine in asymptomatic human immunodeficiency virus infection: A controlled trial in persons with fewer than 500 CD4-positive cells per cubic millimeter. *New England Journal of Medicine, 322,* 941–949.

Wenger, N. S., Linn, L. S., Epstein, M., & Shapiro, M. F. (1991). Reduction of high-risk sexual behavior among heterosexuals undergoing HIV antibody testing: A randomized clinical trial. *American Journal of Public Health, 81,* 1580–1585.

World Health Organization (1990). *Current and future dimensions of the HIV/AIDS pandemic: A capsule summary, September 1990.* Geneva: World Health Organization Global Programme on AIDS, 1990.

Wykoff, R. F., Jones, J. L., Longshore, S. T., Hollis, S. L., Quiller, C. B., Dowda, H., & Gamble, W. B. (1991). Notification of the sex and needle-sharing partners of individuals with human immunodeficiency virus in rural South Carolina: 30-month experience. *Sexually Transmitted Diseases, 18,* 217–222.

13

Interventions for Sexually Active, Heterosexual Women in the United States

JANET S. MOORE, JANET S. HARRISON,
and LYNDA S. DOLL

INTRODUCTION

Existing data suggest an alarming increase in numbers of women heterosexually exposed to human immunodeficiency virus (HIV). Through October 1992, 242,146 adult cases of acquired immunodeficiency syndrome (AIDS) were reported to the Centers for Disease Control and Prevention (1992a). Among these, 25,947 (11%) were adult women, 40% of whom were infected through sexual contact with an infected male partner. Between 1988 and 1990, AIDS had become the sixth leading cause of death among women ages 25 to 44 in the United States (Centers for Disease Control, 1992b). During 1991, the proportion of AIDS cases increased most among women, African Americans, and Hispanics, and persons exposed to HIV through heterosexual contact (Centers for Disease Control, 1992c).

Efforts to target prevention programs for women, particularly women at risk through sexual contact, have lagged behind those for homosexual men and intravenous drug users (IDUs). In this chapter we will first review data on the epidemiology of HIV/AIDS among women and rates of sexual behav-

JANET S. MOORE, JANET S. HARRISON, and LYNDA S. DOLL • Division of HIV/AIDS, National Center for Infectious Diseases, Centers for Disease Control and Prevention, Atlanta, Georgia 30333.

Preventing AIDS: Theories and Methods of Behavioral Interventions, edited by Ralph J. DiClemente and John L. Peterson. Plenum Press, New York, 1994.

iors that put women at risk for HIV. Because most studies report data on women without specifying differences by HIV-risk categories, we do not report separate data on women at risk through heterosexual contact. We will then describe information on interventions and assess both the use and the usefulness of existing behavioral theory and empirical data on psychosocial predictors in the design of interventions for women. Our emphasis throughout the chapter will be on women whose exposure risk is through sexual contact with male partners.

EPIDEMIOLOGY OF AIDS AND HIV INFECTION IN WOMEN

Analysis of data from AIDS case surveillance (Ellerbrock, Bush, Chamberland, & Oxtoby, 1991) and HIV seroprevalence surveys (Burke et al., 1990; Gwinn et al., 1991; St. Louis et al., 1991; Sweeney, Onorato, Allen, Byers, & The Field Services Branch, 1992) suggests a similar epidemiologic profile for women diagnosed with AIDS and for women with less severe HIV disease. Women with HIV infection are likely to be young African-American or Hispanic women living in metropolitan areas, who have been infected through their own injecting drug use or that of a male sex partner. Heterosexual women with AIDS are more likely than heterosexual men (27% vs. 16%) to have been diagnosed in their 20s, although studies of women seeking reproductive health services show HIV seroprevalence rates increase until age 30 (Sweeney et al., 1992). Among applicants for military service between 1985 and 1989, seroprevalence rates among 17- and 18-year-old women exceeded those among male applicants of the same age. Over time, HIV seroprevalence has decreased among 17- to 19-year-old male military applicants, though less so among African Americans. However, seroprevalence rates increased over time among African-American female applicants of the same age (Burke et al., 1990).

Cumulative incidence rates of AIDS cases among African-American and Hispanic women are 13 and 8 times higher, respectively, than those among whites. Similarly, seroprevalence rates in a national survey of child-bearing women were found to be 5 to 15 times higher among African-American women than among whites, with rates for Hispanic women between those of these two groups (Gwinn et al., 1991). Though infected women can be found in all 50 states, they are more likely to live in the Northeast, the District of Columbia, or Puerto Rico. Between 1988 and 1991, the most rapid increase in AIDS cases among heterosexually infected persons occurred among persons from the South (Centers for Disease Control, 1992c).

Heterosexual contact with a male partner who injects drugs remains the most prevalent transmission route for women infected through a male partner, representing nearly 57% of all female heterosexual AIDS cases as of October

1992. However, sexual contact with an HIV-infected male partner whose risk is not specified (26% of all female heterosexual cases) is now the second largest category of heterosexual transmission among women with AIDS (Centers for Disease Control, 1992a). The number as well as the proportion of women infected through heterosexual transmission, regardless of the partner's risk, is expected to continue to rise. Key epidemiologic factors in this continuing heterosexual transmission to women are the greater effectiveness of HIV transmission from men to women than from women to men (European Study Group on Heterosexual Transmission of HIV, 1992) and the greater probability for women to encounter an HIV-infected partner than for men (Centers for Disease Control, 1992a). Key behavioral factors in this continuing transmission are the failure of many heterosexual men and women to adopt safer sex practices (Catania et al., 1992) and the failure of some infected persons to disclose their antibody status to sex partners (Landis et al., 1992).

HIV-RELATED SEXUAL RISK IN HETEROSEXUAL WOMEN

Women are more likely to become infected with HIV through heterosexual contact if they have multiple sex partners, a partner who does not consistently use condoms, or a partner from a geographic location where HIV is endemic. Examination of existing data on recent sex partners suggests that minority women, the population at greatest risk for HIV, may be primarily at risk not because they have multiple partners but because their male partners do. Analyses of data from the National Survey of Family Growth Cycle IV showed that, in 1988, less than 1 in 200 of currently married and less than 1 in 10 of currently unmarried women reported recent multiple sexual partners. In the previous three months, 11% of women reported no sex partners, 85% reported one partner, 4% two partners, and less than 1% three or more partners (Seidman, Mosher, & Aral, 1992). Divorced or separated African-American women were more likely than any other race or marital status group to report two or more recent sex partners, although only 16.4% of this group reported such contacts.

Data collected during 1989 in a national probability household sample (General Social Survey [GSS]) showed that women on average had only 0.91 sex partners during the preceding year (Smith, 1991). Young unmarried participants, men, and residents of central cities were more likely to have had a greater number of sex partners. Analysis of sex partner data from the GSS collected between 1988 and 1990 showed that African-American and white women were equally likely to have had five or more partners in the preceding year (African American: 0.8%; white: 0.4%). In comparison, 11% of African-American and 4% of white men reported five or more partners in the past year (R. T. Michael, personal communication, 1992).

Limited data are available on behavioral changes women and their partners have made in response to AIDS. In a national telephone survey, Catania et al. (1992) found that 71% of respondents with partners at high risk for HIV had not used condoms in the previous six months. Analyses completed by Campbell and Baldwin (1991) using the 1988 Survey of Family Growth Cycle IV showed that 13% of women indicated that their partners used condoms for sexually transmitted disease (STD) prophylaxis and that 75% of this condom use had begun after they heard about AIDS. Thirteen percent also reported limiting their sexual relations to one man. Nearly two-thirds of unmarried women with five or more lifetime partners, the group assumed to be at highest risk, reported some form of behavior change to prevent infection. In this group, behavior change was reported by 65% of both African-American and white women. Those least likely to report behavior change included women with less than a ninth grade education and women residing in the Northeast.

Results from a convenience sample of women surveyed at family planning clinics in Pennsylvania in 1987 showed that 67% with regular partners and 72% with casual partners reported never using condoms (Soskolne, Aral, Magder, Reed, & Bowen, 1991). Higher condom use levels were reported by women younger than 20, nonwhites, those with multiple partners, and those reporting a previous STD. Finally, a study of women in south Florida found that approximately 60% engaged in unprotected sex with their main partners. Hispanic women were most likely and African-American women were least likely to report engaging in sex without a condom. Disturbingly, over 40% of Hispanic and Haitian women and 15 and 20%, respectively, of white and African-American women said they would have sex without a condom with a partner who was HIV seropositive (Harrison et al., 1991).

Because of the limited number of behavioral studies targeting women, assessing the extent of women's sexual behavior change is difficult. Trends are emerging, however, concerning the characteristics of sexual risk behaviors of women. First, studies indicate that women are at risk for acquiring HIV heterosexually because of the risk behaviors of their male partners (i.e., intravenous drug use and multiple sex partners). Second, there is substantial evidence of inconsistent condom use among most women with high-risk partners. There is emerging evidence that some subgroups of women, such as African-American women, are using condoms with male partners at higher rates than are other subgroups.

PSYCHOSOCIAL PREDICTORS OF HIV-RELATED SEXUAL RISK OF HETEROSEXUAL WOMEN

The data reviewed thus far clearly demonstrate that interventions to reduce high-risk sexual behaviors are essential to stem the surge of new HIV infections among women. The most effective way to bring about this behavior change is not yet apparent, however. Typically, interventionists look to theories of behavior change and to empirical findings on determinants of risk behavior as the first steps in determining the contents of an intervention. Identification of predictors is expected to offer clues as to the cause of behavior, and if causes can be identified, interventions can be targeted to address these causes. The following review describes existing research on the psychosocial predictors of sexual risk behaviors of women. This information will be used at a later point in this chapter when describing and reviewing the adequacy of interventions for women.

Studies examining psychosocial predictors of women's risk behavior typically have not looked to theories of behavior change to identify variables for investigation, although many have looked at variables that could be subsumed under one or more influential theories of health behavior. Perception of risk or feelings of vulnerability, beliefs about the effectiveness of safer sex practices, beliefs about the costs of HIV-related protective behavior, beliefs about social norms for safer sex and a desire to comply with these norms, and beliefs about one's ability to successfully implement safer sex practices are all issues that theories of health behavior posit as important for understanding who initiates health protective behaviors. Researchers of women's HIV-related risk behavior have begun to explore these issues, though results from quantitative studies are still quite limited. Thus, much of the literature reviewed below will be qualitative in nature.

HIV Knowledge

All theories of health behavior assume that persons are knowledgeable about health risks and that psychosocial factors then determine who acts on this knowledge. Surveys of women's HIV-related knowledge indicate that even women at highest risk know that HIV is transmitted through sex and intravenous drug use and are aware of effective means of reducing exposure to HIV through these routes (Flaskerud & Nyamathi, 1989; Harrison et al., 1991; Valdiserri, Arena, Proctor, & Bonati, 1989). Several studies have shown, that some groups of women continue to believe that HIV can be transmitted through casual routes such as kissing, drinking from a glass, shaking hands, being bitten by a mosquito, and using dirty toilets (Flaskerud & Thompson, 1991; Harrison et al., 1991; Hobfoll, Jackson, Lavin, Britton, & Shepherd,

1992). Some investigators speculate that a belief in the casual transmission of HIV may lead to the assumption that becoming HIV infected is beyond one's control, and thus, protective action has no value (Marin & Marin, 1990). Although this idea is quite intriguing, it has not been empirically substantiated.

In fact, little is known about the relationship of HIV knowledge to women's risk behavior. Because knowledge is uniformly high among most groups investigated, few studies have attempted to predict women's risk behavior from their level of knowledge. Those studies examining this relationship generally find that knowledge does not influence safer sex behaviors, particularly partners' use of condoms (Flaskerud & Nyamathi, 1989; Hinkle, Johnson, Gilbert, Jackson, & Lollis, 1991; Jemmott & Jemmott, 1991).

What then prevents women from acting on their knowledge of HIV/AIDS to implement safer sex practices? To explore this issue, we examined other psychosocial variables derived from models of health behavior as they relate to sexual risk behaviors of women.

Perceptions of Risk

Both quantitative and qualitative studies have addressed the issue of perceived risk or susceptibility to HIV among women. Research indicates that women who report involvement in a number of sexual risk activities often do not perceive themselves to be at risk for HIV (Bridgers, Figler, Vaughan, & Sawin, 1990; Ehrhardt, Yingling, Zawadzki, Martinez-Ramirez, Stein, 1991; Harrison et al., 1991; Hobfoll et al., 1992; Worth, 1990a).

A variety of reasons have been posited for the failure of women to estimate their risk accurately. Poor urban minority women (i.e., those frequently most at risk) live daily with a variety of risks, including imminent threats to survival for themselves and for their children. In comparison to these risks, HIV/AIDS may appear a distant and relatively unlikely occurrence (Mays & Cochran, 1988). Women who are at greatest risk may also deny or fail to acknowledge risk because they cannot afford to consider their own or their partners' risk behaviors (Hobfoll et al., 1992; Worth, 1989, 1990a). The acknowledgement of risk would result in a confrontation with facets of their lives that are painful (e.g., partner's sexual activity with others), threatening (e.g., loss of partner), or that require a reevaluation of their life-styles (e.g., leaving prostitution and finding alternative employment). For women with few personal and social resources, confrontation with realities in their lives may be an overwhelming experience. Instead, they may overlook or deny the relevance of information to maintain the belief that neither they nor their partners are at risk (Ehrhardt et al., 1991; Wingood & DiClemente, 1992).

Few studies report data on HIV risk perception as a predictor of involvement in risk behaviors. At least one cross-sectional study has found that women who engage in higher levels of risk behavior respond that they feel more vulnerable to HIV/AIDS than women who report lower levels of risk behavior (Bridgers et al., 1990). This finding suggests accurate estimations of vulnerability, at least among some groups of women. Another cross-sectional study, however, has shown perception of risk to be unrelated to reports of risk behavior (i.e., partners' condom use) (Hinkle et al., 1991). Longitudinal studies are needed to determine if women's current or changing perceptions of risk will result in modifications of risk behavior, as several behavioral theories imply.

Beliefs and Skills Related to Safer Sex Practices

Response Efficacy

Women, regardless of race/ethnicity or socioeconomic status, generally report that condom use and abstinence are effective ways to reduce their chances of becoming infected with HIV (Harrison et al., 1991; Hobfoll et al., 1992; Valdiserri, Arena, Proctor, & Bonati, 1989). Several studies, however, demonstrate that women also attribute effectiveness to practices that have no proven efficacy (Harrison et al., 1991; Hobfoll et al., 1992). For example, Hobfoll and colleagues (1992) found that over 50% of the inner city women in their study reported that using a diaphragm or having sex with a man who had a vasectomy were successful measures for avoiding the AIDS virus. Valdiserri et al. (1989) report that 21% of women recruited from family planning clinics thought that withdrawing the penis before ejaculation was as safe as using a condom in reducing the risk of HIV transmission. Studies could not be found that examine the relationship between women's beliefs about the effectiveness of certain safer sex practices and their adoption of these practices.

Perceived Costs of Safer Sex Practice

Perhaps more has been written about the costs women associate with the practice of safer sex than about any of the other determinants. A relatively large qualitative literature suggests that women expect a number of negative consequences to occur as a result of introducing safer sex practices into their relationships with male partners. They anticipate that introducing the topic will displease and anger the partner and, in turn, may cause domestic tensions, possible abuse, and potential loss of the relationship (Mays & Cochran, 1988; Wingood & DiClemente, 1992; Wingood, Hunter, & DiClemente, in press; Worth, 1990a). Given the economic and social conditions in which many women at risk live, these consequences are likely to be perceived as far greater than the costs associated with HIV infection (Mays & Cochran, 1988; Worth, 1989, 1990b). Results from several studies however, challenge the proposition that all poor, minority women perceive that the introduction of safer sex practices will be detrimental to their relationships. In two qualitative studies, low income minority women indicated that they would not be afraid to introduce condoms into their relationships (Fullilove, Fullilove, Haynes, & Gross, 1990; Kline, Kline, & Oken, 1992).

Women perceive costs to safer sex practices, particularly to condom use, other than those associated with partner reactions. Women often report that sex doesn't feel as good with a condom (Stewart, DeForge, Hartmann, Kaminski, & Pecukonis, 1991; Valdiserri et al., 1989), that condoms are inconvenient and reduce spontaneity (Jemmott & Jemmott, 1991; Stewart et al., 1991), and that they are embarrassed about purchasing condoms and introducing them into the relationship (Stewart et al., 1991; Valdiserri et al., 1989). An additional cost to condom use mentioned by women in qualitative studies is the loss of the opportunity to become pregnant (Worth, 1990b). Women who desire children and who see child-bearing as a major part of their identity may be unwilling to incur this loss.

Few studies could be found in which perceived negative effects of practicing safer sex, in this case condom use, were used to predict sexual behavior. In a study of African-American inner-city college students, Jemmott and Jemmott (1991) found that women who perceived more costs to condom use, including inconvenience, embarrassment, and loss of pleasure and spontaneity, were more likely to engage in high-risk sex than were women with more positive attitudes. Valdiserri and colleagues (1989) also found that attitudes about condoms were predictive of condom use. Both of these studies were cross-sectional in nature, and it is possible that attitudes about condoms and condom use are associated because those who use condoms develop a more positive attitude toward them. Additional studies are needed to disentangle cause-and-effect relationships between these variables.

Self-Efficacy

Several behavioral theories suggest that persons who have confidence in their ability to effect changes in their lives are more likely to attempt behavior change and to succeed in making changes than those who have little confidence (Bandura, 1982; Becker et al., 1977). Belief about efficacy to implement safer sex practices has been operationalized as a specific belief that one can initiate condom use with partners. Quantitative studies examining women's specific beliefs about their ability to practice safer sex could not be found in the literature. Instead, work by Jackson, Hobfoll, Justin, Britton, and Shephard (1992) used a general measure of self-efficacy (i.e., a measure of mastery) to predict which inner-city women attending public prenatal clinics would be more likely to practice safer sex. They found that women who scored higher on the mastery scale were more likely to practice safer sex than were women who had lower scores. This relationship was particularly strong for African-American women.

Qualitative research suggests that many women at risk do not feel effi-cacious at implementing safer sex practices because they feel they have little power to negotiate sexual behavior change with their partners (Fullilove et al., 1990; Nyamathi & Lewis, 1991; Wingood & DiClemente, 1992; Wingood, Hunter, & DiClemente, in press). Researchers agree that many women do not have the power to negotiate sexual behavior in their relationships. These researchers call for interventions that help women find nonconfrontational approaches to sexual negotiation while also helping them become empowered in other aspects of their lives (Fullilove et al., 1990).

Very little is known about the characteristics of women who feel most efficacious or powerful in their relationships with male partners or how these characteristics translate into self-protective behaviors. Given the importance ascribed to these constructs in determining safer sex practices, additional re-search is needed to determine the extent to which women feel powerless, the circumstances that contribute to this feeling, and the conditions under which women develop a sense of efficacy, power, or control in their lives.

Social and Cultural Norms for Safer Sex

Qualitative data generally suggest that the sexual norms in many poor minority communities prevent women from initiating safer sex practices. Women are expected to play a passive role, with all sexual decisions made by the man (Fullilove et al., 1990; Worth, 1989, 1990b). Recent quantitative data, however, present a slightly different view of norms concerning women's roles in making sexual decisions. For example, a study by Stewart and col-leagues (1991) found that 90% of women from an urban family planning clinic responded that it is "all right for women to refuse sex"; 99% responded that it is "all right for women to insist on condom use"; and 92% responded that it is "all right for women to carry condoms."

Norms about safer sex practices have also been examined in terms of beliefs about what others in the community are doing. For example, 45% of the women in the study by Stewart et al. (1991) reported that their male friends used condoms when they had sex and 39% reported that their female friends did so. Valdiserri and colleagues (1989) found that 77% of the women in their study indicated that most women they knew thought that using con-doms was a good idea. In terms of the prediction of safer sex practices from normative beliefs about condom use, Jemmott and Jemmott (1991) found that inner-city college women who agreed with the statements, "Most guys do not want to use condoms" and "Most girls do not want to use condoms," were less likely to use condoms than were those who perceived more favorable social norms. Again, few data have been reported on this subject, and no longitudinal studies have been conducted to determine the cause-and-effect relationship between normative beliefs and safer sex practices of women.

INTERVENTIONS FOR WOMEN TO PROMOTE SAFER SEX

The predictors of high-risk sex reviewed in the previous section offer clues as to potential causes of unsafe behavior and, thereby, offer suggestions for the design of interventions for women. The following section will describe interventions that currently exist or are under development. The correspondence between the content of these interventions and the psychosocial findings reviewed earlier will then be discussed.

There is a paucity of published literature describing interventions targeted for women, and even fewer published reports evaluating their effectiveness. Instead, most of the available literature on the subject consists of recommendations for the content of interventions. Thus, in this chapter we will review the limited information published on safer sex interventions for women but also will include personal communications with researchers who are in the process of implementing and evaluating interventions. All the programs described have an evaluation component; however, most are still in the stage of data collection, and therefore, their impact has not yet been determined. Results on the effectiveness of the intervention will be reported when available.

In addition to the research presented in this chapter, many health departments, community-based organizations, churches, schools, and individuals are involved in HIV/AIDS education and prevention on a daily basis. Because these programs often do not have sufficient funds or personnel to support the evaluation of successes and failures, they are not reviewed here. Several publications describe HIV/AIDS interventions for women, however. We refer readers to these publications for a more comprehensive listing of available HIV risk-reduction programs for women (Center for Women Policy Studies, 1991; HDI Projects, 1990; Multicultural AIDS Coalition, 1992; Nova Research Company, 1992).

Dimensions of Interventions for Women to Promote Safer Sex

Interventions designed to increase safer sex activities differ on a number of dimensions. Perhaps the most important dimension on which they vary is the underlying assumption about the causes of unsafe sex (i.e., the theory of behavior driving the intervention). For example, early interventions were based on the belief that lack of information or knowledge was the cause for failure to take protective action. Thus, these interventions attempted to change unsafe behaviors through the provision of information, primarily about routes of transmission and ways to avoid exposure to HIV. It quickly became evident that, although knowledge may be an important element in bringing about women's safer sex practices, it certainly is not sufficient. Despite adequate knowledge, women frequently hold attitudes that are incompatible with changing sex practices, and they often do not have the skills needed to initiate, negotiate, and implement these practices. Thus, more recent interventions have begun to use psychosocial theory and findings, such as those summarized earlier in this chapter, to determine the content of their programs. These recently developed programs attempt to bring about the desired behavior change by modifying attitudes, beliefs, and behaviors through a variety of mechanisms including changing social norms, increasing personal and inter-personal skills, creating feelings of self-efficacy, and providing social and in-stitutional supports to help women initiate and maintain newly developed behaviors. Many programs currently in progress use all of these elements to encourage safer sex practices among women.

Another dimension on which interventions for women differ is in the expected outcome of the intervention. Again, this dimension is related to the theory of behavior underlying the intervention. For some interventions, a change in HIV-related knowledge is all that is expected, whereas others attempt to increase willingness to seek HIV testing and counseling by reducing the stigma associated with HIV. Most interventions, however, attempt to bring about actual change in sex practices (e.g., increased condom use), or at least an intent to modify sexual behavior. Behavior change typically is measured at the individual level, although a small number of interventions are oriented toward behavior and attitude change at the community level.

Interventions vary on other dimensions as well including the population targeted, the places from which women are recruited, and the medium through which interventions are delivered. Populations of women targeted for HIV interventions have varied widely, although poor urban minority women have been the recipients of most programs. Additionally, because of concerns about vertical transmission, pregnant women have often been targeted for behavior change programs. Finally, prostitutes and partners of intravenous drug users constitute two target groups identified as particularly in need of interventions because of the greater probability of exposure in these groups.

The points of access differ widely for various interventions, but generally all assume that one must go to the places women frequent in order to recruit them into programs. Many interventions reach women through clinics, in-cluding prenatal and WIC clinics (Public Health Foundation's Nutrition Program for Women, Infants, and Children). Others attempt to reach them through street recruitment or through outreach services in places that women frequent on a day-to-day basis, such as laundromats and beauty parlors.

Finally, programs differ in terms of the medium through which the intervention is delivered. Techniques for delivering interventions include videos to increase knowledge and teach skills; written material such as brochures and newsletters; individual or group instruction, demonstration, role-playing, and interaction; and an ongoing relationship with a role-model or buddy.

Interventions will be grouped and discussed according to the underlying assumptions (or theory) about the mechanism for changing sexual behavior. For those interventions that utilize several theories of behavior in developing the content of their programs, we will categorize the intervention according to our assumptions about the primary model or theory of behavior change underlying the intervention, but we will describe all facets of the program.

Interventions That Provide Information and/or Referral Services

Interventions by Flaskerud and Nyamathi (1988, 1990) were designed to increase safer sex practices and self-referral to HIV testing and counseling by providing information about HIV/AIDS and mechanisms for protecting oneself. These investigators report a study of Vietnamese women (Flaskerud & Nyamathi, 1988) and one of African-American and Hispanic women (Flaskerud & Nyamathi, 1990) recruited through WIC clinics. All women who attend these clinics routinely participate in monthly education programs on various topics. As one of their monthly education programs, women in the experimental groups in both studies viewed a 12-minute slide presentation on HIV/AIDS and were given an AIDS information brochure and community guide handout. The control groups in both studies received information on nutrition during pregnancy at their monthly education program. Outcome measures included knowledge of the signs and symptoms of AIDS, methods of sexual transmission of HIV, and HIV prevention measures; attitudes about those with HIV infection; and current sex practices. Both studies report changes in knowledge from pretest to posttest for the experimental groups, with no changes in the control group in the study of African-American and Hispanic women. Control group results were not reported for the study of Vietnamese women.

In terms of changes in sex practices between pretest and posttest, women in the experimental groups of both studies reported increasing safer sex practices. Interpretation of these findings is difficult for several reasons, however. First, control group results from the Vietnamese study are not reported. Second, the control group as well as the experimental group in the African-American and Hispanic women's study reported increases in safer sex practices from pretest to posttest. Finally, in both studies the measure of sexual behavior at pretest was actual sex practices, whereas the measure at posttest was intent to practice safer sex. Because neither study attempted to show the link between changes in sex practices and changes in knowledge, it cannot be determined if knowledge was the important element in bringing about the observed behavior change.

An intervention designed to change HIV-related knowledge and attitudes among pregnant women attending a prenatal clinic was described by Mason and colleagues (1991) and evaluated by Berrier and colleagues (1991). The study was designed to increase HIV/AIDS knowledge and to change related attitudes that may prevent women from seeking HIV counseling and testing. Actual changes in sex practices or intent to change these behaviors were not evaluated. During a group orientation session, the experimental group received an educational intervention that included factual information about HIV transmission, risk factors, risk reduction strategies, and HIV testing. The control group attended the standard group orientation session without the HIV component.

At posttest both the intervention and the control group showed an increase in knowledge; however, the increase within the experimental group was significantly greater than that in the control group. There were no changes in attitudes about HIV testing nor was there an increased willingness to be tested. This study is another demonstration of the ability of HIV/AIDS educational programs to change relevant knowledge; however, this study also falls short of evaluating the role of knowledge in bringing about changes in sex practices.

The CDC-sponsored Perinatal HIV Reduction and Education Demonstration Activities Project (PHREDA) conducted in seven high-seroprevalence cities is another example of an intervention study directed primarily at providing education and referral to appropriate services (C. Galavotti, personal communication, November 1992). The goal of this project was somewhat broader than that of the other studies reviewed; its primary intent was to reduce perinatal transmission of HIV among infected women or those at risk for infection by providing HIV-related education and by promoting the use of contraception and family planning services. The methods for achieving these goals varied from site to site but included case management and referral services, group education and skill building, and changing of community norms surrounding risk reduction. Women were recruited through both traditional family planning settings as well as through nontraditional settings such as drug treatment centers and street recruitment. Evaluation of the effectiveness of these interventions to increase safer sex and contraceptive practices has not been completed; however, much has been learned about condom use and other contraceptive behaviors among women at risk (Centers for Disease Control, 1992d, 1992e; Kline et al., 1992; Mitchell, Thompson,

Namerow, Gordon, Carrington, & Williams, 1992). Tunstull, Oliva, Degeles, and Darney (1991) report data from the San Francisco site of the PHREDA project indicating that women at high risk can be reached more successfully through nontraditional settings such as street outreach than through traditional clinics.

In summary, there are a number of reported studies on providing information to and referral services for women at risk for heterosexually acquired HIV. Although outcome evaluations are limited, these studies suggest that on the one hand knowledge about risk behaviors can be increased, while on the other hand there is little evidence that increasing knowledge is a mechanism by which changes in high-risk sex practices can be effected.

Interventions to Change Beliefs and Attitudes and to Increase Skills Needed to Practice Safer Sex

Research on women's failure to implement safer sex has revealed that often they do not have the necessary skills to protect themselves and that they frequently hold attitudes and beliefs incompatible with initiating safer sex. The range of skills needed to practice safer sex includes initiation of the topic of safer sex with partners, negotiation or resolution of conflict with partners who disagree about practicing safer sex, and ability to purchase a condom and to assist partner in correct usage. Not only do women lack these necessary skills, but they frequently are unwilling to attempt behavior change because they lack confidence in their ability to be successful. The following studies take an attitude-change/skills-building approach to changing women's sex practices.

Britton and colleagues (1992) report on an intervention that used skill building and self-empowerment as means for changing high-risk sex practices. Low-income women attending a prenatal clinic were assigned to participate in either an HIV prevention program, a general health promotion program, or no intervention. Participants in all three groups were given a "condom credit card" with which they could acquire free condoms at three local pharmacies.

The content of the HIV prevention program included four group sessions focusing on information on HIV/AIDS and safer sex practices, discussions regarding condom use with partners, role-playing and guided fantasy about negotiating with partner, and practice using condoms on penile models. A pretest, posttest, and six-month follow-up measured HIV/AIDS knowledge, intentions regarding high-risk sex practices, and feelings of power or mastery. Analyses indicated that the HIV intervention group had higher knowledge scores at both posttest and follow-up than did the other two groups. Additionally, they expressed greater intentions to purchase condoms and spermicides, acquired more free condoms with their "credit cards," and reported more use of condoms at posttest and follow-up than women in the other groups. Scores on the mastery scale increased from pretest to posttest for all groups but were maintained at follow-up only in the treatment group.

A group of researchers at the Medical College of Wisconsin (Kelly et al., 1992) have implemented a behavioral intervention for women attending urban primary health care clinics. All women recruited into the study were at risk because of an STD diagnosis, multiple sex partners, or a high-risk male partner. Women were randomly assigned to an HIV/AIDS intervention or a comparison intervention addressing health topics unrelated to AIDS. Participants attended four 90-minute group sessions that included information dissemination, goal-setting, role-modeling of behaviors, and role-playing. The content of the intervention included HIV/AIDS information, enhancing perceptions of risk, condom use, and sexual communication skills training, problem solving regarding risk reduction, and social support for making behavior changes and managing partner resistance. Results of the effectiveness of the intervention showed that women in the HIV intervention group were more knowledgeable about AIDS risk, reported fewer episodes of unprotected vaginal and anal intercourse, and were more consistent in condom use after the intervention than were those in the comparison group.

Researchers will soon begin recruiting women attending health clinics in a small southern city for participation in a study aimed at increasing competencies in a number of areas related to HIV (J. S. St. Lawrence, personal communication, October 1992). Women will be assigned to participate for six sessions in one of three groups. The control group will act primarily as a support group for women at high risk, providing basic information and discussions about HIV. The two treatment groups will receive demonstrations on technical competency (e.g., putting on a condom), and social competency including initiating discussions, developing self-assertiveness, disseminating information, and negotiating with a partner who does not wish to use a condom. The first treatment group will only receive demonstrations of the targeted skills, whereas the second group will practice the skills and receive feedback on their performance.

Outcomes of interest will be measured at pretest, posttest, and two retests (6 and 12 months after the intervention). Measures will include AIDS knowledge, beliefs about risk, feelings of self-efficacy, response efficacy, attitudes toward HIV prevention (particularly condom use), and actual sex practices including condom use.

A study by Exner (personal communication, November 1992), is using a modification of the AIDS Risk Reduction Model (Catania, Kegeles, & Coates, 1990) to develop an intervention for women in a Planned Parenthood Clinic in Brooklyn, New York. By providing information, demonstrations, role-playing, rehearsal, and feedback, this intervention focuses on helping women identify their HIV risk, make HIV risk reduction a priority in their lives, commit to changing behavior and to withstanding frustration in attempting behavior change, reduce negative attitudes and beliefs about condoms, and develop actual skills to negotiate and implement condom use with partners. Women also will be assisted in getting the social services they need to reduce stresses and demands that prevent them from making HIV reduction a priority in their lives. Methods and time frames for evaluating the effectiveness of the intervention are currently being determined through pilot work.

A study sponsored by the Centers for Disease Control, known as Project Cares (R. Cabral, personal communication, November 1992) will provide interventions for women who are at risk for unplanned pregnancy and HIV but who may not attend traditional family planning centers. Women will be recruited through drug treatment centers, homeless shelters, an HIV clinic, and street outreach in high-risk neighborhoods. The goal of the intervention is to reduce both unplanned pregnancies and HIV risk behaviors. The mechanisms for achieving this goal will include increasing women's perception of risk, decreasing misconceptions about HIV/AIDS and safer sex behaviors, developing specific skills needed to purchase condoms and initiate and negotiate condom use, developing concrete plans for changing behavior, and increasing feelings of self-efficacy. Participants' readiness to change behavior (Prochaska, DiClemente, & Norcross, 1992) will be assessed by paraprofessional peer advocates, who will then attempt to engage the women in stage-appropriate activities. A control group will receive standard family planning care. Outcome measures will include condom use with main partner, condom use with other partners, reproductive decisions, and other contraceptive use.

Interventions Promoting Safer Sex through Changes in Social Norms

Interventions that attempt to change social norms related to safer sex have been reported for gay men (S. Kegeles, personal communication, August 1992; Kelly et al., 1991), but only two such projects could be found for women (C. Galavotti, personal communication, December 1992; O'Reilly & Higgins, 1991). As part of a large, multisite demonstration project to prevent HIV among hard-to-reach groups, female prostitutes and female sex partners of drug users have been recruited for a study that is in its fourth year (O'Reilly & Higgins, 1991). Prior ethnographic research revealed locations where female sex workers and partners of drug users could be accessed for the study. Community volunteers, trained to deliver "role-model" stories printed in brochures, posters, and newsletters, discuss the contents with each participant. The role-model in the story, who is similar to the woman recruited in terms of age, race, and life-style, describes the difficulties she has encountered but overcome in implementing safer sex in her life. The stories are expected to change individual sex practices through modeling of the woman described in the story and to reduce sexual risk behavior in the community as a whole by changing social norms about risk behavior. Norm change is expected to occur because the stories convey the message that others in the community are changing their behavior, and thus, such change is socially approved. Persons who directly participate in the study are then expected to convey the information to others, and gradually the message about safer sex becomes diffused throughout the community (Rogers & Havens, 1962).

Currently, the effectiveness of this intervention is being evaluated through multiple cross-sectional surveys of persons randomly recruited through street outreach in both treatment and control communities. Outcome measures include intentions to have sex partners use condoms as well as reported condom use by partners. The investigators are currently analyzing the behavior change data to compare differences in communities that received the intervention and matched communities that did not.

A similar prevention program and study targeted for sexually active women under 35 years of age is being planned in five cities (C. Galavotti, personal communication, December 1992). Participants will be identified in places that young women frequent, such as laundromats and beauty parlors, and will receive "role-model" stories about women similar to themselves. Outreach workers will distribute these stories through newsletters and will provide prevention messages tailored to the woman's readiness to change sexual behavior (Prochaska et al., 1992). Again, outcomes will be compared between treatment and comparison communities since the goal of the intervention is to promote community norms that support risk reduction and thereby change individual behavior.

The results of these studies should offer a great deal of information about the effectiveness of large-scale, community-level interventions in bringing about behavior change among women. Because these studies intervene through many different mechanisms (e.g., role-model stories, individual counseling through a community volunteer, and community norm change through diffusion of information), understanding which of the mechanisms produce behavior change will be challenging.

CONCLUSIONS

Interventions to reduce HIV sexual risk behaviors of heterosexual women are obviously in their infancy. At this time, we have only limited information about the effectiveness of the described interventions in bringing about safer sex practices, and even less information about the impact of the various programs on long-term behavior change. What then can be surmised about the effectiveness of the various interventions for women?

There is evidence that women's knowledge about HIV/AIDS can be increased, but there is little support for the proposition that increasing knowledge will produce the desired change in sexual behavior. Clearly, interventions that provide only information, although important to raise consciousness about the threat posed by HIV, are not sufficient to bring about the needed behavior change.

Evidence is emerging that interventions focusing on changing attitudes and skills related to sexual communication, partner negotiation, and use of condoms increase women's safer sex practices. Data on the effectiveness of this approach, however, have been reported from only a few small studies. Thus, the generalizibility of these findings is unknown.

Evaluation of one component of the skill-building approach has received no attention. Theoretically, increasing skills should produce a sense of self-efficacy or mastery about practicing safer sex which in turn would allow women to encounter new sexual situations with a sense of confidence and power. But limited data are available on the ability of attitude-change/skill-building interventions to affect self-efficacy and there are no data linking self-efficacy with changes in confidence about new sexual encounters.

At this time, we have insufficient data to determine the impact of changing relevant social norms on the sex practices of women. In fact, there is no evidence that current interventions actually change the sexual norms in communities where women at risk live. Data addressing the ability of interventions to produce norm changes in these communities and the relationship between norm changes and women's sexual behavior are sorely needed.

Although data on the effectiveness of interventions are limited, they can be evaluated in terms of their design and ability to produce outcome data in the future. Early interventions suffered from inadequate control groups, difficulties in the definition and operationalization of outcomes, and problems with follow-up. Current studies appear to have dealt with many of these problems in their designs. Researchers of current interventions are likely to encounter problems disentangling the mechanisms by which their interventions are producing behavior change. Most of the interventions contain many components (e.g., skill building, changing attitudes about condoms, individual or group support, etc.). Determining which of these factors mediates behavior change will require careful measurement of the proposed mediator (e.g., beliefs and attitudes about condoms) and linking changes in the mediator produced by the intervention to changes in outcome measures (e.g., condom use).

Determining which components of the intervention mediate behavior change is important for practical and theoretical reasons. In practical terms, only a portion of the intervention may be producing the desired behavior change, and replicating the entire program may be inefficient and expensive. Because different components may be important for different populations (e.g., social norm change for gay men and sexual negotiation for women at high risk), providing all groups with all components may not only be inefficient but also may detract from the credibility of the intervention. Finally, determining the factors that produce the desired outcome offers substantiation for different theories of behavior and thus increases the scientific body of knowledge about behavior change.

Another dimension on which interventions can be evaluated, even at this early stage in their implementation, is their ability to address the potential causes of risk behavior identified through psychosocial research. Recent interventions have had more data on psychosocial determinants from which to draw than did earlier interventions, and thus have incorporated more of the findings into the content of their programs. Increasing women's sense of power or mastery, developing sexual communication and negotiation skills, changing perceptions of condoms and their acceptability to partners, and increasing comfort and skills surrounding condom use are issues dealt with by most current interventions described in this chapter.

An area that psychosocial research indicates is pivotal in women's failure to adopt safer sex practices, but that may receive insufficient attention in current interventions, is that of perceived risk of HIV. Although many interventions deal with this topic, most appear to handle it superficially. Qualitative psychosocial research suggests that women's low evaluation of their risks may represent a defensive maneuver to allow denial of unpleasant realities in their lives (e.g., the risk behaviors of a male partner, the threat of losing one's livelihood). It is possible that only women in the most unempowered situations engage in defensive lowering of risk perception; however, these women may be those most at risk for HIV infection.

What can interventions provide these women? Perhaps Exner's proposal (T. Exner, personal communication, November 1992) to link women with social services that can meet other needs and thus assist women in getting out of their position of powerlessness would allow them to consider their risk in realistic terms. Additionally, social or institutional interventions oriented toward improving the conditions under which poor, minority women live should be mounted and carried out simultaneously with the individual interventions discussed in this chapter. Without changes in the social and economic environment, women are unlikely to experience the feelings of control and choice necessary to seriously consider their risk for HIV infection and the life changes necessary to reduce their risk.

REFERENCES

Bandura, A. (1982). Self-efficacy mechanism in human agency. *American Psychologist, 37,* 122–147.

Becker, M. H., Haefner, D. P., Kasl, S. V., Kirscht, J. P., Maiman, L. A., & Rosenstock, I. M. (1977). Selected psychosocial models and correlates of individual health-related behaviors. *Medical Care, 15,* (suppl. 5), 27–46.

Berrier, J., Sperling, R., Preisinger, J., Evans, V., Mason, J., & Walther, V. (1991). HIV/AIDS education in a prenatal clinic: An assessment. *AIDS Education & Prevention, 3,* 100–117.

Bridgers, C., Figler, K., Vaughan, S., & Sawin, K. J. (1990). AIDS beliefs in young women: Are they related to AIDS risk-reduction behavior? *Journal of the American Academy of Nurse Practitioners, 2,* 107–111.

Britton, P. J., Jackson, A. P., James, T. J., Levine, O. H., Orozco, E. A., Shepherd, J. B., Hobfoll, S. E., & Lavin J. (1992, August). *AIDS prevention among women.* Paper presented at a meeting of the American Psychological Association, Washington, DC.

Burke, D. S., Brundage, J. F., Goldenbaum, M., Gardner, L. I., Peterson, M., Visintine, R., Redfield, R. R., & The Walter Reed Retrovirus Research Group. (1990). Human immunodeficiency virus infections in teenagers. *Journal of the American Medical Association, 263,* 2074–2077.

Campbell, A. A., & Baldwin, W. (1991). The response of American women to the threat of AIDS and other sexually transmitted diseases. *Journal of Acquired Immune Deficiency Syndromes, 4,* 1133–1140.

Catania, J. A., Coates, T. J., Stall, R., Turner, H., Peterson, J., Hearst, N., Dolcini, M. M., Hudes, E., Gagnon, J., Wiley, J., & Groves, R. (1992). Prevalence of AIDS-related risk factors and condom use in the United States. *Science, 258,* 1101–1106.

Catania, J., Kegeles, S., & Coates, T. J. (1990). Towards an understanding of risk behavior: An AIDS risk reduction model (AARM). *Health Education Quarterly, 17,* 53–72.

Center for Women Policy Studies. (1991). *The guide to resources on women and AIDS* (2nd ed.). Washington, DC: Author.

Centers for Disease Control & Prevention. (1992a, October). *HIV/AIDS Surveillance Report.* Atlanta, GA: Centers for Disease Control.

Centers for Disease Control & Prevention. (1992b). Mortality patterns—United States, 1989. *Morbidity & Mortality Weekly Report, 41,* 121–125.

Centers for Disease & Prevention Control. (1992c). Update: Acquired immunodeficiency syndrome—United States, 1991. *Morbidity & Mortality Weekly Report, 41,* 463–468.

Centers for Disease Control. (1992d). Childbearing and contraceptive-use plans among women at high risk for HIV infection: Selected U.S. sites, 1989–1991. *Morbidity & Mortality Weekly Report, 41,* 135–141.

Centers for Disease Control. (1992e). HIV-risk behaviors of sterilized and nonsterilized women in drug treatment programs—Philadelphia, 1989–1991. *Morbidity & Mortality Weekly Report, 41,* 149–152.

Ehrhardt, A. A., Yingling, S., Zawadzki, R., Martinez-Ramirez, M., & Stein, Z. (1991, July). *Barriers to safer sex for women from high HIV prevalence communities.* Paper presented at the 7th International Conference on AIDS, Florence, Italy.

Ellerbrock, T. V., Bush, T. J., Chamberland, M. E., & Oxtoby, M. J. (1991). Epidemiology of women with AIDS in the United States, 1981 through 1990. *Journal of the American Medical Association, 265,* 2971–2975.

European Study Group on Heterosexual Transmission of HIV. (1992). Comparison of female to male and male to female transmission of HIV in 563 stable couples. *British Medical Journal, 304,* 809–813.

Flaskerud, J. H., & Nyamathi, A. M. (1988). An AIDS education program for Vietnamese women. *New York State Journal of Medicine, December,* 632–637.

Flaskerud, J. H., & Nyamathi, A. M. (1989). Black and Latina women's AIDS related knowledge, attitudes, and practices. *Research in Nursing & Health, 12,* 339–346.

Flaskerud, J. H., & Nyamathi, A. M. (1990). Effects of an AIDS education program on the knowledge, attitudes and practices of low income Black and Latina women. *Journal of Community Health, 15,* 343–355.

Flaskerud, J. H., & Thompson, J. (1991). Beliefs about AIDS, health and illness in low-income white Women. *Nursing Research, 40,* 266–271.

Fullilove, M. T., Fullilove, R. E., Haynes, K. E., & Gross, S. (1990). Black women and AIDS prevention: A view towards understanding the gender rules. *The Journal of Sex Research, 27,* 4–64.

Gwinn, M., Pappaioanou, M., George, J. R., Hannon, W. H., Wasser, S. C., Redus, M. A., Hoff, R., Grady, G. F., Willoughby, A., Novello, A. C., Petersen, L. R., Dondero, T. J., & Curran, J. W. (1991). Prevalence of HIV infection in childbearing women in the United States. *Journal of the American Medical Association, 265,* 1704–1708.

Harrison, D. F., Wambach, K. G., Byers, J. B., Imershein, A. W., Levine, P., Maddox, K., Quadagno, D. M., Fordyce, M. L., & Jones, M. A. (1991). AIDS knowledge and risk behaviors among culturally diverse women. *AIDS Education & Prevention, 3,* 79–89.

HDI Projects–National Hispanic Education and Communication Projects. (1990). *Latina AIDS action plan and resource guide.* Grantee 1988–1993 of the U.S. Centers for Disease Control. Washington, DC.

Hinkle, Y. A., Johnson, E. H., Gilbert, D., Jackson, L., & Lollis, C. M. (1991, August). *African-American females who always use condoms: Their attitudes, knowledge about AIDS and sexual behavior.* Paper presented at the meeting of the American Psychological Association, San Francisco, CA.

Hobfoll, S. E., Jackson, A. P., Lavin, J., Britton, P. J., & Shepherd, J. B. (1992, August). *Safer-sex knowledge, behavior, and attitudes of inner-city women.* Paper presented at the meeting of the American Psychological Association, Washington, DC.

Jackson, A., Hobfoll, S. E., Justin, L., Britton, P., & Shephard, B. (1992, August). *The influence of inner-city women's personal and social resources on AIDS risk and health behavior.* Paper presented at a meeting of the American Psychological Association, Washington, DC.

Jemmott, L. S., & Jemmott, J. B. (1991). Applying the theory of reasoned action to AIDS risk behavior: Condom use among black women. *Nursing Research, 40,* 228–234.

Kelly, J. A., Murphy, D. A., Washington, C., Wilson, T. S., Koob, J. J., Kalichman, S. C., Davis, D. R., Ledezma, G., & Davantes, B. (1992, November). *HIV/AIDS prevention groups for high-risk inner-city women: Intervention outcomes and effects on risk behavior.* Paper presented at a meeting of the American Public Health Association, Washington, DC.

Kelly, J. A., St. Lawrence, J. S., Diaz, Y. E., Stevenson, L. Y., Hauth, A. C., Brasfield, T. L., Kalichman, S. C., Smith, J. E., & Andrew, M. E. (1991). HIV risk behavior reduction with key opinion leaders of population: An experimental analysis. *American Journal of Public Health, 81,* 168–171.

Kline, A., Kline, E., & Oken, E. (1992). Minority women and sexual choice in the age of AIDS. *Social Science & Medicine, 34,* 447–457.

Landis, S. E., Schoenbach, V. J., Weber, D. J., Mittal, M., Krishan, B., Lewis, K., & Koch, G. G. (1992). Results of a randomized trial of partner notification in cases of HIV infection in North Carolina. *New England Journal of Medicine, 326,* 101–106.

Marin, B., & Marin, G. (1990). Effects of acculturation on knowledge of AIDS and HIV among Hispanics. *Hispanic Journal of Behavioral Science, 12,* 110–121.

Mason, J., Preisinger, J., Sperling, R., Walther, V., Berrier, J., & Evans, V. (1991). Incorporating HIV education and counseling into routine prenatal care: A program model. *AIDS Education & Prevention, 3,* 118–123.

Mays, V. M., & Cochran, S. D. (1988). Issues in the perception of AIDS risk and risk reduction activities by Black and Hispanic/Latina women. *American Psychologist, 43,* 949–957.

Mitchell, J. L., Thompson, R., Namerow, P., Gordon, T., Carrington, B., & Williams, S. (1992, July). *A comparison of contraceptive usage by HIV infected and non-infected women one year post delivery.* Paper presented at the 8th International Conference on AIDS/III STD World Congress, Amsterdam, The Netherlands.

Multicultural AIDS Coalition. (1992). *Searching for women: A literature review on women, HIV and AIDS in the United States* (3rd ed.). University of Massachusetts, Boston: Law Center, College of Public and Community Service.

Nova Research Company. (1992). *Women at risk: An annotated bibliography.* Prepared for the National Institute on Drug Abuse, Community Research Branch.

Nyamathi, A. M., & Lewis, C. E. (1991). Coping of African-American women at risk for AIDS. *Women's Health Issues, 1,* 53–62.

O'Reilly, K. R., & Higgins, D. L. (1991). AIDS community demonstration projects for HIV prevention among hard-to-reach groups. *Public Health Reports, 106,* 714–720.

Prochaska, J. O., DiClemente, C. C., & Norcross, J. C. (1992). In search of how people change: Applications to addictive behavior. *American Psychologist, 47,* 1102–1114.

Rogers, E. M., & Havens, A. E. (1962). Toward a theory of the diffusion and adoption of innovations. In E. M. Rogers (Ed.), *Diffusion of innovations* (pp. 301–316), New York: The Free Press of Glencoe.

Seidman, S. N., Mosher, W. D., & Aral, S. O. (1992). Women with multiple sexual partners: United States, 1988. *American Journal of Public Health, 82,* 1388–1394.

Smith, T. W. (1991). Adult sexual behavior in 1989: Number of partners, frequency of intercourse and risk of AIDS. *Family Planning Perspectives, 23,* 102–106.

Soskolne, V., Aral, S. O., Magder, L. S., Reed, D. S., & Bowen, G. S. (1991). Condom use with regular and casual partners among women attending family planning clinics. *Family Planning Perspectives, 23,* 222–225.

Stewart, D. L., DeForge, B. R., Hartmann, P., Kaminski, M., & Pecukonis, E. (1991). Attitudes towards condom use and AIDS among patients from an urban family practice center. *Journal of the National Medical Association, 83,* 772–776.

St. Louis, M. E., Conway, G. A., Hayman, C. R., Miller, C., Petersen, L. R., & Dondero, T. J. (1991). Human immunodeficiency virus infection in disadvantaged adolescents. *Journal of the American Medical Association, 266,* 2387–2391.

Sweeney, P. A., Onorato, I. M., Allen, D. M., Byers, R. H., & The Field Services Branch. (1992). Sentinel surveillance of human immunodeficiency virus infection in women seeking reproductive health services in the United States, 1988–1989. *Obstetrics & Gyencology, 79,* 503–510.

Tunstall, C. D., Oliva, G., Kegeles, S., & Darney, P. (1991, November). *Outreach to women at high risk of perinatal HIV transmission presents new challenges to family planning providers.* Paper presented at a meeting of the American Public Health Association, Atlanta, GA.

Valdiserri, R. O., Arena, V. C., Proctor, D., & Bonati, F. A. (1989). The relationship between women's attitudes about condoms and their use: Implications for condom promotion programs. *American Journal of Public Health, 79,* 499–501.

Wingood, G. M., & DiClemente, R. J. (1992). Cultural, gender and psychosocial influences on HIV-related behavior of African-American female adolescents: Implications for the development of tailored prevention programs. *Ethnicity & Disease, 3,* 381–388.

Wingood, G. M., Hunter, D., & DiClemente, R. J. (in press). Sexual communication/negotiation among African-American young adult women: Implications for HIV prevention. *Journal of Black Psychology.*

Worth, D. (1989). Sexual decision-making and AIDS: Why condom promotion among vulnerable women is likely to fail. *Studies in Family Planning, 20,* 297–307.

Worth, D. (1990a). Women at high risk of HIV infection: Behavioral, prevention and intervention aspects. In D. Ostrow (Ed.), *Behavioral aspects of AIDS and other sexually transmitted diseases* (pp. 101–117). New York: Plenum Press.

Worth, D. (1990b). Minority women and AIDS: Culture, race and gender. In D. A. Feldman (Ed.), *Culture and AIDS: The global pandemic* (pp. 1–43). New York: Praeger.

14

HIV Prevention for Gay and Bisexual Men in Metropolitan Cities

ROBERT B. HAYS and JOHN L. PETERSON

INTRODUCTION

The acquired immunodeficiency syndrome (AIDS) epidemic continues to exert a profound toll on urban gay men. As of the end of 1992, more than 150,000 cases of AIDS had been reported in the United States among men who have had sex with other men (Centers for Disease Control, 1993). It is estimated that by the end of 1993, between 240,000 and 280,000 homosexual and bisexual men will have developed AIDS, with between 30,000 and 50,000 men developing AIDS during 1993 alone (Centers for Disease Control, 1990). The majority of U.S. gay and bisexual men with human immunodeficiency virus (HIV) or AIDS reside in major metropolitan areas (Centers for Disease Control, 1993). The National Academy of Sciences Commission on AIDS has predicted that AIDS will "settle in" to gay and minority communities; thus the need for effective preventive interventions for those communities is tremendous. In this chapter, we review the prevalence and predictors of HIV infection and HIV risk behavior among urban gay men, discuss preventive interventions that have been used to reduce HIV risk-taking among urban gay men, highlight strengths and limitations of the existing literature, and present suggestions for future research.

The majority of AIDS cases in the United States still occur among urban gay men (Centers for Disease Control, 1993). Human immunodeficiency virus spread rapidly in the early days of the epidemic, first in cities where gay men

ROBERT B. HAYS • School of Medicine, University of California, San Francisco, California 94143, and Center for AIDS Prevention Studies, San Francisco, California 94105. *JOHN L. PETERSON* • Department of Psychology, Georgia State University, Atlanta, Georgia 30303.

Preventing AIDS: Theories and Methods of Behavioral Interventions, edited by Ralph J. DiClemente and John L. Peterson. Plenum Press, New York, 1994.

tended to live open life-styles. Larger cities favored the creation of neighborhoods where gay-identified individuals could work, live, and love openly according to their sexual orientation. Many U.S. cities include well-established gay neighborhoods with gay-specific organizations, institutions, social structures, and political clout. Ironically, these same centers of gay liberation, with sexual mores emphasizing erotic exploration and experimentation—typified in many ways by the "clone" and bathhouse subcultures (Levine, 1992)—served as ideal breeding grounds for the rapid spread of HIV. Thus, gay men who lived in large urban areas in the late 1970s and early 1980s have the highest rates of HIV infection in the United States.

The relatively high degree of community organization within these urban areas also enabled the mobilization and initiation of the first community-based HIV prevention and risk-reduction campaigns. Gay and bisexual men integrated into the gay communities of major urban areas are now among the most knowledgeable and motivated with regard to HIV prevention and have demonstrated some of the most significant changes in HIV risk behaviors. Human immune deficiency virus seroprevalence among gay men varies by city, region, and behavioral characteristics of the population. This ranges from about 50% among gay men in San Francisco to 38% in New York, to much lower levels in other areas (Curran, Jaffe, Hardy, Morgan, Selik, & Dondero, 1988). For example, 19% of the 301 gay men in the Cleveland Men's Study were found to be infected with HIV (Smucny et al., 1992).

PREVALENCE OF HIV-RELATED RISK BEHAVIOR AMONG URBAN GAY MEN

In response to the AIDS epidemic, gay and bisexual men have made tremendous changes in their sexual behavior (Becker & Joseph, 1988; Coates et al., 1988; Ekstrand & Coates, 1990; Martin, Garcia, & Beatrice, 1989; McCusker, Stoddard, Zapka, Zorn, & Mayer, 1989; Stall, Coates, & Hoff, 1988). These have been described as the most dramatic behavioral changes ever documented in the public health literature (Coates, 1990). Sharp declines have been reported in rates of unprotected anal intercourse, the major route of HIV transmission among gay and bisexual men (Ekstrand & Coates, 1990, Martin, Dean, Garcia, & Hall, 1989; McKusick, Coates, Morin, Pollack, & Hoff, 1990). In a longitudinal survey of 624 New York City gay men, Martin, Garcia, and Beatrice (1989) found reports of condom use to substantially escalate from 2% in 1981 to 62% in 1987. Correspondingly, declining rates of rectal gonorrhea have been documented in several urban areas (Hansfield, 1985; Martin, Dean, Garcia, & Hall, 1989). It is important to note that celibacy is not the preferred strategy of gay men for dealing with the risk of AIDS. Instead, gay men are more likely to reduce their number of sexual contacts outside of primary relationships and to eliminate or modify anal intercourse by use of condoms (Becker & Joseph, 1988). Clearly, recommending abstinence is not a useful approach for risk reduction with gay men.

Unfortunately, these patterns of behavioral change appear uneven given the greater sexual risk behavior observed among gay men outside AIDS epicenters (Ames & Beeker, 1990; Kelly, St. Lawrence, Betts, Brasfield, & Hood, 1990; St. Lawrence, Hood, Brasfield, & Kelly, 1989; Ruefli, Yu, & Barton, 1992), ethnic minority gay men (Peterson, Coates, Catania, Middleton, Hilliard, & Hearst, 1992), and younger gay men (Hays, Kegeles, & Coates, 1990; Stall et al., 1992). For example, younger gay men are consistently found to engage in higher rates of unsafe sex than older gay men (Hays et al., 1990; Stall et al., 1992) and a disproportionate number of the new HIV seroconversions within the gay community are occurring among young men. A 1992 population-based survey of San Francisco gay men aged 18 to 29, found 17% to be HIV-positive (Osmond et al., 1993).

Furthermore, it appears that a substantial percentage of gay men are having difficulty maintaining changes in high-risk sexual behavior (Adib, Joseph, Ostrow, & James, 1991; Ekstrand & Coates, 1990; Stall et al., 1990). For example, Stall et al. (1990) reported that 19% of the respondents in one longitudinal survey of San Francisco gay men had "relapsed" to high-risk sex at least once from 1984 to 1987. Recent reports from the Multicenter AIDS Cohort Study (MACS) in Chicago and the City Clinic and Men's Health Studies in San Francisco suggest that after years of decline, HIV seroconversion rates have increased in these cohorts (San Francisco Department of Public Health, 1989; Kingsley et al., 1990).

It should be recognized, however, that most of the data on risk reduction among gay men is based on intensively studied and extensively retested cohorts in several major AIDS epicenters. These cohorts tend to oversample white gay men who are older, better educated, of higher socioeconomic status, and more motivated concerning HIV/AIDS than the community as a whole. These studies may thus overestimate the degree of changes within the gay community since they underrepresent ethnic minority men, lower social class men, younger men, men who are less integrated within the gay community, and men who have sex with men but do not identify as gay.

PREDICTORS OF RISK-TAKING AMONG URBAN GAY MEN

Understanding the correlates of high-risk behaviors is central to designing effective preventive interventions. A considerable body of literature now exists on the individual, situational, and social factors associated with whether or not gay men engage in safer sex. This body of research is important because it helps us understand gay men's risk taking, but also it provides suggestions for designing behavioral interventions.

Demographic Predictors

Several demographic factors have been found to predict HIV risk reduction among urban gay men, including ethnicity, age, and social class. African-Americans and Hispanics are disproportionately represented among AIDS incidence rates (Peterson & Marin, 1988), and nonwhite gay men tend to engage in higher rates of unsafe sex than white gay men (Peterson et al., 1992). Since 1986, AIDS cases among nonwhite gay and bisexual men have risen more rapidly than among white gay and bisexual men (Rutherford, Barnhart, & Lemp, 1988). Also, younger men have been found to engage in higher rates of unsafe sex than older men (Hays, Kegeles, & Coates, 1990; Kelly et al., 1990; Stall et al., 1992; Valdiserri et al., 1988). Lastly, among gay and bisexual men, lower educational attainment and lower socioeconomic status are associated with engaging in unsafe sex (Calabrese, Harris, & Easley, 1987; Peterson et al., 1992; Van Raden, Kaslow, & Kingsley, 1988).

Psychosocial Factors of HIV Risk Reduction

Relationship Status

Significantly more unprotected anal intercourse occurs within the context of a committed relationship than among casual partners (Hays, Kegeles, & Coates, 1990; McKusick et al., 1990). Gay men tend to use condoms more frequently with casual or secondary partners than with primary partners (Schechter, 1988; Valdiserri et al., 1988). Higher risk behavior has also been found associated with stronger tendencies to engage in sex as an expression of love (Joseph, Adib, Joseph, & Tal, 1991).

Personal Behavior History/Sexual Habituation

Past sexual behavior is the strongest predictor of future sexual behavior (Joseph et al., 1991; McKusick, Horstman, & Coates, 1985; McCusker, Stoddard, Zapka, Zorn, & Mayer, 1989). Subsequent high-risk behavior is associated with higher risk behavior in the past (Joseph et al., 1991). This finding suggests that individuals who are in the process of "coming out" (e.g., young gay men), and whose sexual behavior patterns are less entrenched, may be the most promising audience for safer sex promotion.

Meanings of Sex

Higher risk behavior has been associated with greater personal importance placed on sex, particularly using sex as an expression of love or as a response to a partner's desire (i.e., fulfilling partner's demands [Joseph et al., 1991]). Additionally, those men who report using sex as a way to relieve tension are less likely to have reduced their risk behavior (McKusick, Hortsman, & Coates, 1985). These authors also found that 69% of the men who had three or more sexual partners during the past month agreed with the statement that, "It is hard to change my sexual behavior because being gay means doing what I want sexually."

Integration into Gay Community

Whereas those gay men who were most highly integrated into the gay community were initially most likely to become infected with HIV, they were also more likely to be personally exposed to the prevention campaigns in the gay community. Men who are less integrated into the gay community are now less likely to have made HIV risk reduction changes.

Knowledge of Health Education Guidelines

Knowledge of HIV risks and guidelines is a necessary but insufficient contributor to risk reduction among gay and bisexual men (Becker & Joseph, 1988; Stall, Coates, & Hoff, 1988). Current studies find high levels of knowledge among gay and bisexual men (Centers for Disease Control, 1993; Valdiserri et al., 1987), but the data suggest there is a threshold effect: little new behavior change will be accomplished by providing additional information (Becker & Joseph, 1988). Indeed, a variety of studies have consistently found knowledge to have little or no relation to risk-reduction behavior (Joseph et al., 1987; McKusker et al., 1989; McKusick, Horstman, & Coates, 1985). For example, in an intervention study with gay men in Pittsburgh, Valdiserri and his colleagues (1987) found that gay men were highly knowledgeable about the routes of HIV transmission, but that nonetheless nearly two-thirds reported engaging in unprotected receptive intercourse with more than one partner in the preceding six months. Clearly, factors other than knowledge are major determinants of safer sex behavior. It is possible that knowledge is related to initial behavior change but not to maintenance of behavior change (Becker & Joseph,

1988). While gay men are generally very knowledgeable about basic safe sex guidelines, the main area of confusion now seems to be regarding the risk level of oral–genital sex, but this confusion reflects the lack of definitive epidemiological evidence on this topic.

Perceived Threat

Perceiving oneself as vulnerable to HIV infection may be necessary to motivate one to adopt safe sex behaviors (Catania, Kegeles, & Coates, 1990). For example, the lower levels of risk reduction found among nonwhite men and younger gay men have been explained as due to the stereotyped perceptions that AIDS is primarily a disease of white gay men or older gay men. As in the case of knowledge, a threshold may be reached whereby increased perceptions of threat no longer confer beneficial effects. In an analysis of data from 637 men participating in the Chicago (MACS) study, Joseph et al., (1987) found no observable benefit to an increased sense of risk, and suggested in fact that greater sense of risk may be counterproductive, leading to psychological and social distress that may ultimately reduce adherence to behavioral risk reduction guidelines or disrupt maintenance of established, positive behaviors. Similarly, in comparisons of men who engaged in risky and safe behavior, perceived risk did not distinguish between the two groups (Siegel, Mesagno, Chen, & Christ, 1989).

Response Efficacy

Gay men tend to believe in the efficacy of safer sex guidelines (Joseph et al., 1987; McKusick, Wiley et al., 1985), and this response efficacy appears more associated with the initial adoption of risk reduction behaviors, than with later changes over time (Joseph et al., 1987).

Sexual Enjoyment

The more positive perceived consequences of using condoms, the more likely gay men are to use them (Catania et al., 1991). A potent cost of low-risk sex is the perception of reduced enjoyment of low-risk activities. A variety of studies have found that the perception that high-risk activities are more enjoyable than low-risk activities is inversely related to risk reduction among gay men (Hays, Kegeles, Coates, 1990; McKusick et al., 1990). For example, Valdiserri et al. (1988) found that the sharpest difference between gay men who never used condoms versus those who always used them was the perception of the never users that condoms "spoiled" sex.

Interpersonal Barriers

Feeling that one may offend one's partner, jeopardize one's relationship with him, or lose his affection represent significant interpersonal costs that may reduce one's motivation for engaging in safe sex. Engaging in safer sex requires communicating this desire to one's partner and may necessitate negotiation or assertiveness skills in convincing one's partner or refusing requests for unsafe behavior. For example, in a study of young gay men, those men who engaged in unsafe sex rated their sexual communication skills lower than those men who consistently engaged in safer sex (Hays, Kegeles, & Coates, 1990).

Social Norms and Peer Support

The belief that one's peers engage in and support low-risk sex and disapprove of high-risk sex has been found to be a powerful predictor of risk reduction among gay men (Catania et al., 1991; Emmons et al., 1986; Hays, Kegeles, & Coates, 1992; Kelly, St. Lawrence, Brasfield et al., 1990; Klein, Sullivan, Wolcott, Landsveris, Namir, & Fawzy, 1987; Joseph et al., 1987; McKusick et al., 1990). In addition, gay men report they are most likely to seek help from friends and lovers in trying to change high-risk behavior (Catania, Coates, Kegeles et al., 1988).

Influence of Alcohol/Drugs

The combination of drugs and/or alcohol is associated with engaging in high-risk sex (McKirnan & Peterson, 1989; Stall, McKusick, Wiley, Coates, & Ostrow, 1986; Valdiserri, Lyter et al., 1988). Further, in a longitudinal cohort of gay men in Boston, men who reduced their frequency of alcohol consumption or stopped using marijuana were significantly more likely to have changed to consistently low-risk sexual practices (McCusker et al., 1990).

Self-Efficacy

In addition to possessing the requisite skills for risk reduction, individuals must feel confident that they are capable of making the necessary behavior changes to reduce risk. Feelings of self-efficacy with regard to safer sex have been found to be associated with risk reduction among gay men (Aspinwall, Kemeny, Taylor, Schneider, & Dudley, 1991; Emmons 1986; McKirnan & Peterson, 1989; McKusick et al., 1990).

HIV Antibody Testing/Knowledge of Serostatus

Examinations of the relation between antibody testing and risk reduction have yielded mixed results. In a comprehensive review of the effects of HIV testing on risk behaviors, Higgins et al. (1991) found that changes in risk behavior were generally independent of knowledge of serostatus, though several studies did suggest that being told one is seropositive had a beneficial impact on subsequent risk behavior (Fox, Odaka, Brookmeyer, & Polk, 1987; McKusick et al., 1990; McCusker et al., 1988; Valdiserri et al., 1988).

Difficulty in Controlling Sexual Impulses

Men who perceive greater difficulty controlling sexual impulses are less likely to report having reduced high-risk behaviors (Joseph et al., 1991; Joseph et al., 1987). For example, in a study of 108 gay men in New York City, men who perceived themselves to be lower in sexual self-control reported more occasions of unprotected anal intercourse with ejaculation than men who reported greater control (Exner, Meyer-Bahlburg, & Ehrhardt, 1992).

Coping Style

In an analysis of San Francisco gay men, those men who reported unprotected anal intercourse used sex more of the time to help cope with stressful situations than men who did not engage in unprotected intercourse (Folkman, Chesney, Pollack, & Phillips, 1992).

Predictors of HIV Risk-Taking Will Vary with Subgroup

In a comparison of younger versus older men in San Francisco, Stall et al. (1992) found that the correlates of unprotected anal intercourse were different for older versus younger men. Factors related to initial adoption of safe sex behaviors may be different from those related to maintenance and/or incremental improvement (Ekstrand & Coates, 1990; Joseph et al., 1987). In addition, there may be historical changes in the relationship of variables to risk reduction. For example, early in the epidemic, McKusick et al. (1985) found that having a visual image of a person with AIDS (and knowing people with AIDS) was associated with risk reduction, whereas this association has not held up in later studies. It is possible there is no longer much variance in these dimensions among urban gay men, now that in AIDS epicenters virtually all gay men have had personal contact with friends or acquaintances with AIDS. Thus provision of information and communication about risk may have been critical at early stages of the epidemic, but at this stage of the epidemic it is necessary to move beyond those goals.

It is extremely important to remember that the "gay community" is not a monolithic, static entity. There will always be new men who come out as gay and enter the gay community (e.g., young gay men, men who migrate to urban areas from small towns or other countries, older men who have only recently recognized or accepted their homosexuality), who have not been exposed to the prevention campaigns of previous years and who do not have the high level of knowledge and AIDS awareness of the "general" gay community, and have not yet been socialized into the norms of the gay community. For this reason, HIV prevention programs must be ongoing within the gay community, despite the general trends toward safer sex which have occurred within the gay community as a whole.

In their review of the HIV risk reduction literature, Becker and Joseph (1988) suggested that more research was needed on factors associated with whether or not high-risk individuals adopt risk reduction behaviors. That suggestion has been heeded for older cohorts of urban white gay men given the volume of data on this strata of homosexual men. There is, however, a conspicuous absence of survey research on risk-taking among minority gay men, including older men in AIDS epicenters.

HIV PREVENTION AMONG URBAN GAY AND BISEXUAL MINORITY MEN

After a decade of the AIDS epidemic, there is very limited behavioral research on gay and bisexual nonwhite men. Most studies in large urban cities have included only small samples of gay and bisexual minority men, although these men account for over 30% of all AIDS cases among men who have sex with other men (Centers for Disease Control, 1993). In one of these studies, ethnic minority men were found to have significantly higher HIV seroprevalence rates than white gay men (Samuel & Winkelstein, 1987). Nonetheless, there are still few data on the extent of HIV risk behaviors and determinants of these behaviors among homosexually active nonwhite men. Recently, however, data from one AIDS epicenter indicate that high-risk sexual behavior is still inflated among gay and bisexual African-American men.

HIGH-RISK SEXUAL BEHAVIOR AMONG GAY/BISEXUAL AFRICAN-AMERICAN MEN

The behavioral research available on gay and bisexual African-American men is not derived from probability samples of homosexually active men in the African-American general population. This limitation results largely from the fact that these ethnic gay men are more diverse, hidden, or "closeted" populations than their white cohorts, especially in urban areas. Therefore, the results from these studies are based on convenience samples and warrant caution if generalized to representative samples of white gay men.

A recent study by Peterson et al. (1992) examined high-risk sexual behavior and condom use among gay and bisexual African-American men in the San Francisco Bay Area. Peterson and his colleagues conducted anonymous interviews of 250 respondents recruited in 1990 from bars, bathhouses, erotic bookstores, and through African-American newspapers, health clinics, and personal referral from study participants. Of the men (73%) who engaged in anal intercourse within the past six months, over half reported having had unprotected anal intercourse, 22% with primary and 35% with secondary male partners. Also, a small proportion of the total sample reported that they had engaged in unprotected vaginal intercourse with primary (7%) or secondary (12%) female partners. High-risk sexual behavior was most strongly associated with marginal status (e.g., low income, being paid for sex, and/or injection drug use [IDU]); discomfort with public disclosure of one's homosexuality; perceiving oneself as being at risk of HIV infection; and lack of social support for concerns about one's unsafe sex. Men who were more likely to use condoms had stronger beliefs that condom use was normative, stronger beliefs that they could practice safe sex, and more positive expectations about using condoms. Also, men with marginal status were less likely to use condoms.

These data indicate that gay and bisexual African-American men in San Francisco have a substantially higher prevalence (52%) of risk behavior than the levels of risk behavior (15–20%) found for white gay and bisexual men during similar time periods (Ekstrand & Coates, 1990; McKusick et al., 1990; Winkelstein et al., 1987). This evidence suggests that, in the second decade of the AIDS epidemic, gay and bisexual African-American men have maintained higher HIV risks than their white cohorts in San Francisco. It is unclear to what extent these risk levels are comparable for white and nonwhite samples because of differences in sampling techniques. Studies on white gay men in San Francisco are derived from two samples, one a population-based sample and the other a convenience sample largely recruited from gay men who patronize bars. The African-American sample is also a convenience sample but is not largely recruited from gay bars.

FACTORS RELATED TO HIV RISK REDUCTION AMONG GAY AFRICAN-AMERICANS

Gay and bisexual African-American men may differ from white gay men in characteristics that affect their levels of HIV risk and the types of intervention programs needed to change their high-risk behavior. While these differences may not exist for all gay and bisexual African-American men, several characteristics should be considered in developing HIV prevention programs for this population.

Social Status

Many gay and bisexual African-American men at high risk of HIV may be low income and engage in prostitution or injection drug use. The social status of these men increases the difficulty of reaching them during the delivery of risk reduction campaigns. Economic differences between white and African-American men may require that financial incentives be offered to recruit eligible participants for these intervention programs. Alternatively, job training and job referrals may be sufficient incentives to attract low-income high-risk men to prevention programs. Also, vouchers for drug treatment could be useful to recruit gay and bisexual men who are injection drug users.

Social Networks Different for White and African-American Gay Men

Unlike gay white men, gay and bisexual African-American men will not be reached if prevention programs rely on targeting identifiable gay urban neighborhoods. These men are less likely to be involved in mainstream gay white culture in urban cities throughout the United States. Consequently, they frequently lack the institutions available in mainstream gay culture, such as gay newspapers, gay political and social organizations, and gay businesses. Without formal gay institutions, the opportunity to reach them is likely to depend on informal social networks which are more discrete and amorphous. While formidable, these obstacles can be overcome if appropriate HIV prevention strategies are developed relevant to the life-styles of gay and bisexual African-American men. Interventions may need to use outreach and street intercept techniques to reach many of these men at risk. It may be more useful to reach high-risk men in the sociosexual venues in which sexual activity occurs (e.g. public restrooms, parks, adult bookstores, steam baths). Outreach campaigns need to be developed based on ethnographic information about these men's social networks and locales for sexual activity. Also, prevention campaigns for bisexual men may require different strategies than those for men who engage exclusively in homosexual behavior. The HIV prevention efforts should consider aspects of these men's sexual relationships with their female partners, such as gender roles, power differences, and control in sexual decision making.

Dual Identity and Antigay Sentiment

Gay and bisexual African-American men confront strong antihomosexual attitudes in the African-American community if they publicly disclose their homosexuality. This antigay sentiment largely results from the influence of the Judeo-Christian views in African-American religion and traditional gender roles in African-American culture. Despite antigay sentiment toward white gay men, African-American gay men may be more reluctant to resist gay prejudice because such resistance may create conflict between their racial membership and sexual identity. If they publicly identify as gay, they risk the possibility of alienation from the mainstream African-American community. Also, there is limited organizational support from African-American gay men to overcome homophobia because of the lack of a formal gay subculture. Efforts will need to be made to improve these men's acceptance of public awareness of their same-sex behavior and identity, such as the use of popular role-models who publicly self-identify as gay.

Limited Prevention Resources

While there are numerous AIDS prevention organizations funded to serve white gay men, few AIDS prevention organizations are available for gay and bisexual African-American men. Even in AIDS epicenters, such as San Francisco and New York, most minority community organizations are inadequately equipped to provide effective prevention campaigns for gay and bisexual African-American men. Also, there are few gay organizations in African-American communities to provide HIV prevention campaigns. Therefore, mainstream minority organizations with HIV prevention programs will need to develop greater awareness of and sensitivity to gay and bisexual populations. These programs will need to employ gay and bisexual African-American men who are knowledgeable about AIDS risk reduction and who are familiar with the subculture of these men.

Limitations of Perceived Risk

Typically, white gay men in AIDS epicenters have become aware of their HIV risks, through widespread deaths of friends and lovers, and this perception of their HIV risks has influenced them to modify their HIV risk behaviors. However, many African-American gay men may still deny their risks if they reside outside AIDS epicenters or outside white gay neighborhoods. Even in urban cities, such as San Francisco, gay and bisexual African-American men who correctly perceived themselves to be at risk for HIV infection had not discontinued high-risk sexual behavior. Therefore, campaigns to increase risk perceptions are not enough to cause behavior change.

HIV PREVENTION PROGRAMS FOR GAY MEN IN URBAN CENTERS

Despite the abundance of survey data, it is surprising that there are only a few studies that have examined the impact of HIV prevention programs on urban gay men. The most urgent need for research now is in the design and evaluation of interventions that incorporate previous findings on patterns of risk-taking into on-going community programs for gay men (Coates, 1990; National Research Council, 1993). Effective strategies will need to be innovative in their approach for gay men to pay attention to them, because many men in AIDS epicenters are already knowledgeable about AIDS and may be "burned out" hearing about it. Also, the involvement of peers may offer the most promising approach to delivery interventions for these men in view of evidence that both white and nonwhite men are most likely to turn to peers and rate them as the most helpful source of help in dealing with AIDS risk reduction and HIV-related concerns (Hays, Catania, McKusick, & Coates, 1990; Peterson et al., in press). The paucity of intervention data among urban gay men becomes immediately apparent when it is recognized that most prevention programs have been designed and implemented for gay men by community-based organizations but have rarely been evaluated. Since the science on HIV interventions is still in its infancy, the design of rigorous methodological evaluations of these programs present formidable challenges.

HIV prevention programs that have been used with urban gay men may include approaches that employ individual-level interventions or community-level interventions. Individual-level interventions have utilized: personal information and counseling (e.g., clients at public health clinics, HIV antibody test sites, telephone hotlines); face-to-face groups (e.g., small-group meetings and workshops); media approaches, involving mass media (e.g., television, radio, billboards, posters) and/or small media (e.g., pamphlets, brochures); safer sex videos, community forums, outreach to settings where gay men congregate socially (such as bars, social organizations, neighborhood settings); or for sex (public sex environments, bathhouses, sex clubs). Community-level approaches have employed a combination of these strategies. Many of the prevention programs for urban gay men were designed and implemented quickly in response to urgent need. As we enter the second decade of the epidemic, it is essential that a research base is developed that identifies those strategies that are effective and efficient in facilitating and maintaining safer sex behaviors among gay and bisexual men in metropolitan cities. In the following section, we discuss the limited evaluation data that exist on interventions for these men.

Individual-Level Interventions

Some data have been reported on the effectiveness of individual counseling for reduction of high-risk sexual behavior and promotion of condom use (Centers for Disease Control, 1992). Individual counseling sessions for homosexual/bisexual men in Denver were provided as part of the Centers for Disease Control (CDC) Community Demonstration Projects for HIV Prevention, between 1988 and 1991. Participants were recruited through referrals from community organizations, public clinics, and other health care providers; advertising campaigns and word-of-mouth communication. Study participants made two visits at study entry, then made follow-up visits every six months. During initial visits, participants (1) completed self-administered questionnaires regarding knowledge, attitudes, beliefs, and sexual behaviors; (2) received HIV-antibody testing; (3) received counseling on the natural history of HIV infection, modes of transmission, and ways to prevent infection; and (4) received skills training, including techniques for effective condom use. At each follow-up visit, participants completed questionnaires and received HIV-antibody testing and reinforcement of educational messages. From 1988 through 1991, 298 men completed questionnaires at both initial and 12-month visits. At the 12-month follow-up, between 17% and 29% of the men reported they had discontinued anal intercourse. For those men who continued anal intercourse, condom use significantly increased from 63% at initial visits to 71% after 12 months. Unfortunately, this research design did not employ a control group so it is not known whether factors outside the risk-reduction program may have accounted for these changes.

In a primarily observational study of the effects of antibody testing on homosexually active men in Boston, McCusker et al. (1988) offered HIV antibody testing with individual counseling regarding the meaning of the HIV antibody test, an explanation of the results, and information on HIV risk reduction. The 270 participants were recruited through advertisements in the waiting area of a Boston community health clinic and direct mailings to health center clients, and were predominantly white, college-educated, and between the ages of 20 and 34. At the initial visit, participants completed a written questionnaire which assessed sexual behavior during the previous six months and received a physical examination and HIV antibody testing. Men who chose to learn their antibody test results returned within three months to receive their result and be counseled. At six-month and one-year follow-up visits, participants again completed questionnaires about their sexual behaviors. Compared to men who did not know their HIV status and men who learned they were HIV negative, those who learned they were HIV positive decreased their frequency of unprotected insertive anal intercourse at six-month and one-year follow-ups. No change in unprotected receptive intercourse was found.

Research in other areas of health promotion has documented that context may be as important as content to induce health-related behavior change. Valdiserri and his colleagues (1987) have suggested that group formats may be more successful in promoting HIV risk reduction than media campaigns or individual counseling sessions because such a format can affect group social norms. Likewise, Shernoff and Bloom (1991) suggest that groups provide the opportunity for individuals to experience themselves as part of a larger community struggling together and to help create or strengthen their ties to that community. Using peers to deliver the information may also increase their effectiveness, as has been observed in smoking prevention programs for adolescents.

Valdiserri and his colleagues have reported a series of investigations which examined the effects of small group risk-reduction sessions with gay and bisexual men (Valdiserri et al., 1988). Beginning in 1985, participants in the Pittsburgh cohort of the MACS were invited through direct mail to participate in an AIDS prevention educational session. The intervention consisted of an informal group educational session led by a gay male health educator. Groups consisted of 5 to 10 participants and lasted 60 to 75 minutes. The goals of the session were to (1) increase knowledge about HIV transmission and natural history; (2) increase understanding of the relative HIV risks of specific sexual practices; (3) improve skills in the appropriate use of condoms; and (4) increase knowledge about interpreting HIV antibody tests.

Self-administered questionnaires were completed at three time intervals: one to two weeks before the intervention, two weeks after the intervention, and four to six months after the intervention. One-third of the men accepted the invitation to participate in the intervention and over four hundred actually attended the sessions. Although the vast majority of those invited to attend did not, there were no differences found in the risk-taking behaviors between those who attended and those who did not. Also, those who attended the sessions were more likely to have a college degree. The immediate postintervention follow-up revealed significant increases in attitudes favoring AIDS prevention, such as: more agreement with the value of safer sex practices and condom use, higher perceived vulnerability to AIDS, greater intention to discuss AIDS prevention with sexual partners, and greater perceptions of peer acceptance of safer sex. Although this study demonstrated a positive impact on factors that may influence behavior change, immediate behavior changes were not assessed and long-term changes were not reported.

Another study by the same research team (Leviton et al., 1990; Valdiserri et al., 1988) used a randomized trial to compare two different types of small-group interventions. Most participants (N = 584), recruited from the metropolitan Pittsburgh area from 1986 to 1987, were white and over half had some college education. They were randomly assigned to attend either of two interventions. Intervention I was a single 90-minute lecture/discussion educational session providing information on the following topics: transmission and pathogenesis of HIV infection; the clinical outcomes of HIV infection; safer sex guidelines; proper use of condoms; and interpretation of HIV antibody tests. This session was led by a gay health educator.

Intervention II included two components. The first component was identical to Intervention I, the second component included skills-training, using role-playing, psychodrama, and group process techniques. The goals of this component were to: promote acceptability of safe sex; teach behavior modification strategies for safe sex; stress legitimacy of safe sex as an alternative; and explore nonerotic functions of sex for gay men. The investigators theorized that through group processes, participants explored their own beliefs and opinions about options for safer sex, and learned that their peers in the group supported the idea. Through role-playing, men learned appropriate skills to assert themselves with potential partners, and to insist on safer alternatives to unprotected anal intercourse. In the group they gained feedback about their behavior, support from others, and information about the consequences of their assertiveness. Intervention II lasted 140 minutes and was led by a gay therapist.

Evaluation data were obtained through self-administered questionnaires (assessing attitudes regarding risk reduction and safer sex, knowledge and sexual behaviors) completed prior to the intervention and at two six-month follow-ups. The results showed that Intervention II, which included social skills training and peer support, was superior to the lecture/discussion method in impacting both risk behaviors and safer sex attitudes. At both six-month and one-year follow-ups, participants in Intervention II significantly increased condom use during insertive anal intercourse relative to participants in Intervention I. Men in Intervention II increased their use of condoms with partners from 36% preintervention to 80% one year later, compared to men in Intervention I who increased condom use from 44% to 55%.

The authors concluded that the effect of skills training on condom use for insertive anal intercourse represented a 33% improvement. It is unclear why the effects were not also found for receptive anal intercourse; the ability of the receptive partner to assert himself may require more intensive intervention. With regard to attitudes, Intervention II caused greater reduction of value placed on ejaculating inside the partner, increased overall endorsement of protective sex, increased intentions to use condoms, and reduced negative attitudes toward condom use (Leviton et al., 1990). No effect was found for knowledge which was high prior to intervention. These results suggest that interventions which teach men how to negotiate safer sexual encounters as part of the intervention can result in benefits above and beyond the mere dissemination of information.

In an interesting follow-up to their intervention, Silvestre, Lyter, Valdiserri, Huggins, and Rinaldo (1989) identified 24 men from the Pittsburgh Men's Study who later seroconverted despite participation in the intervention and examined the factors related to their seroconversions. Based on interviews with 13 of those men, the authors suggested that future interventions also include information and counseling about the impact of emotions on risk perceptions and risk behavior, negotiation and assertiveness training for dealing with partners who may exert pressure for unsafe sex, and more detailed information on condom use, lubricants, and how to avoid condom breakage. More intensive counseling for substance abusive, depressed, and self-destructive individuals may also be necessary. Further, follow-up "booster" sessions may be advisable to reinforce changes.

Stop AIDS discussion groups have been widely used as an AIDS prevention strategy by many communities. During its first two years of operation in San Francisco from 1985 to 1987, over 7,000 gay and bisexual men attended a Stop AIDS group. Though Stop AIDS has been credited with success in changing community norms in San Francisco, there is a lack of evaluation data on the effects of this program, but, some researchers (Miller, Booraem, Flowers, & Iverson, 1990) have undertaken evaluations of Stop AIDS groups in Southern California (Orange County). Participants were recruited from community settings, where gay and bisexual men were known to congregate, by trained volunteers who engaged potential participants in conversation about AIDS prevention and offered invitations to attend a Stop AIDS discussion group. Participants were later scheduled for discussion groups consisting of 4 to 15 participants, conducted on weeknights in private homes. The one-time groups lasted 3-1/2 hours and were led by trained peer facilitators. The structured discussion groups focus on the impact the AIDS epidemic has had on one's life; HIV transmission and safer sex guidelines; the role of alcohol and drugs as contributors to unsafe sex; HIV antibody-testing; changes in the gay community due to AIDS; visions for the future of the gay community; and ways participants can be involved to end the epidemic. At the end of each group, participants completed personal commitment cards, verbal declarations of their commitment, and a questionnaire immediately before and after the discussion group. The results showed significant improvements in AIDS-related knowledge, attitudes, and behavioral intentions.

The same research design was subsequently used to evaluate the Stop AIDS groups in three other communities: Chicago, Orange County, and Phoenix (Flowers et al., 1991). Similarly, participants completed pre- and postquestionnaires regarding knowledge, attitudes, and behavior intentions immediately before and after attending a Stop AIDS group. The results showed participants increased their knowledge and behavioral intentions following the group intervention. While these studies are promising in demonstrating immediate benefits of the Stop AIDS group, they are limited by their lack of longer term follow-up and no assessment of actual risk behavior. In a previous report (Miller et al., 1990), it was found that intention to reduce high-risk behavior was associated with actual reduced risk behavior at a three-month follow-up, as reported by both the participant and a sexual partner qualified to rate him.

The small-group format can also be extended to multiple sessions. Theoretically, multiple session groups have a number of advantages over single session groups. They are able to address more intensively the particular issues targeted and they allow an opportunity for the participants to assimilate the material learned and incorporate it into their daily lives between sessions, and then bring those experiences back into later sessions. Yet, multiple sessions require more time and motivation from participants, and it may be difficult to recruit the men who would most benefit to actually attend them.

Roffman and his colleagues are currently investigating the possibility of providing a small-group HIV prevention intervention via telephone conference calls. In preliminary research in which men were offered the choice of face-to-face or telephone counseling, those men who selected telephone counseling were more likely to describe themselves as bisexual, to be more closeted, and to indicate that it was important for them to conceal their sexual orientation from others, but they did not differ in terms of HIV risk behavior (Roffman et al., 1989). Using a telephone conference call format, participants were afforded the benefits of group counseling while being permitted to maintain their anonymity. In a preliminary analysis to test the feasibility of this approach, Roffman and his associates found that participants decreased their frequency of high-risk behaviors and increased low-risk behaviors, with risk reduction maintained over one-month follow-up assessments. In addition, participants perceived norms among friends as more safe-sex affirmative and showed increases in self-efficacy. However, no control group was included in these results.

Community-Level Interventions

Since gay bars often provide the setting where sexual contacts are made and patrons have been found to have high rates of risky sex (Stall, Ekstrand, Hoff, Paul, Catania, & Coates, 1993), HIV prevention interventions centered at gay bars can be very valuable. Honnen and Kleinke (1990) report a relatively simple intervention aimed at promoting condom use among bar patrons. Specifically, they examined whether signs in bars would prompt gay bar patrons to take free condoms. The experiment was conducted in three gay bars in Anchorage, Alaska, and used an ABAB experimental design with a two-week baseline and intervention intervals. A sign placed in each bar said, "In the state of Alaska, 38 people have died of AIDS. Many more have tested positive. Condoms can reduce the spread of AIDS." This message was chosen to help customers appreciate the risk of contracting HIV without using a strong fear appeal that might cause denial. The researchers compared the number of free condoms taken from containers in the bar during the time periods when the signs were present and absent. They found that 748 condoms were taken when signs were present versus 510 taken when signs were absent. Thus, the signs resulted in 47% increase in number of condoms taken. Though the researchers did not assess whether the condoms were in fact used, this study does show that a relatively simple prompt can influence a necessary antecedent behavior for HIV risk-reduction. The use of an unobtrusive behavioral measure (number of condoms taken) is also praiseworthy, given the questionable validity of self-report data. Interestingly, the authors report that signs were kept up voluntarily after the study was over, suggesting that bar owners can be cooperative and supportive of prevention activities.

Within recent years, increased concern has been devoted to the need to reduce the rate of unsafe sex among young gay and bisexual men. This concern prompted Kegeles, Hays, and Coates (1992) to develop and evaluate a community-level HIV prevention program tailored specifically to the needs of young gay and bisexual men. The goals, framework, activities, and materials for this study were guided by previous research with this population and through an extensive process of social marketing and focus groups with young gay and bisexual men. This preliminary research identified the critical issues and guiding principles for designing the intervention. First, it was recognized that AIDS prevention is not in itself sufficiently motivating or captivating for young gay men. Many young gay men perceive AIDS to be a problem mainly of older gay men. For example, in focus groups conducted with young gay men, participants expressed the view that those who were likely to have AIDS were "older gay men with mustaches who go to leather bars." Consequently, young gay men tend not to seek out AIDS prevention services. Community organizations consistently report that very few young men come to their AIDS prevention activities, such as safer sex workshops. Further, AIDS is only one threat among many that young gay men confront in a homophobic society where gay-bashing, discrimination, and battles over gay rights are commonplace, and young gay men may be dealing simultaneously with issues such as self-esteem, alienation, social identity, and family problems. Therefore, a successful AIDS prevention intervention for young gay men would need to relate HIV risk-reduction to the satisfaction of other needs, such as the development of one's social network, enjoyment of social interactions, and enhancement of self-esteem. Through focus groups, it became clear that various social concerns were highly motivating for young gay men (i.e., how to meet and have fun with other men of their age) and a social focus was adopted as the central theme of this intervention study.

A second key issue guiding the development of the intervention was the recognition of the power of peer influence for young gay men and the value of developing a peer-based intervention. For example, in preliminary longitudinal research with young gay men, increases in perceptions that the social norms of one's peers favored safe sex was the strongest predictor of young men changing, over the course of a year, from high- to low-risk behaviors (Hays et al., 1992). A third guiding principle was the desire that the intervention serve a mobilizing and empowering function within the young gay men's community. Providing young gay men with a mechanism to design and implement the intervention activities seemed more likely to foster a sense of personal commitment to HIV prevention among the young men and a sense of ownership of the prevention activities. Finally, the intervention design used the theory of diffusion of innovations (Rogers & Shoemaker, 1983), which posits that members of a social system are most likely to adopt new behavioral practices (i.e., safer sex) based on favorable evaluations of the innovation conveyed to them by other similar and respected individuals. Therefore, community change occurs through a process of informal communication and modeling by peers within their interpersonal networks. The intervention was designed to create such a process through which young gay and bisexual men would actively communicate with each other about safer sex and encourage each other to practice it so that it would become the mutually accepted norm.

The intervention was implemented in Eugene, Oregon, a medium-sized community, and lasted for eight months. The program, called the Mpowerment Project, was designed for gay and bisexual men aged 18 to 29, and sought to promote a norm for safer sex through a variety of social, outreach, and small-group activities designed and run by peers. Consistent with the empowerment philosophy of the intervention, the project was administered by a "core group" of 12 to 15 young gay men in the community who, with other volunteers, coordinated and conducted all project activities. The core group, which met weekly, was empowered to make all project decisions, including the project name, the types of activities the project sponsored, the types of outreach activities they did, and the project materials developed. The core group was assisted by a Community Advisory Board, comprised of men and women from the AIDS, gay and lesbian, public health, and university communities, who met monthly with the core group to give advice about project activities. The community advisory board members also provided a link between the project and their respective organizations and generated ideas and support for continuing the project when the study ended.

The program included four main components: (1) formal peer outreach; (2) small-group sessions; (3) informal peer outreach; and (4) an ongoing publicity campaign. Formal outreach was conducted by the outreach team which was comprised of young gay male volunteers and was led by a peer outreach coordinator. The outreach team developed enjoyable, entertaining, and motivational activities in which to educate and encourage young men about safe sex, which they regularly performed at a gay bar and other community events for young gay men, such as university dances or the local gay pride festival. They also developed materials for distribution at their performances which included safe sex information, condoms, graphic images designed to give ideas for eroticizing low-risk activities, and invitations to Mpowerment activities. All outreach materials were designed by the young men themselves and used their natural language with explicit, erotic images. The outreach team continually changed its repertoire of activities.

Unlike older gay men, there are few social settings where young gay men can socialize. Therefore, a major aspect of the intervention's formal outreach was to create new settings and events that would attract young gay men at which safe sex could be promoted. The research project sponsored a wide variety of events designed to appeal to each segment of the young gay men's community. These activities included rap groups, picnics, weekly video parties, house parties, hikes, and so on, and a series of large dance parties, called "Club M," which each attracted two hundred to three hundred young gay men. These events were designed to be enjoyable social events but each event emphasized safe sex promotion (i.e., a theatrical performance). The project office, which was centrally located in a convenient and accessible part of town, served as a community drop-in center for young gay and bisexual men. Regular office hours were maintained and young gay and bisexual men were encouraged to socialize there and were invited to volunteer to be active in working on some component of the project.

The second major component of the project was to offer small-group sessions, which were called "M-groups." These groups were peer-led, single-session meetings of 8 to 10 young gay or bisexual men that lasted two to three hours. Group sessions were usually held at the project center but occasionally they were held in participants' homes or other locations convenient for young men. Preliminary research identified several factors that contributed to unsafe sex among young gay and bisexual men and these factors were targeted as variables to influence in the small groups: clearing up misconceptions about safer sex; increasing the enjoyment of safer sex; building communication skills for negotiating safer sex; and addressing interpersonal issues that may interfere with safe sex. In addition, since it was recognized that not all high-risk-taking men were likely to attend a group session, the groups also provided training in how the participants might informally communicate with their friends outside the group to encourage them to practice safer sex. The format of the group session, developed through a series of focus groups with young gay and bisexual men, was designed to be fun and interactive, and included structured exercises, informal discussion, and role-plays. The groups were promoted as a enjoyable way for young gay and bisexual men to meet other young men, find out about the project, and hear how other young men were dealing with social issues of importance to them, such as sex, dating, and relationships. All men who were interested in being involved were encouraged to attend a group as entry into the project.

Also, the small-group sessions were designed to motivate and train participants to encourage their friends to have safer sex through informal peer outreach. Similar to previous studies (Kelly, St. Lawrence, Hood, & Brasfield, 1989), an attempt was made to develop a process of social diffusion that promotes safer sex among gay men in the community. The facilitators introduced the topic by stating the importance of encouraging their friends to engage in safer sex, and then discussed with the group specific ways they could encourage their friends. Participants then role-played two scenarios that gave the opportunity to practice encouraging friends. The facilitators asked the participants to each make a commitment to invite several of their friends to an M-group and provided them with M-group invitations and safer sex packages to give to their friends. The facilitators concluded the groups by inviting the participants to become involved with the Mpowerment Project and announced upcoming project events and volunteer opportunities. Participants were given badges with the project logo which they were asked to wear to show their support for the project and its mission. It was hoped that wearing the badges might also trigger conversations among their acquaintances about the project and also serve as a reminder for young men about the norm for safer sex that the project was seeking to establish.

The fourth component of the program was an ongoing publicity campaign about the project and its activities within the gay community, which included articles and advertisements in the gay newspaper, posters and fliers in settings frequented by young gay men, and "word of mouth" among core group members and their informal social networks. The publicity campaign was intended to establish an awareness and legitimacy of the program, invite young men to become involved with the program and its activities, and provide a continual reminder of the norm for safer sex within the young gay men's community. The program was not advertised via publicity channels of the mainstream community (e.g., local newspaper, radio, television, etc.) because it was felt that if the project became known within the general community as a program for young gay men, young men who were not comfortable being associated with a publicly gay-identified organization would be reluctant to become involved.

The community mobilization process was designed to be self-perpetuating and set in motion an ever-widening diffusion process by which young men communicated with each other about HIV risk-reduction. Given the ongoing and multifaceted nature of the intervention activities, it was hoped that virtually all young gay men in the community would be reached via at least one of the intervention activities. Ideally, the majority of young gay men would be reached with several risk-reduction messages through several sources, thus increasing the likelihood that the message would ultimately be internalized. The intervention lasted for eight months.

To evaluate the intervention, a longitudinal cohort of young gay and bisexual men from Eugene (n = 193) and a control community, Santa Barbara, California (n = 110) was assessed pre- and postintervention via mail-back surveys (73% return rate). Participants were recruited into the cohort by teams of local young gay men who distributed surveys in social settings frequently visited by young gay and bisexual men, including bars, university and community settings, and through their informal social networks. Follow-up surveys were mailed to the participants, who were asked to complete the questionnaire at their convenience and mail it back in the self-addressed, stamped envelopes provided. They were reimbursed $10 each time they completed the survey, which was widely publicized within the gay community to establish its legitimacy. It was presented as focusing on a broad range of topics of importance to young men, including coming out, relationships, sexuality, and AIDS. Of particular relevance to the intervention evaluation were measures of: sexual behavior in the previous two months; psychosocial variables that have been found to be causally related to HIV risk-taking among young gay and bisexual men; and participation in various project activities.

Following the intervention, rates of unprotected anal intercourse in the intervention community were found to decrease from 40% to 31%, while rates remained stable in the control community (39% and 40%). In addition, important psychosocial mediating variables demonstrated improvements in the intervention community compared to the control community. After the intervention, young men in the intervention city reported decreased enjoyment of unprotected anal intercourse, greater ability to avoid high-risk sex when aroused, and improved sexual communication skills with sexual partners than young men in the control city. Also, analyses were conducted to determine which of the various intervention activities actually reached the most high-risk men. The greatest proportion of high-risk-taking men (those who reported engaging in unprotected anal intercourse at the baseline assessment) were reached by formal outreach events conducted at bars and community events, by the large social events, and by receiving informal outreach from friends of theirs who attended small-group sessions. As might be expected, the high risk men were less likely to attend a safe sex workshop or to become actively involved in the project by volunteering. Nevertheless, the small groups were effective in increasing the degree to which participants encouraged their friends to engage in safer sex.

CONCLUSIONS

Despite remarkable reductions in the HIV risk behaviors of urban gay men, there are few intervention studies to identify the causes responsible for those changes. Of those available, interventions that are broader in scope and attempt to influence information, motivation, and behavioral skills appear to produce behavior change. It is difficult, however, to compare across studies due to the lack of consistency in the measurement of high-risk behavior and the varying time periods assessed. It would facilitate cross-comparisons if all researchers would report the combined total percentage of their participants engaging in unprotected anal intercourse, in addition to percentages engaging in insertive and receptive intercourse. Studies involve many limitations such as: lack of a theoretical basis; neglect of elicitation research; self-selection bias in subject recruitment; absence of data on men who are ethnic minority, lower-income, young, or outside AIDS epicenters; inadequate control groups to assess historical trends; reliance on self-report measures; failure to measure presumed mediating factors; and susceptibility to demand characteristics.

Despite these problems, some convincing findings are evident. Peers have been shown to be highly effective in conveying HIV-related information and serve as credible behavior change models. Approaches that use peers also tap into the enhanced credibility, identification, and normative influence of peers as persuasive sources and are consistent with research in the community and organizational literature on the value of involving people in the solutions to their own problems. The importance of targeting social norms, including skills-training, is clear, and peer support appears superior to information only approaches.

Risk reduction campaigns have been designed at both a community- and individual-level. Community-level interventions provide individuals with information and skills through channels of influence indigenous to a community. Diffusion approaches have the potential to reach large numbers of high-risk men with cost-effective, inexpensive, community-wide campaigns. The underlying assumption is that individuals are more likely to initiate and maintain healthful behaviors when: (1) a variety of avenues are used to inform and motivate; (2) specific strategies are used to teach skills needed for low-risk activities; (3) specific health-diminishing behaviors become less socially acceptable in the community; and (4) perceived social sanctions are persistent, inescapable, and provided on a sufficiently regular basis. Small-group interventions provide an intensive, individual approach that can be useful to impact information, personal risk assessment, and skills training and may be especially useful for individuals who lack a gay community or formal gay institutions.

In the second decade of the HIV epidemic, risk reduction programs are still needed for urban gay and bisexual men. The difficulty of sustaining behavioral change prompts the need to continue prevention efforts for urban gay men to avoid relapses of unsafe sexual behavior. These men experience a wide range of profound stressors, including their own illness; sickness and death of friends and acquaintances; and decisions to take the HIV antibody test, which may influence their coping ability to avoid HIV high-risk behaviors. Also, urban gay men who are young or members of an ethnic minority are especially in need of risk reduction campaigns to help them modify their sexual life-style to prevent HIV infection. Those campaigns are warranted because of the high level of unsafe sex found in this group of men and their neglect in earlier prevention studies in large cities. Despite the decline in HIV seroconversions, the epidemic is far from over in the gay community and neither is the need for prevention services.

REFERENCES

Adib, S. M., Joseph, J. G., Ostrow, D. G., & James, S. A. (1991). Predictors of relapse in sexual practices among homosexual men. *AIDS Education & Prevention, 3,* 293–304.

Ames, L. J., & Beeker, C. (1990). *Gay men in small cities: How risky are they?* Paper presented at 6th International Conference on AIDS, San Francisco.

Aspinwall, L. G., Kemeny, M. E., Taylor, S. E., Schneider, S. G., & Dudley, J. P. (1991). Psychosocial predictors of gay men's AIDS risk reduction behavior. *Health Psychology, 10*, 432–444.

Becker, M. H., & Joseph, J. G. (1988). AIDS and behavioral change to reduce risk: A review. *American Journal of Public Health, 78*, 394–410.

Calabrese, L. H., Harris, B., & Easley, K. (1987). *Analysis of variables impacting on safe sexual behavior among homosexual men in an area of low incidence for AIDS.* Paper presented at 3rd International Conference on AIDS, Washington, DC.

Catania, J. A., Coates, T. J., Kegeles, S. M., Ekstrand, M., & Guydish, J. (1988). Implications of the AIDS risk reduction model for the gay community: The importance of perceived sexual enjoyment and help-seeking behaviors. In V. Mays, G. Albee, J. Jones, J. Schneider (Eds.), *Psychological approaches to the prevention of AIDS* (pp. 242–261). Beverly Hills: Sage.

Catania, J. A., Coates, T. J., Stall, R., Bye, L., Kegeles, S. M., Capell, F., Henne, J., McKusick, L., Morin, S., Turner, H., & Pollack, L. (1991). Changes in condom use among homosexual men in San Francisco. *Health Psychology, 10*, 190–199.

Catania, J. A., Gibson, D., Chitwood, D., & Coates, T. J. (1990). Methodological problems in AIDS behavioral research. *Psychological Bulletin, 108*, 339–362.

Catania, J. A., Kegeles, S. M., & Coates, T. J. (1990). Toward an understanding of risk behavior: An AIDS risk reduction model. *Health Education Quarterly, 17*, 53–72.

Centers for Disease Control and Prevention (1993). *HIV/AIDS Surveillance: Year-End Edition.* Washington, DC: U.S. Public Health Service.

Centers for Disease Control (1990). Estimates of HIV prevalence and projected AIDS cases: Summary of workshop, October 31–November 1, 1989. *Morbidity and Mortality Weekly Report, 39*, 10–119.

Coates, T. J. (1990). Strategies for modifying sexual behavior for primary and secondary prevention of HIV disease. *Journal of Consulting & Clinical Psychology, 58*, 57–69.

Coates, T. J., Stall, R. D., Catania, J. A., & Kegeles, S. M. (1988). Behavioral factors in the spread of HIV infection. *AIDS, 2*(suppl. 1), 239–246.

Cochran, S. D., Mays, V. M., Ciarletta, J., Caruso, C., & Mallon, D. (1992). Efficacy of the theory of reasoned action in predicting AIDS-related sexual risk reduction among gay men. *Journal of Applied Social Psychology, 22*, 1481–1501.

Curran, J. W., Jaffe, H. W., Hardy, A. M., Morgan, W. M., Selik, R. M., & Dondero, T. J. (1988). Epidemiology of HIV infection and AIDS in the United States. *Science, 239*, 610–616.

Doll, L. S., Byers, R. H., Bolan, G., Douglas, J. M., Moss, P. M., Weller, P. D., Joy, D., Bartholow, B. N., & Harrison, J. S. (1991). Homosexual men who engage in high-risk sexual behavior: A multi-center comparison. *Sexually Transmitted Diseases, 18*, 170–175.

Doll, L. S., Peterson, L. R., White, C. R., Johnson, E. S., Ward, J. W., & The Blood Donor Study Group (1991). Homosexually and nonhomosexually identified men who have sex with men: A behavioral comparison. *Journal of Sex Research, 29*, 1–14.

Ekstrand, M. L., & Coates, T. J. (1990). Maintenance of safer sexual behaviors and predictors of risky sex: The San Francisco Men's Health Study. *American Journal of Public Health, 80*, 973–977.

Emmons, C., Joseph, J. G., Kessler, R. C., Wortman, D. B., Montgomery, S. B., & Ostrow, D. G. (1986). Psychological predictors of reported behavior change in homosexual men at risk for AIDS. *Health Education Quarterly, 13*, 331–345.

Exner, T. M., Meyer-Bahlburg, H. F., & Ehrhardt, A. A. (1992). Sexual self control as a mediator of high risk sexual behavior in a New York City cohort of HIV+ and HIV− gay men. *The Journal of Sex Research, 29,* 389–406.

Flowers, J. V., Booraem, C., Miller, T. E., Iverson, A. E., Copeland, J., & Furtado, K. (1991). Comparison of the results of a standardized AIDS prevention program in three geographic locations. *AIDS Education & Prevention, 3,* 189–196.

Folkman, S., Chesney, M. C., Pollack, L., & Phillips, C. (1992). Stress, coping and high risk sexual behavior. *Health Psychology, 11,* 218–222.

Fox, R., Odaka, N. J., Brookmeyer, R., & Polk, B. F. (1987). Effect of HIV antibody disclosure on subsequent sexual activity in homosexual men. *AIDS, 1,* 241–246.

Hansfield, H. H. (1985). Decreasing incidence of gonorrhea in homosexually active men—minimal effect of risk of AIDS. *Western Journal of Medicine, 143,* 469–470.

Hays, R. B., Catania, J. A., McKusick, L., & Coates, T. J. (1990). Help-seeking for AIDS-related concerns: A comparison of gay men with various HIV diagnoses. *American Journal of Community Psychology, 18,* 743–755.

Hays, R. B., Kegeles, S. M., & Coates, T. J. (1990). High HIV risk taking among young gay men. *AIDS, 4,* 901–907.

Hays, R. B., Kegeles, S. M., & Coates, T. J. (1991). Understanding the high rates of HIV risk-taking among young gay and bisexual men: The young men's survey. Paper presented at the 7th International Conference on AIDS, Florence, Italy.

Hays, R. B., Kegeles, S. M., & Coates, T. J. (1992). Changes in peer norms and sexual enjoyment predict changes in sexual risk-taking among young gay men. Paper presented at 8th International Conference on AIDS, Amsterdam, The Netherlands.

Higgins, D. L., Galavotti, C., O'Reilly, K. R., Schnell, D. J., Moore, M., Rugg, D. L., & Johnson, R. (1991). Evidence for the effects of HIV antibody counseling and testing on risk behaviors. *Journal of the American Medical Association, 266,* 2419–2428.

Honnen, T. J., & Kleinke, C. L. (1990). Prompting bar patrons with signs to take free condoms. *Journal of Applied Behavioral Analysis, 23,* 215–217.

Joseph, J. G., Montgomery, S. B., Emmons, C., Kiracht, J. P., Kessler, R. C., Ostrow, D. G., Wortman, C. B., & O'Brien, K. (1987). Perceived Risk of AIDS: Assessing the behavioral and psychosocial consequences in a cohort of gay men. *Journal of Applied Social Psychology, 17,* 231–250.

Joseph, K. M., Adib, S. M., Joseph, J. G., & Tal, M. (1991). Gay identity and risky sexual behavior related to the AIDS threat. *Journal of Community Health, 16,* 287–297.

Kegeles, S. M., Hays, R. B., & Coates, T. J. (1993, June). *A community-level risk reduction intervention for young gay and bisexual men.* Paper presented at 8th International Conference on AIDS, Amsterdam.

Kelly, J. A., St. Lawrence, J. S., Brasfield, T. L., Stevenson, Y. L., Diaz, Y. Y., & Hauth, A. C. (1990). AIDS risk behavior patterns among gay men in small southern cities. *American Journal of Public Health, 80,* 416–418.

Kelly, J. A., St. Lawrence, J. S., Hood, H. V., & Brasfield, T. L. (1989). Behavioral intervention to reduce AIDS risk activities. *Journal of Consulting & Clinical Psychology, 57,* 60–67.

Kelly, J. A., St. Lawrence, J. S., Betts, R., Brasfield, T. L., & Hood, H. V. (1990). A skills-training group intervention model to assist persons in reducing risk behaviors for HIV infection. *AIDS Education & Prevention, 2,* 24–35.

Kingsley, L. A., Bacella, H., Zhou, S. Y. J., Rinaldo, C., Chmiel, J., Detels, R., Saah, A., Van Raden, M., Ho, M., Armstrong, J., & Mernoz, A. (1990, June). *Temporal trends in HIV seroconversion: A report from the Multicenter AIDS Cohort Study (MACS).* Paper presented at the 6th International Conference on AIDS, San Francisco.

Levine, M. (1992). The life and death of gay clones. In G. Herdt (Ed.), *Gay culture in America: Essays from the field* (pp. 68–86). Boston: Beacon Press.

Leviton, L. C., Valdiserri, R. O., Lyter, D. W., Callahan, C. M., Kingsley, L. A., Huggins, J., & Rinaldo, C. R. (1990). Preventing HIV infection in gay and bisexual men: Experimental evaluation of attitude change from two risk reduction interventions. *AIDS Education & Prevention, 2,* 95–108.

Martin, J. L., Garcia, M. A., & Beatrice, S. T. (1989a). Sexual behavior changes and HIV antibody in a cohort of New York City gay men. *American Journal of Public Health, 79,* 501–503.

Martin, L., Dean, L., Garcia, M., & Hall, W. (1989b). The impact of AIDS on a gay community: Changes in sexual behavior, substance use and mental health. *American Journal of Community Psychology, 17,* 269–293.

McCusker, J., Stoddard, A. M., Mayer, K. H., Zapka, J., Morrison, C., & Saltzman, S. P. (1988). Effects of HIV antibody test knowledge on subsequent sexual behaviors in a cohort of homosexually active men. *American Journal of Public Health, 78,* 462–467.

McCusker, J., Stoddard, A. M., Zapka, J. G., Zorn, M., & Mayer, K. H. (1989). Predictors of AIDS-preventive behavior among homosexually active men: A longitudinal study. *AIDS, 3,* 443–448.

McCusker, J., Westenhouse, J., Stoddard, A. M., Zapka, J. G., Zorn, M. W., & Mayer, K. H. (1990). Use of drugs and alcohol by homosexually active men in relation to sexual practices. *Journal of Acquired Immune Deficiency Syndromes, 3,* 729–736.

McKirnan, D. J., & Peterson, P. L. (1989). AIDS-risk behavior among homosexual males: The role of attitudes and substance abuse. *Psychology & Health, 3,* 161–171.

McKusick, L., Coates, T. J., Morin, S., Pollack, L., & Hoff, C. (1990). Longitudinal predictors of reductions in unprotected anal intercourse among gay men in San Francisco: The AIDS Behavioral Research Project. *American Journal of Public Health, 80,* 1–8.

McKusick, L., Horstman, W., & Coates, T. J. (1985). AIDS and sexual behavior reported by gay men in San Francisco. *American Journal of Public Health, 75,* 493–496.

McKusick, L., Wiley, J., Coates, T. J., Stall, R., Saika, G., Morin, S., Charles, K., Horstman, W., & Conant, M. (1985). Reported changes in the sexual behavior of men at risk for AIDS, San Francisco, 1982–1984: The AIDS Behavioral Research Project. *Public Health Reports, 100,* 622–629.

Miller, T. E., Booraem, C., Flowers, J. V., & Iverson, A. E. (1990). Changes in knowledge, attitudes, and behavior as a result of a community-based AIDS prevention program. *AIDS Education & Prevention, 2,* 12–23.

National Research Council (1993). *The social impact of AIDS in the United States.* Washington, DC: National Academy Press.

Osmond, D. H., Page, K., Wiley, J., Garrett, K., Sheppard, H. W., Moss, A. R., Schrager, L., & Winkelstein, W. (1993, June). Human immunodeficiency virus infection in homosexual/bisexual men, ages 18–29. The San Francisco Young Men's Health Study. Paper presented at the 9th International AIDS Conference, Berlin, Germany.

Peterson, J., Coates, T., Catania, J., Hilliard, B., Middleton, L., & Hearst, N. (in press). Help-seeking for AIDS high risk behavior. *AIDS Education and Prevention.*

Peterson, J. L., Coates, T. J., Catania, J. A., Middleton, L., Hilliard, B., & Hearst, N. (1992). High-risk sexual behavior and condom use among gay and bisexual African American men. *American Journal of Public Health, 82,* 1490–1494.

Peterson, J. L. & Marin, G. (1988). Issues in the prevention of AIDS among Black and Hispanic men. *American Psychologist, 43,* 871–877.

Roffman, R. A., Gordon, J. R., Beadnell, B. A., Stern, M., Craver, J. N., Douglass, F., & Simpson, D. (1989, November). *Reaching gay and bisexual men who continue to engage in unsafe sexual activity: A comparison of subjects recruited for in-person or telephone counseling formats.* Paper presented at the 23rd Annual Convention of the Association for Advancement of Behavior Therapy, Washington, D.C.

Rogers, E. M. (1983). *Diffusion of innovations* (3rd Ed.). New York: Free Press.

Ruefli, T., Yu, O., & Barton, J. (1992). Sexual risk-taking in smaller cities: The case of Buffalo, New York. *The Journal of Sex Research, 29,* 95–108.

Samuel, M., & Winkelstein, W. Jr. (1987). Prevalence of human immunodeficiency virus infection in ethnic minority homosexual/bisexual men. *Journal of the American Medical Association, 257,* 1901–1902.

San Francisco Department of Public Health (1989). Continued seroconversion for HIV antibody among homosexual and bisexual men. *San Francisco Epidemiology Bulletin, 5,* 35–37.

Schechter, M. T. (1988). Patterns of sexual behavior and condom use in a cohort of homosexual men. *American Journal of Homosexual Men, 78,* 1535–1538.

Shernoff, M., & Bloom, D. J. (1991). Designing effective AIDS prevention workshops for gay and bisexual men. *AIDS Education & Prevention, 3,* 31–46.

Siegel, K., Mesagno, F. P., Chen, J. Y., & Christ, G. (1989). Factors distinguishing homosexual males practicing risky and safer sex. *Social Science & Medicine, 28,* 561–569.

Silvestre, A. J., Lyter, D. W., Valdiserri, R. O., Huggins, J., & Rinaldo, C. R. (1989). Factors related to seroconversion among homo- and bisexual men after attending a risk-reduction educational session. *AIDS, 3,* 647–650.

Smucny, J., Hom, D., Ellner, J. J., Carey, J. T., Houser, H. B., Calabrese, L. H., Edmonds, K., Bowerfind, E., Proffitt, M., Yen-Lieberman, B., Rehm, S., Wilson, T. R., & Lederman, M. M. (1992). Risk factors for HIV infection in homosexual men: The Cleveland Men's Study of Risks in a Low-Prevalence Area. *Cleveland Clinic Journal of Medicine, 59,* 573–580.

St. Lawrence, J. S., Hood, H. V., Brasfield, T., & Kelly, J. A. (1989). Risk knowledge and risk behavior among gay men in high vs. low AIDS prevalence areas. *Public Health Reports, 104,* 391–396.

Stall, R., Barrett, D., Bye, L., Catania, J., Frutchey, C., Henne, J., Lemp, G., & Paul, J. (1992). A comparison of younger and older gay men's HIV risk-taking behaviors: The Communication Technologies 1989 Cross-Sectional Survey. *Journal of Acquired Immune Deficiency Syndromes, 5,* 682–687.

Stall, R. D., Coates, T. J., & Hoff, C. C. (1988). Behavioral risk reduction for HIV infection among gay and bisexual men: A comparison of published results from the United States. *American Psychologist, 43,* 859–864.

Stall, R. D., Ekstrand, M., Hoff, C., Paul, J., Catania, J., & Coates, T. (1993, June). *Early interventions for HIV infection among gay men in two secondary AIDS epicenters.* Paper presented at 9th International Conference on AIDS, Berlin.

Stall, R. D., McKusick, L., Wiley, J., Coates, T., & Ostrow, D. (1986). Alcohol and drug use during sexual activity and compliance with safe sex guidelines for AIDS: The AIDS Behavioral Research Project. *Health Education Quarterly, 13,* 359–371.

Valdiserri, R. O., Lyter, D. W., Kingsley, L. A., Leviton, L. C., Schofield, J. W., Huggins, J., Ho, M., & Rinaldo, C. R. (1987). The effect of group education on improving attitudes about AIDS risk reduction. *New York State Journal of Medicine, 87,* 272–278.

Valdiserri, R. O., Lyter, D., Leviton, L. C., Callahan, C. M., Kingsley, L. A., & Rinaldo, C. R. (1988). Variables influencing condom use in a cohort of gay and bisexual men. *American Journal of Public Health, 78,* 801–805.

Valdiserri, R. O., Lyter, D. W., Leviton, L. C., Callahan, C. M., Kingsley, L. A., & Rinaldo, C. R. (1989). AIDS prevention in homosexual and bisexual men: Results of a randomized trial evaluating two risk reduction interventions. *AIDS, 3,* 21–26.

Van Raden, M., Kaslow, R., & Kingsley, L. (1988). Incidence and nonsexual risk factors for recent HIV infection in homosexual men. Paper presented at the 4th International Conference on AIDS, Stockholm.

Winkelstein, W. (1988). The San Francisco Men's Health Study: Continued decline in HIV seroconversion rates among homosexual/bisexual men. *American Journal of Public Health, 78,* 1472–1474.

Winkelstein, W., Samuel, M., & Padian, N. (1987). The San Francisco Men's Health Study, III: Reduction in human immunodeficiency virus transmission among homosexual/bisexual men, 1982–86. *American Journal of Public Health, 77,* 685–689.

15

HIV Prevention among Gay and Bisexual Men in Small Cities

JEFFREY A. KELLY

INTRODUCTION

One consequence of the emergence of the human immunodeficiency virus (HIV) epidemic over a decade ago among homosexually active men in the largest American cities is that most behavioral research on acquired immunodeficiency syndrome (AIDS) involving gay and bisexual men has been conducted primarily in urban centers. To a very large extent, what we know about gay men's HIV risk patterns and changes made in behavior in response to AIDS is based upon studies conducted in New York, San Francisco, Chicago, Los Angeles, and a handful of other urban areas traditionally considered as "AIDS epicenters." Further, behavior change conclusions are often based upon a relatively small number of volunteer cohorts longitudinally followed in those cities. While it is understandable, and was certainly appropriate, to intensively study gay men's risk behavior in areas where the HIV epidemic struck earliest and most harshly, a byproduct of this focus is that we still know very little about behavior patterns, behavior changes, and intervention approaches pertinent to HIV prevention in other geographical areas. To a large extent, behavioral research to date on HIV risk among gay men is in fact behavioral research among gay men from San Francisco, New York, and Chicago. These findings from urban gay men may or may not be generalizable to homosexually active men who live in smaller cities.

Approximately 59% of AIDS cases diagnosed to date in the United States have occurred in areas of the country *other than* the 10 largest American

JEFFREY A. KELLY • Department of Psychiatry and Mental Health Sciences, Medical College of Wisconsin, Milwaukee, Wisconsin 53226.

Preventing AIDS: Theories and Methods of Behavioral Interventions, edited by Ralph J. DiClemente and John L. Peterson. Plenum Press, New York, 1994.

cities plus San Francisco (Centers for Disease Control, 1993b). Thus, while AIDS is widely considered an enormously serious threat in our largest urban cities, the HIV epidemic is also an enormously serious but often unrecognized threat in our moderate size and smaller cities. Human immunodeficiency virus seroprevalence is believed to be approximately 50% among gay men in San Francisco and approximately 40% among gay men in New York (Anderson & Levy, 1985; Curran et al., 1988; Martin, Garcia, & Beatrice, 1989), and has remained essentially at that level for a number of years. By contrast, limited data from samples of gay men in smaller cities indicate that HIV seroprevalence is still considerably lower; seroprevalence estimates range from 9% upwards among homosexually active men in small to moderate size American cities (Curran et al., 1988; Kelly et al., 1992), with the lowest rates usually found in the smallest cities. As we will discuss shortly, there is considerable reason to believe that high-risk sexual behavior rates also remain elevated among many gay men in smaller cities. In the context of high but stable HIV seroprevalence and reduced rates of sexual risk behaviors among urban gay men, and moderate rising HIV prevalence but high rates of sexual risk behaviors among smaller-city gay men, we face the prospect of a sharp increase in new HIV infections among gay and bisexual men in areas not traditionally considered AIDS epicenters. The front line for HIV primary prevention among gay men may now have shifted from large urban centers to smaller cities where, if infection prevalence is to remain relatively low, behavior change prevention efforts are now urgently needed.

At the outset in any discussion of HIV prevention in smaller cities, there arises the question of what constitutes a small city. One consideration is a city's population size, although this leads to relative judgments about the meaning of "small." The population level at which a city becomes small is often in the eye of the beholder. Beyond and probably more important than population size, HIV prevention efforts among gay men outside our largest cities is likely to be influenced by the AIDS prevention resources available in a community, cohesiveness of an identifiable gay community or the social networks within that community; and the presence and nature of social meeting places. Other factors include the adequacy of gay-sensitive public health and community-based HIV prevention programs; level of community empowerment or social structures; geographic proximity to urban centers; and local experience with AIDS including AIDS deaths, gay community perceptions about HIV/AIDS, and HIV seroprevalence. There are undoubtedly cities with relatively small populations but with the social characteristics of cities much larger in size, and there are undoubtedly cities with relatively large populations that appear, in terms of AIDS-pertinent social characteristics, much like smaller cities. Rather than arbitrarily setting size criteria for what constitutes a small city, this chapter will simply focus on behavior change interventions that have been undertaken in geographical areas not traditionally considered to be AIDS epicenters.

HIV RISK BEHAVIOR LEVELS AMONG SMALL-CITY GAY MEN

Cohorts of gay men were established in the early 1980s and have been intensively followed in longitudinal AIDS behavioral research studies for over 10 years in several large cities. By contrast, almost all research examining the HIV risk characteristics of homosexually active men in smaller cities has relied on cross-sectional sampling of convenience groups. This is probably attributable to a lack of resources for constructing cohorts derived by representatively sampling gay men, as well as the much more dispersed, hidden, and often closeted nature of gay men in many nonurban areas that makes it very difficult to locate and engage truly representative community samples in long-term cohort studies. Results of studies derived from convenience samples must be interpreted cautiously, especially when attempting to generalize to different community subsets.

A series of studies by Kelly and colleagues has examined HIV risk behavior patterns among men patronizing gay bars in both small and moderate sized American cities. Kelly, St. Lawrence, Brasfield, Stevenson et al. (1990) administered risk behavior questionnaires to men entering gay bars in three small southern cities. Twenty-four percent of respondents reported having had unprotected anal intercourse in the past two months; of those men who engaged in high-risk behavior, unprotected anal intercourse occurred an average of six times in the two-month retrospective period. A similar survey conducted in late 1988 in somewhat larger cities (including Seattle, Tampa, and Mobile) found that 37% of respondents had engaged in unprotected anal intercourse in the previous three months, with risk level most strongly predicted by peer norms concerning the social acceptability of safer sex practices, AIDS health locus of control, age, and accuracy of personal risk estimation but not personal HIV serostatus knowledge (Kelly, St. Lawrence, Brasfield, Lemke et al., 1990). Similar predictors of risk were found by Kelly, Kalichman et al. (1991) in a study of 470 gay men in convenience samples drawn from community social organizations and bars in Memphis, Tampa, Mobile, and Biringhampton, New York; 45% of these men reported having unprotected anal intercourse in the previous six months. To ascertain whether these high rates of risk behavior might be attributable to the behavior of men involved in primary relationships or relationships between partners of known serostatus, questions in these areas were also included. Nearly 60% of men reporting unprotected anal intercourse said it occurred with a nonexclusive partner, and in only 17% of cases did the respondent have firsthand knowledge that both he and the partner were tested and were HIV negative.

In the most extensive study to date examining HIV risk among gay men in small cities, nearly 2,000 men entering gay bars in 16 cities with populations under 200,000 in four different regions of the country were surveyed in 1992 to assess risk behaviors and HIV serostatus testing history (Kelly, Murphy, Roffman et al., 1992). Eighty-five percent of all men entering clubs completed the measures. Nearly one-third of respondents indicated that they had engaged in unprotected anal intercourse an average of eight times in the past two months, usually outside of exclusive long-term relationships. High-risk behavior was associated particularly with beliefs that insistence on safer sex practices would not be well accepted by peers, weak intentions to use condoms, underestimation of personal risk, younger age, and higher overall levels of sexual activity. Approximately 68% of the small-city men reported that they had been tested for HIV antibodies, and approximately 9% of the men tested said they were seropositive.

These data establish risk behavior levels among small-city gay men much higher than those reported among participants in AIDS behavioral research cohorts during approximately the same period of time (Ekstrand & Coates, 1990; Martin et al., 1989). For example, approximately 10% of San Francisco gay men enrolled in risk behavior study cohorts reported engaging in unprotected anal intercourse over the past year (Ekstrand & Coates, 1990) at about the same time period when the prevalence of risk behavior was 24 to 45% in the past two to three months among small-city gay men in the studies just described. This provides evidence that gay men in small and moderate sized communities remain at much higher HIV risk than their large-city counterparts who have exhibited substantial behavior changes over the past decade.

Major sampling and methodology differences complicate these comparative interpretations. Because studies of risk behavior among small-city gay men have typical relied heavily on sampling in bars—often the only organized center of open socializing for gay men in smaller cities—it is not clear to what extent the high-risk levels found among men in those studies are characteristic of all gay men in these cities or only those men who patronize bars. Stall, Ekstrand, Paul, McKusick, and Coates (1993) surveyed both gay bar patrons and gay men sampled through household telephone surveys in Tucson, Arizona and Portland, Oregon in 1992 and found significantly higher risk levels among gay men sampled from bars than those sampled from household telephone calls. For example, 24% of Portland gay men recruited in bars reported having unprotected anal intercourse with a nonprimary partner in the past year compared to 15% among men sampled in the household survey (Stall, et al., 1993). Even within bar samples, risk levels appear related to a city's geographical proximity to a major AIDS epicenter. St. Lawrence, Hood, Brasfield, and Kelly (1989) found HIV risk behavior levels lowest (and risk knowledge highest) among gay men surveyed in large-city bars, and established increasing rates of risk behavior among bar patrons sampled and assessed in the same way in cities progressively smaller and more geographically distant from the large epicenter city. For example 35% of all sexual acts in the past two months reported by small-city gay men involved unprotected anal intercourse, while only 13% of the sexual activities of AIDS epicenter men involved this activity. The most commonly occurring homosexual activity reported by AIDS epicenter men was mutual masturbation, a very low-risk practice. In contrast, one of the most common homosexual behaviors among small-city men was unprotected anal intercourse.

The question of how much higher risk behavior levels are among gay men in small cities relative to their counterparts in New York or San Francisco, will be conclusively answered only by further studies which employ comparable sampling methods, survey items, and risk definitions, and retrospective time frames for assessing risk behavior. Until such studies are conducted, conclusions about risk behavior levels of gay men in small and moderate size cities must be interpreted recognizing the different sampling methods used. At present, we can conclude that sexual risk behavior levels are very high among gay men in small and moderate size cities who patronize bars, but are not yet as well established among other segments of the homosexually active population.

FACTORS INFLUENCING HIV PREVENTION IN SMALL CITIES

Small and moderate size cities often differ from large urban areas in ways that influence both HIV risk and the development of intervention programs intended to reduce risk among gay men. While all cities are not alike, we will discuss here several characteristics that appear common and must be taken into account when planning HIV prevention programs.

Level of Perceived Risk

In the gay communities of New York, San Francisco, and other cities with high prevalence of HIV infection for many years, most men know many people with AIDS and have lost many friends and acquaintances to the disease. The threat of the HIV epidemic is close, undeniable, and carries pervasive personal impact. Within the gay community of many smaller cities, HIV prevalence is lower and HIV infection was introduced later. As a result, gay men often know fewer peers with AIDS, are less continually reminded of its personal impact, and may perceive HIV/AIDS as a more distant threat.

Community Networks are Different in Small Cities than in Urban Centers

Within many large cities, there are extensive and established networks of gay community organizations and social meeting places, an active press and communication channels, and quite often neighborhoods with large gay residential concentrations. Particularly in San Francisco and New York, a history of community empowerment, visibility, and activism has resulted in political, health, and social structures responsive to needs of the gay community. These community networks, resources, and structures are rarely present in smaller cities where gay communities are often hidden, dispersed, and unorganized, and where the primary and sometimes only community structure is a gay bar. In the absence of tight cohesive social and communication networks, there are less efficient avenues for the dissemination of health and prevention information, mechanisms to change and disseminate social norms to promote risk behavior reduction, and methods to support behavior change efforts. Too often, political and public health entities in small city areas—especially in conservative regions of the country—appear unaware that there is a gay community, are disdainful of it, or are disinterested in HIV prevention. Several years ago, the author made contact with an AIDS task force in a southern city concerning development of an HIV prevention trial for gay men. Although the city had at least three gay bars, the directors of the local AIDS task force said the organization did not like to undertake HIV prevention programs with "homosexuals." Even when AIDS prevention efforts are initiated, the often closeted and unempowered nature of the gay community in some small cities limits the effectiveness of these efforts. The author also knew of an instance when a health department speaker in a small city gave a talk on AIDS in a bar with only a few people present. Although the event had been well publicized, many people were apparently unwilling to attend and be identified as gay by a health department official in a town where such public knowledge could result in considerable stigma and harassment.

Inadequate Prevention Resources

In contrast to the large, visible, and well-funded AIDS prevention and service organizations long established in our largest cities, few smaller cities have major organizations with the resources or expertise to mount effective and sustained community HIV prevention campaigns. Funding for HIV prevention programs has been concentrated in large urban centers, and community-based small-city AIDS prevention organizations have typically had to rely primarily on proceeds from occasional bake sales, car washes, and drag shows to support their efforts.

Differing Community Value Systems

Many small or moderate size communities are located in regions with social and political values more conservative or traditional than are typical in larger urban centers. The dominant social values of a city are often also reflected within its gay community, so it would not be unexpected for many small-city gay men to have values regarding openness in social, political, and sexual matters that are relatively more conservative than those of their counterparts living in more urban areas. These factors, combined with intolerant general public attitudes, may contribute to a lack of community openness and cohesion within small-city gay populations. The level of conservatism within a gay community can also influence how various prevention approaches will be received. Some explicitly erotic safer sex campaigns appropriate and effective in a liberal and tolerant community may be considered awkward, embarrassing, or offensive, even to gay men, in more traditionally conservative areas.

Although these factors can constitute obstacles to the development of HIV prevention programs for gay men in smaller cities, they are not insurmountable and, in fact, present opportunities for innovative primary prevention campaigns which take into account the social characteristics of small and moderate size communities. For example, while there are rarely visible, organized gay residential and commercial neighborhoods, there are often close-knit social networks based on friendships, shared social activities, and places for socializing. Unlike in large urban areas, it is often possible to enumerate and identify almost all areas in a smaller city where gay men meet to socialize or seek sexual partners, and to construct ethnographic portrayals of the major social networks that operate these settings. These characteristics permit the focusing of HIV prevention campaigns within identified settings and social networks. To the extent that a community has very close-knit circles of friends and acquaintances, these social networks may carry considerable influence over the behavior of their members. For that reason, efforts to change risk behavior norms may be particularly efficient in such communities.

Finally, in urban areas hard hit by AIDS, gay communities have long been saturated with HIV educational campaigns and, we suspect, many people have become fatigued by AIDS prevention messages. Within many small and midsized cities, AIDS is still not "taken for granted" and there remains much interest in the gay community for learning about and taking part in HIV prevention efforts. In 1990, almost a decade after AIDS was first diagnosed, and after many years of sustained HIV prevention campaigns underway in large cities, members of the author's research group met to discuss development of an HIV prevention study with gay community leaders in a city with a population of nearly 100,000 people, a university, two gay bars, and a location only several hours from a major metropolitan center. In those initial meetings, we sought information on the history of AIDS prevention programs already undertaken in the city and were told that—to the best of anyone's knowledge— no public health authorities had ever offered HIV prevention program assistance in the city's gay community. As much as any experience we have had, this illustrated the urgent importance of developing HIV prevention efforts directed toward small city gay men.

INTERVENTIONS AND THEIR EFFECTIVENESS

In spite of the enormous quantity of behavioral research on AIDS published over the past decade, it remains striking that there have still been only a small handful of studies describing the behavior change impact of *any* HIV prevention intervention in a controlled evaluation. Clearly, AIDS prevention activities of many kinds are being undertaken in communities, large and small, throughout the county and the world. For the most part, however, these programs are being developed and undertaken without the benefit of a research base that has established the effectiveness of the approaches used and, as service efforts, community-based programs are rarely evaluated to determine behavior change outcomes. The paucity of outcome studies evaluating risk reduction interventions appearing to date in the literature would indicate that the behavioral science research community has yet to adequately address the most urgent and critical question in HIV primary prevention: What interventions most effectively help people make and maintain behavior changes to reduce their risk for contracting HIV infection?

In this section, behavior change intervention outcome research undertaken with gay or bisexual men in small cities will be reviewed. Although the number of controlled outcome trials is not large, results of this work have been relatively conclusive and can inform the development of new and more expanded trials. Intervention research to date can be subsumed under two general categories: interventions undertaken in face-to-face contact with individuals or groups and interventions that focus on community level change.

Face-to-Face Behavioral Interventions

The first report of a controlled outcome trial of a group behavioral risk reduction intervention for gay and bisexual men was reported by Kelly, St. Lawrence, Hood, and Brasfield (1989) and was conducted with 104 men living in a southern city with a population size of about 200,000. In the research, materials describing the availability of an AIDS risk reduction program were distributed in gay bars, at health department HIV testing clinics, and in talks given to informal gay-oriented social and community groups. Participants were men over age 21 who reported any high-risk sexual practices occurring during the past year. Men recruited in the study had a mean age of 31 years; 87% were white and 13% African-American or Hispanic. Participants reported an average of 16 same-sex partners in the previous 12 months, with a mean of 19 occurrences of unprotected anal insertive, and 18 occurrences of unprotected anal receptive, intercourse. Thus, the community sample recruited was at very high risk for HIV infection.

Prior to intervention, all participants completed individual assessments that included measures of AIDS risk knowledge, sexual practices occurring over the past four months, the same sexual practices occurring over the past two weeks, and role-play tests of behavioral skill for handling high-risk sexual coercion and pressure. Men were then randomly assigned to either an immediate intervention group or to a brief waiting list comparison condition. Men in the intervention condition attended a series of 12 weekly 75-minute group sessions. Following intervention, all participants from both conditions were reassessed and for ethical reasons the intervention was offered to men who had formerly been in the comparison group. Participants in the original intervention group continued to be followed for eight months to determine their maintenance of behavior change.

The intervention model tested in this research was based on social learning and cognitive–behavioral principles applied to the issue of high-risk sexual behavior change. In groups of 8 to 15 members, study participants first received HIV risk education intended to identify high-risk practices, to encourage risk reduction changes, and identify misconceptions about risk. This was followed by training in cognitive and behavioral strategies to manage potential risk triggers and guide self-change efforts. These efforts included making practical life routine changes (such as avoiding sex when drinking, avoiding settings associated with past risky encounters, keeping and carrying condoms, and practicing condom use) and practicing cognitive self-statements to guide and reinforce one's own change efforts. Participants also practiced sexual assertiveness and communication skills in role-play rehearsal exercises in which confederates simulated coercive risk pressures. The role-play situations practiced were based upon past situations reported as difficult by the men. The final intervention component employed group discussion and problem-solving strategies concerning themes related to the social context of change including establishing stable and steady relationships characterized by low-risk practices, pride and responsibility to protect others and to protect the gay community, involvement in affirmative community organizations, peer support for change, and dating. Most sessions employed skills training procedures including modeling, behavior rehearsal, feedback, and assignments to practice risk-reduction skills in real life with discussion of success or problems in the next group session. Over 80% of men who began the intervention completed all 12 sessions.

Kelly et al. (1989) found that, relative to persons who had been assigned to the comparison group, men in the intervention program showed a significant increase in risk knowledge, as well as improvement in objectively rated assertiveness and social skill in role-play enactments simulating response to coercive pressures to engage in unprotected intercourse or unwanted sex. Most important, intervention participants reduced their frequency of unprotected anal intercourse to near zero levels and increased their condom use from 23% to approximately 75% of all intercourse occasions. These changes, well maintained through eight-month follow-up, were corroborated by both reports of sexual behavior occurring over four-month retrospective intervals and before, after, and at follow-up to the intervention, and by ongoing self-monitoring records completed by each participant. Men also evaluated the program favorably with respect to its perceived usefulness and benefit.

Kelly, St. Lawrence, Betts, Brasfield, and Hood (1990) conducted a small-scale replication trial of an intervention similar to the project just described but in a more abbreviated seven-session group format and with a higher representation (20%) of ethnic minority participants. The study was also conducted in a small southern city, and employed entry criteria and outcome measures similar to those in the Kelly et al. (1989) research. This replication trial produced pre- to postintervention behavior changes comparable in nature and magnitude to the earlier 12-session intervention study: unprotected anal intercourse decreased from an average of 0.9 to 0.2 occurrences in four-month periods from before to after intervention; condom use increased from 72 to 90% of all intercourse occasions; and mean number of partners with whom high-risk practices occurred declined by 50% among intervention participants from baseline to follow-up. These findings indicate that cognitive–behavioral intervention at least relatively briefer (7 sessions) than the 12-session group program evaluated in the original study are also capable of producing substantial levels of behavior change.

While these studies confirm the efficacy of multiple-session group intervention for promoting sexual risk behavior change, our research team later conducted long-term, 24-month follow-up of original participants in the 12-session group intervention program to identify the proportion of small-city gay men who maintained change versus those who had risk behavior lapses, and to examine characteristics of successful change maintainers and of those men who were unsuccessful in their behavior change maintenance (Kelly, St. Lawrence, & Brasfield, 1990). Of positive significance was the fact that 60% of men originally at very high risk when entering the intervention study had no occurrences of unprotected anal intercourse even two years following their participation. However, 40% of men had experienced lapses during the two-year follow-up period. Men who were unsuccessful in maintaining change were younger, less well-educated, had more extensive histories of high-risk sexual behavior with multiple partners before intervention, and ascribed higher levels of enjoyment to past unprotected anal intercourse than those men who had successfully maintained behavior change (Kelly et al., 1990).

The studies just described offered risk reduction assistance to groups of gay men who attended intervention sessions. In an innovative variation of this approach, Roffman and his colleagues (Roffman, Beadnell, & Ryan, 1992; Roffman, Beadnell, Stern, Gordon, Downey, & Siever, 1991) are investigating the impact of a similar type of group cognitive–behavioral intervention but with services offered over the telephone. The rationale for risk reduction intervention by telephone is that it affords anonymity, can reach gay or bisexual men too closeted to attend face-to-face sessions, and—important from the perspective of this chapter's focus—allows men even from rural and isolated areas to participate in group intervention. In contrast to traditional AIDS education and information hotlines that focus primarily on basic education or answering caller questions, the approaches being tested in the Roffman et al. (1991, 1992) study involve caller participation in an ongoing, multiple-session cognitive–behavioral group intervention focused on making risk reduction change, with groups "meeting" together on multiple occasions by means of conference call technology. Although behavior change outcomes from the telephone counseling intervention have not yet been reported, the investigators have found that the intervention attracts a number of small-city rural men at high behavioral risk for HIV infection including those who are bisexual and report that they would be unwilling or unable to attend group intervention programs face to face.

Taken together, these findings indicate that small-city gay men in the study samples, who were engaged in cognitive–behavioral group intervention based on skills training principles, applied to sexual risk behavior reduction, made substantial and meaningful changes in their risk level. Even homosexually active men at very high initial risk due to patterns of having unprotected anal intercourse with multiple partners, were found in several of these studies to make very great levels of change. A relatively large subset of men also had difficulty sustaining those changes when followed for two years after intervention, and all HIV prevention intervention studies that rely on recruited volunteer participants may be enrolling persons who are unusually motivated and ready to make change.

In large urban areas hard hit by AIDS and subjected to ongoing HIV prevention and safer sex messages for many years, there has undoubtedly been a pervasive shift in gay community social norms toward safer sex as an expected behavior standard. In much the same way as shifts in social norms to discourage cigarette smoking have produced gradual declines in smoking rates in the general population, safer sex has become a predominant norm among many, but not all, urban gay men. Young gay men, those who are homosexually active but do not self-identify as gay, and ethnic minority homosexually active men still exhibit higher rates of unsafe sex even in large cities (Centers for Disease Control, 1993; Hays, Kegeles, & Coates, 1990; Peterson, Coates, Catania, Middleton, Hilliard, & Hearst, 1992). Nonetheless, change in social or peer norms driven by fear of AIDS, loss of friends to AIDS, and sustained educational campaigns in most urban gay communities have been associated with widescale reductions in risk behavior.

Within smaller cities, it is likely that sexual behavior norms have not yet changed to the same extent. In addition to the strong predictive relationships found between beliefs about the social acceptability of safer sex insistence and perceived risk behavior of peers with one's own level of sexual risk behavior among gay men in small city samples (Kelly, St. Lawrence, Brasfield, Lemke et al., 1990; Kelly, Murphy, Roffman et al., 1992), this research has also shown that small city gay men often have perceptions that safer sex is not yet an accepted social norm. For example, 54% of the men surveyed by Kelly, St. Lawrence, Brasfield, Lemke et al. (1990) said that their friends "talk about safer sex more than they practice it" and only 58% agreed with the statement that "safer sex is completely accepted by my friends." Consequently, and moving beyond face-to-face group interventions which are time-intensive and likely to reach only a relatively small number of people who volunteer to attend sessions, there is also a pressing need to develop more broad-based community-level interventions that can reach larger numbers of persons. Interventions that change norms within the gay communities of small cities to discourage high-risk behavior and encourage preventive behavior changes appear particularly important. In contrast to urban centers where norms favoring safer sex changed only after a large proportion of gay men had already contracted HIV infection and many had died of AIDS, behavior and sexual norm changes—if they can be produced quickly enough—may have greater potential to limit the prevalence of infection among gay men in small cities where HIV levels are still lower.

Community Level Interventions

Across a set of recent studies, the author's research team has conducted evaluated trials of community-level interventions intended to produced risk behavior change among populations of gay men in smaller cities. The work has been undertaken in small cities for reasons of both public health significance and research evaluation methodology. Since HIV risk behavior levels are often high, and HIV prevalence is increasing among homosexually active men in smaller cities, community intervention trials in these areas are of pressing public health importance. In addition, small cities that are geographically isolated from urban centers and that have relatively stable and non-transient populations, constitute environments in which change in community member behavior can be assessed with considerable reliability and sensitivity.

Earlier in the chapter, we noted that while small and moderate size cities usually lack the identifiable geographical "gay neighborhoods" and formal social organizational structures found in some urban centers that can serve as a focus for HIV prevention interventions, there are clearly many informal social influence and friendship networks. These networks often intersect at a gay bar. Although bars are places where people drink, small-city gay bars also constitute organized, stable, and genuine social communities probably to a much greater extent than most heterosexual bars, precisely because they are one of the only settings where gay men can gather freely to socialize. Because high rates of risk behavior have been established among men who patronize gay bars (Kelly, St. Lawrence, Brasfield, Stevenson et al., 1990; Kelly et al., 1991; Kelly, Murphy, Roffman et al., 1992; St. Lawrence et al., 1989; Stall et al., 1993), they also constitute relevant and ecologically valid settings in which to conduct community-level HIV prevention activities.

To the extent that gay men in small cities are linked within informal social influence networks rather than visible and identifiable geographic communities, prevention approaches that make use of social influence networks appear especially viable. In this regard, social diffusion models to promote behavior change are particularly promising. As articulated by Rogers (1983), diffusion is a process in which behavior changes or innovative trends are initially adopted by popular and well-regarded trend-setters; are modeled and communicated by trend-setters to those with whom they interact and who adopt the innovation early; and gradually but predictably diffuse throughout the population. How efficiently or quietly innovations diffuse depends upon the nature, complexity, and perceived benefits of the innovation; characteristics of trend-setters including their popularity and social credibility; and characteristics of the population including the tightness, cohesiveness, and efficiency of social influence networks linking population members (Bandura, 1986). As Bandura and as Fisher and Misovich (1990) have pointed out, the processes that lead population members to adopt innovations or new behaviors initially exhibited by trend-setters and early adopters, include social modeling, a desire to conform to the norms of members of one's peer reference group, and the expectation that behavior change adoption will produce social benefits and reinforcement. Although social diffusion theory has been used to explain how changes occur in a variety of behavioral phenomena ranging from farmers' adoption of new agricultural practices to trends in new clothing style and fashion, the model also appears logical for the development of community-level HIV prevention campaigns in which one seeks to encourage the adoption of new or innovative risk reduction behavior (such as avoiding anal intercourse, using condoms during intercourse, or engaging only in other forms of safer sex) that is not a strongly accepted present standard of behavior (cf. Bandura, 1986; Fisher & Misovich, 1990; Kelly & Murphy, 1992). In essence, this model holds promise for prompting the initiation of behavior change; creating a social environment in which maintenance of change efforts will be reinforced; and producing new reference group sexual behavior norms that make these risk reduction changes socially accepted, expected, and durable.

An early test of this model was undertaken by Kelly, St. Lawrence, Diaz et al. (1991). In three small cities in Mississippi and Louisiana, risk behavior surveys were administered to all men entering popular gay bars over two three-night survey periods separated by four-month intervals. The cities were selected because prior research had established high-risk behavior levels among gay men in them (Kelly, St. Lawrence, Brasfield, Stevenson et al., 1990), because each had one or two gay bars eager to cooperate with the HIV prevention study, and because the cities were geographically isolated and had relatively stable, nontransient patron populations. These factors permitted a close analysis and tracking of intervention effects on population risk behavior levels.

Following surveys to establish baseline population risk behavior levels among gay men patronizing bars in each city, a community intervention based on diffusion principles was introduced in one city. Bartenders in each club in the intervention city were asked to observe the crowd of people patronizing their bar over 10-day periods and to generate lists identifying those people each bartender felt was most popular and well-liked among gay men. Criteria of popularity were based on the bartenders' observations of how often potentially popular people were greeted by gay male peers, how much gay men in the clubs seemed to like or trust the individual, and the individual's perceived popularity standing among peers. Bartender nomination lists were cross-matched to identify those people who received multiple high popularity nominations, and this core group of popular people was recruited for participation in the intervention. The cadre of opinion leaders included both men and women, included approximately the same proportion of African-American men as those who patronized the clubs, and totaled about 15% of the number of all men present in the clubs during the baseline surveys.

The popular opinion leaders attended a series of four group sessions that taught effective ways to correct friends' misconceptions about risk, communicate practical behavior change recommendations to friends and acquaintances, and personally endorse to others the importance and social desirability of making safer sex behavior changes. For example, the key opinion leaders were taught to convey to others specific advice on ways to implement risk reduction steps such as carrying condoms and keeping them readily available, talking with any potential sexual partner in advance of sex to establish shared safer sex commitment, avoiding sex when intoxicated, and assertively resisting coercion from others to engage in high-risk practices. Because their role was conceptualized as being that of diffusion agents rather than simply "peer educators," the popular opinion leaders were also intensively taught how to initiate conversations with friends or acquaintances that would convey the leader's personal endorsement and personal subscription to the norm of safer sex. This was accomplished by intensive role-play practice of conversations in which the popular opinion leaders incorporated such elements as noting that AIDS is a genuine concern to small-city gay men; stressing that risk is avoidable; explicitly identifying high-risk practices, risk reduction steps, and recommendations for change implementation; using "I" statements to describe changes that the popular opinion leader was also attempting; and specifically and personally endorsing the benefits and social desirability of behavior change.

As opinion leaders became proficient in their practice of these conversations, each was asked to initiate increasing numbers of conversations of a kind that had been practiced with friends and acquaintances each week. The opinion leader cadre were encouraged to think of themselves as trendsetters who could help set a new pattern of safer behavior in their community and perhaps reach friends who would otherwise contract HIV infection. To facilitate opportunities for conversations with peers, the opinion leaders were given small buttons with a traffic light logo (but no text) which matched large posters with the same ambiguous logo placed earlier in the bars. When friends would ask about the meaning of the logo—it was intended to depict the importance of caution—the opinion leaders were afforded additional new opportunities to recommend and endorse behavior change to others. Wearing a button with the traffic-light logo also served to visibly and immediately identify the popular people as endorsers of safer sex and risk avoidance.

In our initial study (Kelly, St. Lawrence, Diaz et al., 1991), population member risk behavior changes in response to the intervention were examined by conducting a follow-up survey at three-month intervals of all men patronizing gay bars in the city where the diffusion intervention had been conducted and, for comparison purposes, in the two other cities that had not received the intervention. From baseline to follow-up survey points in the intervention city, substantial reductions were found in population-wide risk behavior levels. These included 25% to 30% reductions from baseline levels in the proportion of population members who reported any occurrence of unprotected anal intercourse during the past two months; a 16% increase in proportion of intercourse occasions protected by condoms; and an 18% decrease in proportion of population members reporting multiple sexual partners in the two preceding months. Little behavior change was observed in the comparison city populations when surveyed over the same period of time.

In order to extend the intervention and replicate its effects, our research team then focused attention on the two cities that has served as comparisons in the original study. At intervals of approximately six months, and with risk behavior surveys repeated periodically of all men patronizing bars in all study cities, the diffusion intervention just described was introduced in the second of the three study cities and, finally, in the third city. In this multiple baseline or staggered intervention design, population member behavior change should be evident following the point when the community intervention is conducted in a city relative to population member risk levels before it, and the same cause–effect pattern should be replicated as intervention is brought sequentially to each city. As we have previously reported (Kelly, St. Lawrence, Stevenson et al., 1992), this pattern of effects was found. Risk behavior levels—including the proportion of population members who reported any occurrence of un-protected anal intercourse and the proportion of intercourse occasions when condoms were used—changed in the direction of reduced risk from between 15 and 29% of average baseline levels following conduct of the diffusion in-tervention (Kelly, St. Lawrence, Stevenson et al., 1992). In addition, survey data revealed that population members in each city were more likely to per-ceive safer sex as an accepted norm within their peer reference group of gay male friends following intervention than before it.

Taken together, these findings provide evidence for the utility of community-level intervention models based on social diffusion theory to pro-mote the adoption of risk reduction behavior changes among gay men who live in small cities. Specifically, it was possible to produce generalized changes in sexual risk behavior within an entire community population—men pa-tronizing gay bars in a city—by enlisting the efforts of popular opinion leaders to visibly and demonstratively recommend, endorse, and support the behavior change efforts of their friends and acquaintances. In this sense, a relatively small cadre of key popular opinion leaders were able to shift the behavior practices of a much larger group of people. The specific mechanisms by which this process took place remain to be identified. Opinion leader behavior change recommendations and endorsements may have functioned primarily to fre-quently remind or "prompt" others to practice safer sex; they may have made more visible to others the importance of AIDS prevention or reminded them of the local threat of AIDS; they may have produced a norm change facilitating behavior change efforts; or may have operated through a combination of these mechanisms. Regardless, the diffusion intervention produced changes that were more accelerated and of greater magnitude than would have occurred without the intervention.

METHODOLOGICAL ISSUES AND RESEARCH NEEDS

The behavior change interventions discussed in this section show that both face-to-face and community-level diffusion approaches can produce reductions in high-risk sexual behavior practices among gay men who live in small cities not traditionally considered AIDS epicenters. Although undertaken in small cities, these intervention approaches are not uniquely suited only to small-city gay men. Similar skills training interventions have been undertaken with gay men in larger, more urban areas (Valdiserri et al., 1989); with urban minority women (Kelly, Murphy, Washington et al., 1992); and with high-risk adolescents (Jemmott, Jemmott, & Fong, 1992; Rotheram-Borus, Koopman, & Haignere, 1991). Programs such as "Stop AIDS" (Bye, 1990), which incorporate a combination of educational, skills training, and diffusion components, have long been underway in large urban centers. Thus, there is little reason to believe that the basic principles underlying successful risk behavior change interventions are different in small cities than large ones. Nevertheless, the format of interventions, the delivery of prevention programs, and strategies for reaching the less visible gay community in smaller communities, are factors that must be addressed with this target population. In addition, and as discussed earlier in the chapter, gay men outside our largest cities may be less threat sensitized, perceive AIDS as a more distant threat, and perceive fewer peer norms to support risk reduction behavior changes than their urban counterparts who have been strongly and personally affected by AIDS and have had the benefit of receiving support from sustained HIV prevention campaigns for many years. This suggests that intervention elements stressing accuracy of perceived risk, correction of critical risk misconceptions, and induction skills of norm changes, and supports related to sexual behavior change, will be of particular importance in prevention efforts among small-city gay men.

As the author has noted elsewhere (Kelly & Murphy, 1992), it is fortunate that community AIDS prevention campaigns in large and small cities—and with gay men as well as all other populations threatened by the HIV epidemic—have been launched *without* patiently waiting for the results of behavioral research on AIDS community prevention. There have been very few reports of evaluated trials of HIV risk behavior change interventions published to date with any population, and research in this area has clearly lagged far behind the need for and the development of HIV community prevention service programs. Intervention research on AIDS prevention has not yet been undertaken quickly enough or on a scale large enough to stay ahead of the need for intervention strategies by community organizations concerned about AIDS prevention. This is in contrast to many areas of behavioral medicine, health behavior, and community psychology, where community programs have been developed based upon findings of the research literature.

One suspects that many innovative and probably effective grassroots HIV prevention programs have been undertaken by local AIDS service organizations, including those focused on gay men in smaller cities. It will be of immense importance to foster the necessary collaboration between behavioral researchers and applied AIDS service organizations to identify and evaluate promising current or new community prevention programs; to base intervention outcome research on prevention needs that have been identified by community organizations; and to initiate "second generation" HIV prevention programs that reach gay men in small and moderate-size communities and extend beyond providing AIDS education alone to more specifically address social, psychological, and behavioral factors that influence risk behavior.

There is growing concern that HIV prevention efforts in large urban centers have failed to adequately reach "hidden" population segments which remain at elevated risk, including homosexually active men who do not self-identify as gay, ethnic minority gay men, and young gay men (Hays et al., 1990; Centers for Disease Control, 1993; Peterson et al., 1992). Because of the hidden and closeted nature of the life-style among many men who have sex with men in smaller cities, these factors probably operate to an even greater extent among small-city gay men than their urban counterparts. Research is needed to identify potential risk level differences among subgroups of homosexually active men in smaller cities based on ethnicity, age, self-identification in sexual orientation, and connectedness to settings such as bars or settings associated with casual sex, and, most importantly, to rapidly develop and test behavior change interventions that can reach these community subgroups.

Finally, when effective behavior change approaches have been identified, there is an urgent need to "package" them in formats that can actually be used by public health, AIDS prevention, and gay community organizations. Especially within smaller cities in which AIDS prevention organizations lack extensive social or financial resources, translation of interventions from the research or small-scale demonstration project arena to an applied level will require considerable ingenuity and outreach. Some of the intervention approaches discussed this chapter—including the Roffman et al. (1991; Roffman, Beadnell, & Ryan, 1992) risk reduction telephone counseling model and the Kelly, St. Lawrence, Diaz et al. (1991; Kelly, Murphy, Roffman et al., 1992) model of teaching popular people to serve as behavior change endorsement and diffusion agents to their peers—appear well-suited and cost-efficient for HIV prevention efforts among small-city gay men. Face-to-face cognitive–behavioral group interventions, capable of producing perhaps the greatest behavior change impact for their participants, require integration into service and community settings in order to reach large numbers of people. One can envision group behavior change interventions conducted in bars and adaptations of Stop AIDS programs designed to reach small-city gay men as promising approaches for implementation and evaluation.

Most HIV prevention research has relied primarily on self-reports of participant sexual practices to assess intervention effectiveness. Given the private and unobservable nature of sexual behavior, these self-reports are likely to always constitute major measures by which to judge the success of behavior change programs. Nevertheless, to the extent that participant self-reports of sexual practices are potentially influenced by social desirability, responses bias, or inaccurate recall, they may also overestimate the behavior change effects of AIDS prevention interventions. Several of the intervention studies reviewed in this chapter employed other indices to corroborate change including measures of risk knowledge, change intentions and attitudes, and behavioral ratings of role-played sexual assertiveness skill (Jemmott et al., 1992; Kelly et al., 1989). Especially in the context of larger-scale intervention outcome trials, it will be important to examine change in other indices of risk reduction independent of participant self-reports of behavior. Examples of potential corroborative measures include condom taking and condom purchases; rates at which small-city gay men seek HIV antibody testing; and incidence of sexually transmitted disease among gay men. Change found in such indices will serve to confirm the validity and impact of behavior change interventions.

SUMMARY

Although the HIV epidemic in the United States and many western countries was originally concentrated among gay men in large urban areas, the epidemic is not static; new populations are increasingly threatened by HIV and the epidemic will increasingly affect smaller communities distant from original epicenters. The aim of HIV primary prevention is to curtail the rate of new infections and, to do this, prevention efforts must remain ahead of the epidemic's course rather than trailing behind it. We have now a unique opportunity to limit HIV infections among gay men in small and moderate-sized cities to levels lower than those that have already devastated the gay communities of our largest cities. How well we do that will depend how quickly we act.

REFERENCES

Anderson, R. E., & Levy, J. D. (1985). Prevalence to antibodies to AIDS-associated retrovirus. *Lancet, 1,* 217.

Bandura, A. (1986). *Social foundations of thought and action: A social cognitive theory.* Englewood Cliffs, NJ: Prentice-Hall.

Bye, L. L. (1990). Moving beyond counseling and knowledge-enhancement interventions: A plea for community-level AIDS prevention strategies. In D. G. Ostrow (Ed.), *Behavioral aspects of AIDS.* New York: Plenum.

Centers for Disease Control & Prevention (1993a, January 15). Condom use and sexual identity among men who have sex with men. *Morbidity and Mortality Weekly Report, 42,* 12–13.

Centers for Disease Control. (1993b, February). *HIV/AIDS Surveillance.* Atlanta, GA: U.S. Public Health Service.

Curran, J. W., Jaffe, H. W., Hardy, A. M., Morgan, W. M., Selik, R. M., & Dondero, T. J. (1988). The epidemiology of HIV infection and AIDS in the United States. *Science, 239,* 610–616.

Ekstrand, M. L., & Coates, T. J. (1990). Maintenance of safer sexual behaviors and predictors of risky sex. *American Journal of Public Health, 80,* 973–977.

Fisher, J. D., & Misovich, S. J. (1990). Social influence and AIDS preventive behavior. In J. Edwards, R. S. Tindale, L. Heath, & E. J. Posavac (Eds.), *Social influence processes and prevention.* New York: Plenum.

Hays, R. B., Kegeles, S. M., & Coates, T. J. (1990). High HIV risk taking among younger gay men. *AIDS, 4,* 901–907.

Jemmott, J. B., Jemmott, L. S., & Fong, G. T. (1992). Reductions in HIV risk-associated sexual behaviors among Black male adolescents: Effects of an AIDS prevention intervention. *American Journal of Public Health, 82,* 372–377.

Kelly, J. A., Kalichman, S. C., Kauth, M. R., Kilgore, H. G., Hood, H. V., Campos, P. E., Rao, S. M., Brasfield, T. L., & St. Lawrence, J. S. (1991). Situational factors associated with AIDS risk behavior lapses and coping strategies used by gay men who successfully avoid lapses. *American Journal of Public Health, 81,* 1335–1338.

Kelly, J. A., & Murphy, D. A. (1992). Psychological interventions with AIDS and HIV: Prevention and treatment. *Journal of Consulting and Clinical Psychology, 60,* 576–585.

Kelly, J. A., Murphy, D. A., Roffman, R. A., Solomon, L. J., Winett, R. A., Stevenson, L. Y., Koob, J. J., Ayotte, D. R., Flynn, B. S., Desiderato, L. L. Hauth, A. C., Lemke, A. L., Lombard, D., Morgan, M. G., Norman, A. D., Sikkemas, K. J., Steiner, S., & Yaffe, D. M. (1992). Acquired immunodeficiency syndrome/human immunodeficiency virus risk behavior among gay men in small cities: Findings of a 16-city national sample. *Archives of Internal Medicine, 152,* 2293–2297.

Kelly, J. A., Murphy, D. A., Washington, C. D., Wilson, T. S., Koob, J. J., Kalichman, S. C., Davis, D. R., Ledezma, G., & Davantes, B. (1992, November). *HIV/AIDS prevention groups for high-risk inner-city women: Intervention outcomes and effects on risk behavior.* Paper presented at the Annual Meeting of the American Public Health Association, Washington, DC.

Kelly, J. A., St. Lawrence, J. S., Betts, R., Brasfield, T. L., & Hood, H. V. (1990). A skills training group intervention to assist persons in reducing risk behaviors for HIV infection. *AIDS Education & Prevention, 2,* 24–35.

Kelly, J. A., St. Lawrence, J. S., & Brasfield, T. L. (1990). Predictors of vulnerability to AIDS risk behavior relapse. *Journal of Consulting & Clinical Psychology, 59,* 163–166.

Kelly, J. A., St. Lawrence, J. A., Brasfield, T. L., Lemke, A., Amidei, T., Roffman, R. A., Hood, H. V., Smith, J. E., Kilgore, H., & McNeill, C. (1990). Psychological factors that predict AIDS high-risk versus AIDS precautionary behavior. *Journal of Consulting & Clinical Psychology, 58,* 117–120.

Kelly, J. A., St. Lawrence, J. H. S., Brasfield, T. L., Stevenson, L. Y., Diaz, Y. E., & Hauth, A. C. (1990). AIDS risk behavior patterns among gay men in small southern cities. *American Journal of Public Health, 80,* 416–418.

Kelly, J. A., St. Lawrence, J. S., Diaz, Y. E., Stevenson, L. Y., Hauth, A. C., Brasfield, T. L., Kalichman, S. C., Smith, J. E., & Andrew, M. E. (1991). HIV risk reduction following intervention with key opinion leaders of a population: An experimental analysis. *American Journal of Public Health, 81,* 168–171.

Kelly, J. A., St. Lawrence, J. S., Hood, H. V., & Brasfield, T. L. (1989). Behavioral intervention to reduce AIDS risk activities. *Journal of Consulting & Clinical Psychology, 57,* 60–67.

Kelly, J. A., St. Lawrence, J. S., Stevenson, L. Y., Hauth, A. C., Kalichman, S. C., Diaz, Y. E., Brasfield, T. L., Koob, J. J., & Morgan, M. G. (1992). Community AIDS/HIV risk reduction: The effects of endorsements by popular people in three cities. *American Journal of Public Health, 82,* 1483–1489.

Martin, J. L., Garcia, M. A., & Beatrice, S. T. (1989). Sexual behavior changes and HIV antibody in a cohort of New York City gay men. *American Journal of Public Health, 79,* 501–503.

Peterson, J. L., Coates, T. J., Catania, J. A., Middleton, L., Hilliard, B., & Hearst, N. (1992). High-risk sexual behavior and condom use among gay and bisexual African American men. *American Journal of Public Health, 82,* 1490–1494.

Rogers, E. M. (1983). *Diffusion of innovations.* New York: Free Press.

Roffman, R. A., Beadnell, B., & Ryan, R. (1992, July). *Telephone counseling in the reduction of barriers to AIDS prevention.* Paper presented at the 2nd International Congress on Behavioral Medicine, Hamburg, Germany.

Roffman, R. A., Beadnell, B. A., Stern, M., Gordon, J. R., Downey, L., & Siever, M. (1991, August). *Phone counseling in reducing barriers to AIDS prevention.* Paper presented at the Annual Meeting of the American Psychological Association, San Francisco.

Rotheram-Borus, M. J., Koopman, C., & Haignere, C. (1991). Reducing HIV sexual risk behavior among runaway adolescents. *Journal of the American Medical Association, 266,* 1237–1241.

St. Lawrence, J. S., Hood, H. V., Brasfield, T. L., & Kelly, J. A. (1989). Differences in AIDS risk knowledge and behavior patterns in high and low AIDS prevalence cities. *Public Health Reports, 104,* 391–395.

Stall, R., Ekstrand, M. L., Paul, J., McKusick, L., & Coates, T. J. (1993). *Primary prevention needs among gay and bisexual men in Tucson.* Paper presented at the Cascade AIDS Project, San Francisco.

Valdiserri, R. O., Lyter, D., Leviton, L., Callahan, C., Kingsley, L., & Rinaldo, C. (1989). AIDS prevention in homosexual and bisexual men: Results of a randomized trial evaluating two risk reduction interventions. *AIDS, 3,* 21–26.

16

Lessons Learned from Behavioral Interventions
Caveats, Gaps, and Implications

*JOHN L. PETERSON and
RALPH J. DiCLEMENTE*

INTRODUCTION

Since behavior change remains the only means available for the primary prevention of human immunodeficiency virus (HIV), behavioral interventions are critically needed to alter the course of the HIV/acquired immunodeficiency syndrome (AIDS) epidemic. However, researchers face unprecedented challenges in their efforts to develop effective behavior change interventions. One challenge is to address the methodological limitations of previous research. Another challenge is to eliminate the gaps in behavioral intervention research. A final challenge is to understand the implications of previous research for the development of more innovative behavioral interventions. In this chapter, we identify some limitations of, gaps in, and implications of behavioral research interventions to change HIV/AIDS risk behaviors.

CAVEATS OF INTERVENTION RESEARCH

Among the methodological limitations of behavioral intervention research, two are especially prominent. One is that there are few carefully eval-

JOHN L. PETERSON • Department of Psychology, Georgia State University, Atlanta, Georgia 30303. *RALPH J. DiCLEMENTE* • School of Public Health, Department of Health Behavior and School of Medicine, Departments of Medicine and Pediatrics, and Center for AIDS Research, University of Alabama, Birmingham, Alabama 35294.

Preventing AIDS: Theories and Methods of Behavioral Interventions, edited by Ralph J. DiClemente and John L. Peterson. Plenum Press, New York, 1994.

nated outcome studies that have been designed as controlled intervention trials (Fisher & Fisher, 1992; Kelly & Murphy, 1992). Ethical constraints not withstanding, rigorous assessment of behavior change is reduced by the limited use of experimental designs. The absence of random assignment and comparable control groups impedes efforts to determine the impact of these interventions on behavior change. Also, the lack of controlled intervention trials limits the possibility of precisely identifying the components of interventions responsible for the behavior change.

The other major limitation is the reliance on participants' self-reports of behavior change as outcome measures. It is not possible to directly measure changes in HIV risk behavior because of the difficulties involved in assessing privately occurring behavior. Consequently, researchers are dependent on the use of self-report assessments of risk behavior, which may be inaccurate because of problems associated with recall or social desirability bias (Catania, Gibson, Chitwood, & Coates, 1990; Hingson & Strunin, 1993). Whenever possible, additional outcome measures which avoid these limitations should be employed in behavior change interventions. These include such measures as biological markers for sexually transmitted diseases and indicators of related preventive behaviors; for example, possession of condoms or bleach and clean injection needles.

GAPS IN INTERVENTION RESEARCH

The epidemiology of HIV/AIDS has changed substantially over the course of the epidemic. Remarkable changes have been observed in some populations, notably among urban white gay men in AIDS epicenters. Other populations, such as young or minority homosexually active men, heterosexual women, and ethnic minorities in poor urban areas, have not demonstrated similar changes in HIV risk behaviors. Therefore, it is critically important to develop and evaluate risk-reduction interventions for these populations.

There are a number of obstacles to the development of effective behavior change interventions in these urban populations (Cochran & Mays, 1989; Mays & Cochran, 1988; Murphy & Kelly, in press; Peterson & Marin, 1988). These populations experience a wide spectrum of related social problems which are equally if not more salient than the threat of AIDS, including limited health care resources, high unemployment, high rates of drug abuse, and inadequate housing. In addition, cultural and gender differences regarding sexuality and sex roles can be a formidable barrier to effective behavior change (Airhihenbuwa, DiClemente, Wingood, & Lowe, 1992; Chavkin, Cohen, Ehrhardt, Fullilove, & Worth, 1991; Fullilove, Boyser, Haynes, & Gross, 1990; Fullilove et al., 1990; Wingood, Hunter, & DiClemente, 1993; Wingood

& DiClemente, 1992). Information about these factors is critical to the development of effective behavior change interventions tailored to the needs of these specific populations.

IMPLICATIONS FOR FUTURE INTERVENTION RESEARCH

Despite the paucity of research on behavior change interventions, the data suggest at least two behavior change approaches that appear promising. One approach uses cognitive–behavioral interventions to promote social and self-management skills for changing high-risk behavior. A second approach involves the development of community interventions to promote the adoption of social norms which encourage low-risk behavior through channels of influence indigenous to the community (Coates, 1990; Kelly, Murphy, Sikkemas, & Kalichman, 1993).

Another implication for future research is the need for behavior change interventions which demonstrate an ability to maintain initial changes in high-risk behaviors (Stall, Ekstrand, Pollack, McKusick, & Coates, 1990; Ekstrand & Coates, 1990). While the long-term maintenance of low-risk behavior is clearly necessary to limit the occurrence of new HIV infections, it may be substantially more difficult to maintain people's low-risk behavior following their initial behavior change. Therefore, a major issue is to distinguish those factors responsible for initial risk-reduction from those associated with long-term maintenance.

The urgency of the HIV epidemic demands that behavior change interventions should be rapidly developed to curb new HIV infections. The most effective research interventions should also be conducted on a scale broad enough to yield direct public health benefits (Kelly et al., 1993). Ultimately, preventing HIV infections will not only depend on the development and evaluation of innovative behavior change approaches, but also on the translation of intervention research into credible community programs.

REFERENCES

Airhihenbuwa, C. O., DiClemente, R. J., Wingood, G. M., & Lowe, A. (1992). HIV/AIDS education and prevention among African-Americans: A focus on culture. *Journal of AIDS Education & Prevention, 4,* 251–260.

Catania, J. A., Gibson, D. R., Chitwood, D. D., & Coates, T. J. (1990). Methodological problems in AIDS behavioral research: Influences on measurement error and participation bias in studies of sexual behavior. *Psychological Bulletin, 108,* 339–362.

Chavkin, W., Cohen, J., Ehrhardt, A. A., Fullilove, M. T., & Worth, D. (1991). Women and AIDS. *Science, 251,* 359–362.

Coates, T. J. (1990). Strategies for modifying sexual behavior for primary and secondary prevention of HIV disease. *Journal of Consulting & Clinical Psychology, 58,* 57–69.

Cochran, S. D., & Mays, V. M. (1989). Women and AIDS-related concerns: Roles for psychologists in helping the worried well. *American Psychologist, 44,* 529–535.

Ekstrand, M. L., & Coates, T. J. (1990). Maintenance of safer sex behaviors and predictors of risky sex: The San Francisco Men's Health Study. *American Journal of Public Health, 80,* 973–976.

Fisher, J. D., & Fisher, W. A. (1992). Changing AIDS-risk behavior. *Psychological Bulletin, 111,* 455–474.

Fullilove, M. T., Fullilove, R., Bowser, B. P., Haynes, K., & Gross, S. A. (1990). Black women and AIDS: Gender rules. *Journal of Sex Research, 27,* 47–64.

Fullilove, M. T., Weinstein, M., Fullilove, R. E., Crayton, E. J., Goodjoin, R. B., Bowser, B. P., & Gross, S. A. (1990). Race/gender issues in the sexual transmission of AIDS. In P. Volberding & M. A. Jacobson, (Eds.), *AIDS clinical review.* (pp. 25–62). New York: Marcel Dekker.

Hingson, R., & Strunin, L. (1993). Validity, reliability, and generalizability in studies of AIDS knowledge, attitudes, and behavioral risks based on subject self-report. *American Journal of Preventive Medicine, 9,* 62–64.

Kelly, J. A., Murphy, D. A., Sikkemas, K. J., & Kalichman, S. C. (1993). Psychological interventions are urgently needed to prevent HIV infection: New priorities for behavioral research in the second decade of AIDS. *American Psychologist, 48,* 1023–1034.

Kelly, J. A., & Murphy, D. A. (1992). Psychological interventions with AIDS and HIV: Prevention and treatment. *Journal of Consulting & Clinical Psychology, 60,* 476–485.

Mays, V. M., & Cochran, S. D. (1988). Issues in the perception of AIDS risk and risk reduction activities by Black and Hispanic/Latina women. *American Psychologist, 43,* 949–957.

Murphy, D. A., & Kelly, J. A. (in press). Women's health: The impact of the expanding AIDS epidemic. In V. Adesso, D. Reedy, & R. Fleming (Eds.), *Psychological perspectives on women's health.* New York: Hemisphere.

Peterson, J. L., & Marin, G. (1988). Issues in the prevention of AIDS among Black and Hispanic men. *American Psychologist, 43,* 871–877.

Stall, R., Ekstrand, M., Pollack, L., McKusick, L., & Coates, T. J. (1990). Relapse from safer sex: The next challenge for AIDS prevention efforts. *Journal of Acquired Immune Deficiency Syndromes, 3,* 1181–1187.

Wingood, G. M., & DiClemente, R. J. (1992). Cultural, gender and psychosocial influences on HIV-related behavior of African-American female adolescents: Implications for the development of tailored prevention programs. *Ethnicity & Disease, 2,* 381–388.

Wingood, G. M., Hunter, D., & DiClemente, R. J. (1993). A pilot study of sexual communication and negotiation among young African-American women: Implications for HIV prevention. *Journal of Black Psychology, 19,* 190–203.

Index